The Danny Diaries

The Danny Diaries

Overcoming Schizophrenia

ANN CLUVER WEINBERG

Order this book online at www.trafford.com
or email orders@trafford.com

Most Trafford titles are also available at major online book retailers.

In South Africa this book is available from Ann Weinberg, (011)485-1189
Email: sapler.press@artslink.co.za

Sponsor: Christine Allen
Cover artist: Greta Sadur
Copyeditor: Mary Hazelton

Printed in Victoria, BC, Canada.

ISBN: 978-1-4269-1960-2 (Soft)

*Our mission is to efficiently provide the world's finest, most comprehensive
book publishing service, enabling every author to experience success.
To find out how to publish your book, your way, and have it available
worldwide, visit us online at www.trafford.com*

Trafford rev. 01/27/2010

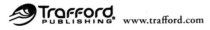

www.trafford.com

North America & international
toll-free: 1 888 232 4444 (USA & Canada)
phone: 250 383 6864 ♦ fax: 812 355 4082

For Nicola and Danny

CONTENTS

INTRODUCTION

This is the true story of what happened to our family and in particular to my son, Danny. I kept diaries of my children talking. I would write these diaries immediately or in the evenings – and my written words were as close as I could get to the spoken words.

The story starts with the happy child Danny in his artistic family attempting to make sense of his world and his feelings, and ends with Danny, a sane adult, writing letters home. Between these two is his psychotic breakdown. He developed too quickly and successfully into a teenage pop star and was drawn into the world of sex, drugs and rock 'n' roll.

The story tells of his total collapse, followed by partial recovery and further collapse. I, with the support of my husband, did not give in. I listened to the experts, but rejected them when their advice didn't work. In the end it was a clear framework with definite rules which helped him more than psychology. And lots of love.

I have changed the names of the immediate family to give Danny a degree of privacy—and some distance as a sane adult from his disturbed younger self. Danny agreed to me writing this book, but does not want me to write about his later life. So I have finished the story with him in Florida, independent and self-supporting.

The story is mostly set in South Africa, where the school year starts in January.

The school years when Danny was at school were: Grade 1, Grade 2, and then Standards 1 to 10. (We now have the American system of Grades 1 to 12.)

Chapter One

THE FAMILY IN LONDON 1960-1969 (DANNY'S BIRTH 1967)

THE YELLOWBRICK HOUSE

I am Lucy. On an optimistic springtime day in 1960, I married Oliver at Hampstead registry office in London. We each had passionate goals and were committed to helping each other achieve these goals: mine was to have children; Oliver's was to become a flute-player. But we thought we might have started too late: a gynaecologist told me that if I didn't have babies soon I wouldn't be able to have them. I then had two miscarriages. Oliver had only started studying music as an adult. However, he had now completed two years of the best flute teaching available—in Paris.

We lived in one room in Kilburn, north London—a thick-walled, solidly warm room. We shared the bathroom with another tenant, and we had a little kitchen down a few stairs and around a corner. Oliver made contact with all the amateur orchestras in London. When they gave concerts they often didn't have a flute player who could play all the notes, so Oliver would get paid for filling in on the night. Miraculously he was then called to Stratford-on-Avon to play the recorder whenever there was a stage musician in a Shakespeare play. Because he dressed up and played on stage, he was paid double—as a musician and as an actor. (Sometimes he only played three notes, so he joked that he was the highest paid musician per note in England.)

I worked a mile's walk away at a warehouse which stored Italian foods. I and my boss shared a sunny corner office. I often brought home pasta and antipasto and tomato paste—it all helped.

During my third pregnancy I had a threatened miscarriage at five months and had to go to hospital. But on 21 March 1962, Nicola was born and she was healthy and we lived with her for a few more months in our Kilburn room. She slept in a carrycot on the chest of drawers, or in an ancient pram in the doorway downstairs. As soon as she could sit up I pushed her to the cemetery nearby, which we both enjoyed.

My passion for children endured. My moments of peak joy in the next twelve years, apart from during love-making or at a very occasional theatre visit, came in interactions with my young children.

But where were we to live? I had some money left over from a twenty-first birthday present, which was just enough for a small deposit on a house or a flat. But in the small flats we could afford in north London we would be on top of others—who would complain of the practising noise, and where Oliver could not escape from little Nicola, and little Nicola could not escape into the garden. We dipped into our capital for a three-wheeled Italian Isetta, and off Oliver drove to south London. Houses were cheaper in the south, so Oliver made contact with an estate agent and was taken all over the place—mostly to houses which required too much fixing-up. Then one day, sighing, but really liking Oliver and wanting to please him, the estate agent took him to a squashed plot in Brockley. He had himself bought this little plot and had planning permission for it, and also a plan. Oliver brought me and Nicola to see the plot and to look at the plan. We bought both. Our north London landlady said, "If you were English you would not dream of having a Brockley address."

Brockley was a grey place in south-east London. There was a long, wide street with big houses on each side which was Breakspears Road. The houses were semi-detached Victorian mansions, identical in style and height, and they were all the colour of dried-out mould. But what went on in those houses was no longer uniform. There were a few houses which were owned and lived in by elderly widows of a different era, but many others were broken up into flats, and often lived in by West Indian railwaymen and their families.

However, if you zoomed up to the west end of Breakspears Road, which was our end, the uniformity disappeared, for this was where the German bombs fell in the Second World War. After the rubble was cleared, the council had put up three skyscraper-high unornamented blocks at a slight angle to each other—blocks which would be much criticized for their social stupidity: mothers with young children living high in those blocks would have to stop their housework, go down in the lift and supervise their children in the small concrete playground below. They housed many people, but I thought it might have been better to be a slum child, able to run in and out.

Next to these blocks was a solid square house lived in alone by an Indian lecturer in his fifties. He taught at Goldsmiths College in Lewisham and later became friendly with Oliver, my husband.

Opposite this house was our empty plot, so thin and squashed that no one had thought of building on it. Its neighbours—a row of garages on one side and the first of the Victorian mansions on the other side—had moved their fences into this plot, slowly, inch by inch, until those fences seemed always to have been there.

I looked at the plan with astonishment. What possibilities! I quickly established that I was allowed to change anything except the basic shape. The plan went across the plot, from fence to fence, with three big south-facing rooms on top of each other, and little rooms on the other sides. Jutting out of the first and second floors on the north were little balconies—overlooking Breakspears Road. Three big noisy roads met at that point so the balconies would not be private or quiet. But more than that: they faced north! I knew the mistake that Herbert Baker had made in South Africa—making his houses face south as they had in England! I had lived in one of those freezing houses. Here in Britain, to get the sun: face south. I took off the north-facing balconies and put great glass windows in the big rooms on the south. The ground floor was an open-plan kitchen and living-room, with black linoleum flooring. The top floor was Oliver's domain—there he could practise and teach in private. Nicky knew from the time she could climb stairs that the little gate to the top was out of bounds. There was a little gate at the bottom too. This meant that she and I could do different things safely and I would not have to watch her all the time. All breakable things I put too high for her to reach, so I didn't have to say, "Don't touch!" all the time.

So we had these three big rooms in the house. But we also had two spaces outside which were the same size as the rooms: five big spaces! The room-sized space in the front was concreted over. Two beautiful lime trees grew there, losing their leaves in winter in a clear seasonal way (unlike back home), and when the new leaves started to come the next spring, we found tiny snowdrops growing round the trunks. The room-sized space at the back was old grass and earth. It sloped down and at the bottom was a tap. Nicky used it for making wonderful muddy child-sized pools. Five good spaces we had. We had South African friends with a similar income. They lived in a "better" area with their two small children in a flat without a garden. Chaos!

The family thrived in Brockley. Our greatest need was to be far from the tyranny of apartheid South Africa. Like our South African friends who had fled with us we were socialist, atheist and anti-bourgeois: I put no curtains on our great glass windows. Electricity was half-price at night and we had underfloor heating which heated up the whole house at night. We were warm and happy and forgot to be guilty. One day I shouted at two yelling four-year-old twins who were rushing around the table. That night I wondered whether I had been right to shout at them. Then I realized that I had not thought of them as "black". We had lost our liberal sensitivities.

The council blocks were some pastel colour I think—too bland to be memorable. But our house was made of yellow London brick—second-hand brick but of recent origin—as yellow as the day it was born. The Brockley children called our house "the witch's house"—because it was so tall and thin and had a little peaked roof.

This house was all I wanted. We had the philosophy of "enough". Oliver went searching for second-hand furniture and found some good-enough things for very little. The very last thing he bought with our last bit of capital was a piano which cost almost nothing but which worked perfectly well.

We were socialists in a world that still believed in socialism. We voted for the Labour Party and our candidate got elected. We seemed hardly aware that we ourselves were benefiting from socialism—with our subsidised mortgage from the Greater London Council, and me having my babies on the National Health. Our bible was *The Little Pete Stories*: about a four-year-old boy who had classless adventures in London, chatting to all who lived and worked there.

My aunt from South Africa visited us. "Don't you envy your friends back home who have beautifully furnished homes and big gardens and lots of servants?"

"Good heavens no! I would hate that."

BRINGING UP NICOLA

We never discussed our principles for bringing up children. The old ways were gone—no punishments, nor even calling a child "naughty"—and no sermons about morality. We believed in love and reason—and Nicky was easy to love and reasonable to talk to. No one in our families had hit, spanked or beaten since the nineteenth century.

I had no career. This was my career. I created a home for Nicola's delight and she was an immensely rewarding child. She was natural and responsive, and loved by everyone. She was beautiful too, but we were not in the culture of looks and stardom, and I don't think she was aware of it. What she liked to do was to dress up and dance and act—and she liked people to respond to her. Aged three she said, "I love all the people who love me."

She would go up to strangers and start a conversation, and she would often give away her own things to them.

My style was to watch and be in the background of her life. I didn't rush up and suggest things and explain things, but waited for her to ask spontaneously.

Discipline was a non-issue. When she was little and wanted to touch some inappropriate thing I would just take her away and show her a flower. She was easily distractible, and she adored flowers.

Bedtime was bedtime—I was clear about that. Occasionally I had to carry her up screaming when she wanted to stay downstairs. I remember thinking that this would be difficult to do with a teenager! Once upstairs there would be teeth-brushing and getting into pyjamas. Then I would get into bed with her and tell her a story and sing her a song. Then she would say, "You can go downstairs now and talk to my daddy."

One day she was playing in the front courtyard and decided to go out of the gate for a walk up the pavement. Oliver saw her, and brought her angrily in. Nicky came to me and said, "I won't do that again. I don't like that cross!"

I was not so successful with shouting at her. A friend phoned. "I don't know what to do about Debbie. Every time I shout at her she bursts into tears."

"Oh well. That's exactly what I used to do when my parents shouted at me. But when I shout at Nicky she just shouts back!"

It was better to prepare her in advance for some new thing. Then she would cooperate and try her best.

In our back patch of garden, Nicky and I dug for treasure. We found bits of green tiles and bits of blue cups. We washed the treasure and put it on a shelf. I didn't tell her about the bombs and the war. I just hoped we never found a bone, and we never did. She had her own ideas about death: "Then the lorry will bump me and break me into lots of pieces. Then I will be a pink flower and you will pick me. Then you will have to make a new Nicola: arms, legs, tummy. No head!"

I never saw Nicky "doing nothing". She had immense ongoing stamina, and that meant that I, who did not, was often tired and sometimes ill, and sometimes desperate for an adult conversation or a book. To help this I invented "Resting Time", when I went to lie down after lunch and she played in her little bedroom. When I went to fetch her she had a whole story project laid out on the floor with her little wooden people, and shoes and buttons as props.

In her ABC book she pointed to a letter and said, "What's that?" I made the sound of the letter. She laughed and wanted it again and again. Oliver was away for six weeks. When he came back, Nicky, aged one-and-a-half, knew all the sounds. Oliver was astounded! By two she could read easy words, and by three she could read books. I told no one. It was against socialist principles to turn your child into a genius. But it was another way for me to get much-needed rest. She was a reader for life.

Feelings, even bad ones, could be put into words: "I thought that I would hit you, cos I couldn't understand why the light wasn't on. That's whys I was crying."

And on another day, very frustrated, she said, "I don't like you, Mummy." I replied cheerfully, "Well not liking me won't get the lunch made," and she laughed.

Dorothy Baruch's child-rearing book said, "They should be allowed to *say* anything, but not to *do* anything." There was still a great fear of children becoming neurotic if they repressed their bad feelings.

And then came Tina. Tina was a blonde eight-year-old who latched on to us when we went for walks. I still put Nicky into a pushchair for longer walks up to Hilly Fields. This was the green top of a hill, with trees and grass and no flowerbeds and no fences. From there you could hardly see the ugly Victorian houses. The children would run around and roll down the slopes.

One day Tina's mother rang on our doorbell. She asked us if we would have Tina to stay for a week so that she could go and discuss something with her husband in Bournemouth. We agreed without even thinking about it. I was so naive that I didn't even ask for Tina's surname or her mother's contact address.

Tina inside our house was a different person from Tina on the walks. As soon as Oliver sat down, Tina climbed on top of him and behaved like a teenage tart, flirting and licking. Oliver prised her loose and put her down and went upstairs. Then Tina lay on the floor and had a tantrum, lying on her back and kicking and screaming like a two-year-old. All this time Nicky sat in her high chair, silent and still and wide-eyed.

Tina had daily tantrums, mostly because we didn't buy her an ice-cream at the very moment when she wanted it. When the week ended, Tina's mother did not come and fetch her. Another week went by, and another. Then Tina's mother rang the doorbell and thanked us, but gave no explanation for the delay. She and Tina disappeared for ever from our lives.

This was our first experience of "out-of-control" behaviour. We never expected our own children to behave like that. Ours had happily married parents and they were doted on and given love, stability, comfort and encouragement.

Psychology ruled. But some of it I had stopped believing. I was Aristotle, wanting to see for myself. I watched to see if "Freudian things" happened. Which they did, but with no anxiety attached. Nicky said, 'I'm going to marry Daddy.'"

"But you need him to be your daddy."

"Oliver will be my husband. Then I will grow two tiny boys in my tummy. Two more Olivers. One will be for my daddy and one will be for your husband."

She stood in the garden with her feet apart and did "up-wees"—like the boys did—just to show she could.

For toilet-training I had taken off her nappy and let her walk around on the linoleum which covered the whole ground floor. She could then get the feeling of it happening and she would stop and watch in wonder. She also watched me doing it with great interest upstairs in the bathroom—and then did it herself. No problems.

"Pumpy" she flushed down the toilet very merrily. "Bye-bye pumpy!" she would say. She knew perfectly well that it was not "a part of her" any more than the food that went in was a part of her, until some of it made blood. All that had been endlessly talked about.

Religion too was talked about openly. (In my own childhood I had atheist parents who were inhibited about religion.) Nicky, aged four, said, "Heaven isn't real is it?"

"No, it's make-believe."

"Well they won't make me believe it!"

One day Oliver was there when the issue of church came up. He said, "She wouldn't understand that—she doesn't even know why people go to church."

"Of course I do!" said Nicky indignantly.

"Why do they?"

"They go to fall in love with God so that he will give them food."

In our area there were many West Indians. Some we liked, some we didn't. Two doors down lived the Clarke family from British Guyana. Mr Clarke was very tall, very thin, very black and very formal. He would invite me in for gin and Ribena—the blackcurrant vitamin C drink we all bought below cost at the clinic. Then he and I would try to solve local problems. Some we got started on—like a crossing for the local pensioners to fetch their pensions from a post office on the other side of a very busy street. But one we failed to solve was that of a four-year-old West Indian boy who got beaten every afternoon by his unemployed father. We phoned the Social Welfare department, but they said they couldn't interfere because "It's their culture".

Mrs Clarke was browner and rounder, and very reticent. The three children were simply brown Londoners, watching the same children's television as Nicky did, sometimes all at their house and sometimes at ours. The programmes were:

Magic Roundabout

Bill and Ben the Flowerpot Men
Blue Peter

Neither the Clarkes nor we ever thought of leaving the television on during the day when adult programmes were showing.

We had a Woody Guthrie record. He put ordinary sentences into songs, so I did that with Nicky. I sang to her more than I talked to her, and then she did the same.

One day I was singing, "All you need is love, love; all you need is love". Nicky said, "You don't only need love; you need food and sense as well."

At five she went to a gym class, and one day came home weeping. "They called me a fatty!" she said. "I didn't like that." She was a little plump, but we ate no junk food, so what was causing it? She and I explored all the cupboards in the kitchen. We found dried fruit—luscious, chewy, dark-orange apricots. She had sat there eating plenty of it and I had seen no reason why not. Now we threw it away, and she got thin again.

At six, she and Kevin, the youngest Clarke child, who was about to turn six, fell in love. Nicky told us, "I'm going to be the queen at Kevin's party and cut the cake. Then I have to kiss Kevin, but I'm not scared of that. Lots of girls are scared to kiss boys. After all he's not my father or my uncle or anything."

We didn't talk about morals as such; but one day she said after a story: "The moral is: Never do what your friends tell you to; always do what you think is right."

One day I had been annoyed with her for grumbling. "Mum," she said, "when you don't want me to grumble you must say: 'Oh Nicky! Don't forget to sing!' Now let's try it out."

Boys in the neighbourhood could be frightening or nice. One day she had been playing at Roland's house and brought him home with her saying, "Can Roland come and watch television?—because he's a nice tame boy."

I found a letter written by Nicky at about five. *Sory mummy I'me a little bit ashamd but you see I get a bit mad for two days love Nicky.*

This seems unusual, since neither Oliver nor I would have used words like "shame" and "ashamed". I think now, looking back, that I would have used the words "right" and "wrong" more often so that the children had an explicit moral structure to refer to. I found a card with a list of ten things for her to remember. "Wash hands after pumpy" was one. And there among the hygiene things was "Don't tell lies". We thought she mostly told stories to entertain us, but later she didn't seem to know the difference between these stories and a lie to get out of something.

Oliver was a fun person for her to be with. He was often away, doing temp jobs on the flute in orchestras far from home. But when he was home he was completely home. He would take Nicky to distant parks with water and ducks, or take over completely if I was tired or ill. He was a very good cook.

So that was the family that Danny was born into.

LITTLE LONG DANNY (1967-1969)

Alas, Stratford was now gone. When Nicky was two or three the Shakespeare Company had its grant for live music withdrawn: no longer could Oliver be paid for being both an actor and a musician—they had to use recordings.

Oliver had an agent. He was sent all around for a few days or a few weeks to play with professional orchestras who were touring or staying put and who were short of a flautist. He went to Ireland and Portugal, but mostly he went to the wet and wintry Midlands of Britain. At first we didn't mind—he was at least playing and getting paid for it. But the time between jobs could be many weeks, and he often had to pay his own travelling expenses.

We were not covering our expenses. So we let out our big room on the middle floor to a disabled ex-civil servant, Rosemary, who lived there and had all her meals with us, and who paid well. For Nicky she was an ideal granny who stayed put. She would bounce in with her latest dance or painting or outfit and find appreciation.

I started giving piano lessons, as I had done back in Johannesburg. But in our area the pupils couldn't pay much. I taught tunes and chords, not classical and reading music. It was a very relaxed way to bring in a bit of extra money.

One long hot summer when Oliver was out of work he made friends with an elderly Hungarian painter: he had simply talked to her at the shops and she had invited him to see her paintings—she lived just around the corner from us.

And one day Oliver, who had never drawn or painted in his life before, started to paint. His Hungarian friend showed him how, but she refused to charge him for formal lessons. He was friendly company and she enjoyed his enthusiasm and progress.

He practised the flute less and less and painted more and more. At first he copied photos or postcards; then went out and painted a bridge or a building from life; and then experimented with imagined scenes and with reality newly shaped. He painted for the love of colour and form and texture—not for mood or meaning. But he never painted pure abstracts. Most of his paintings he sold or gave away as gifts, so I have too few here today. The one I am looking at now is a sort of cubist still life: sharp pointed table legs shoot out in a flat primitive way, and then on a red table-cloth there is a yellow vase with dry branches coming vertically out with thistles at the end of them; and splodgy blue sky all around.

Green Park in London is between Buckingham Palace and Hyde Park—less well known than either. There all day on Sundays, amateur painters show their works and hope to sell them. One Sunday Oliver took three of his paintings there and put them next to the fence. At the end of the day he had sold one! We hugged and giggled—it seemed so unlikely. But he didn't sell another for another three weeks. This went on in the same way through the summer.

And then he met a Spanish artist named Luiz. Luiz really was an artist—he had a painting hanging in the Prado in Madrid, along with El Greco and Goya. But he was now living in London with his girlfriend and he had to earn, so he did popular paintings for Sunday selling. He and Oliver became close friends. Oliver used to go to Luiz' flat after they packed up on Sunday evenings. I didn't mind. I had British television—at its best on Sunday evenings—and British television in the 1960s is said to have been the best television at any time in any place. Richard Dimbleby on Panorama perhaps—interviewing someone, with that glorious bit of Berlioz' *Le Corsair* as introduction.

But apart from all that, Luiz, in a sense, gave us Danny.

He taught Oliver how to do factory paintings: ten canvasses, ten seas, ten skies, and then a slightly different fishing-boat on each one.

Suddenly we were wealthy! Oliver sold ten paintings every week—I think at twenty pounds a painting. An absolutely reliable income at last.

Nicky, aged four, was happy at a nearby state nursery school. My sister Hilary phoned me to say she was pregnant with her second child. Oliver and I decided instantly—and conceived instantly. I had a wonderful pregnancy this time: Oliver said he had never seen me so well and that I should always be pregnant. Nicky watched me growing, fascinated. One night we were having guests, so she was having supper in bed—luckily seen as a treat. She said, thoughtfully, "Ask Jill to bring up my supper. You have such a lot of climbing up and down the stairs to do, and you would be carrying two things—your baby and my supper."

We had friends with three small children in north London. The mother couldn't just put them to bed. They would call and whine and she would rush upstairs to them. This was so disruptive for us that we stopped going to dinner with them.

We were all "child-centred" I think, but Oliver and I could be definite and "authoritative"—a very different word from "authoritarian". We were very confident parents of young children.

I walked to Hilly Fields and back every day right up to the very end of my pregnancy. Two weeks after the due date there was no sign of the baby. It was mid-winter. I remember giving one of my last piano lessons to a huge West Indian man—and me so huge myself. A good painting it could have been.

We were all getting impatient. Nicky said, "I don't think this baby wants to come out."

I worried slightly that I could not love a second child as much as I loved her. I was to have this baby at home. But when I went for a check-up at Lewisham Hospital the pains suddenly came on strongly and I was taken upstairs to give birth. I phoned Oliver; he took Nicky to the Clarkes and came at once to the hospital. He had not been allowed to see Nicky being born, so this was his chance. Everything was very quick this time, but Oliver did arrive during the last ten minutes. Then the baby came out with the cord wrapped all around his long neck. Oliver was so shocked that he went to a basin and vomited. I watched the cord being unwound and the baby wriggling out like a long squiggle. He was a tall, thin baby boy—and he became a tall, thin man.

Danny was born at 7 pm (January 24, 1967). I was taken to a small room for the night and given tea. Danny was put in a cot next to me and Oliver went home to Nicky. I lay in that bed all night, not sleeping. I don't remember Danny crying at all, but I was too excited to sleep. At midnight I asked for a sleeping pill, but this was refused.

After my night of not sleeping I started to doze off at dawn. But now the hospital system got going, and I was powerless to switch off the constant interruptions. The last was the weirdest: Oliver was to fetch me at noon, but this woman came in to find out what I wanted to eat for lunch and supper. I told her I wouldn't be there, but she made my exhausted self fill out my desires none the less.

Oliver fetched me at noon. At home I walked up to the top of the house carrying Danny—very proud to be able to do this so soon after the birth. The big room at the top which was Oliver's flute room or painting room was now my lie-in room.

As soon as I was settled in, Nicky rushed in and looked at him and said, "He's a real little human live earth boy!"

In the twenty hours I had lived with a miniature human, Nicky had grown like Alice: she looked like a child on a giant poster.

But I was in bliss with my two children. I loved them both equally.

My first night home I slept through the night on the top floor while Oliver comforted Danny at the bottom. He had truly woken up now, and he screamed whenever Oliver was not walking him or cuddling him or singing to him. So the second night was daddy's awake night.

After that things settled down. Danny was a good sucker, and I loved breast-feeding, and never had baby blues.

Danny was a calm happy child most of the time, but there were two states which showed themselves from early on: one was of extreme exuberance—joyful and expressive; the other was a state of exhaustion or depression where he looked pale-faced and half-dead: Nicky had never looked pale. Danny had frequent mild infections which tended to linger: Nicky never had a cold for more than a day.

Early exuberance came from Danny when he bounced in the open cupboard door: a baby seat hung from a spring attached to the top of the doorframe. I would put him in and off he would go, in an ecstasy of bouncing bliss.

Nicky adored Danny and showed no signs of jealousy. To check this I asked her whether she was jealous of Danny:

"No, I'm jealous of you."

"Why?'

"Because you can make Danny laugh and I can't."

She tended to swing him around as if he were a large rag doll; so that had to be stopped. But mostly I don't remember problems.

I had written diaries on and off since I was twelve, but I didn't think of it with Nicky until she was two-and-a-half. With Danny I started as soon as he put two words together, which he started doing at 16 months. I would say, "Goodnight Danny" and he would answer, "Bye-bye night."

Or he would request, "More more Mummy" or "More more Daddy", which meant he wanted to be with one of us for longer. He was already using words to express feelings and needs.

When we lay down together he would say, "Off garses!" (Take your glasses off now) and when seeing me up and about without glasses he would command: "Garses on!"

One day, when Danny was 17 months old, he walked over to the closed piano. I was nearby, watching and listening. He touched the lid, then requested, "Un-La". This meant, "Please un-do the piano lid so that I can play la-la-la on it." I was very impressed. He had heard me saying "undo" and "untie" and had taken off the "un" and used it. I wrote it straightaway in my Danny book, which was in a drawer near me.

When anything was new or strange to him he would say with a wonderful lilting intonation, "Look-a-that!"

He fell down the stairs and cut his lip. Sitting on my lap he asked, "What happened a-blood?" Answering himself he said, "Blood fall out a-lip a-downstairs."

When we went for our slow little walks he noticed pipes of every sort: water-pipes, drain-pipes, big pipes, small pipes. In the kitchen I told him how the water came down into the sink. A week later he wanted to hear it all again:

"Pipe down down down a-water Mummy please show me."

He took to Resting Time, when I put him in his cot with his favourite things. By 18 months he knew all the nursery rhymes and would go through his cardboard book of them, singing or reciting each one. One day Oliver put a tape recorder in there, so we have Danny doing that on tape: "Jack-a-Jill-a-up-a-hill-a-fetch-a-pail-a-wor-TU!"

Danny loved his bottles and rejected the idea of my holding him while he sucked. He would lie on his back on the floor, boldly intense, like a trumpeter.

When he was two years old the first picture of baby Bess, his cousin from far away, arrived. Danny looked at it for about five minutes, giving little smiles and not saying anything. When we went upstairs at bedtime he fetched the photo and said, "Take my baby".

A month later Bess and her mother, my sister Jenny, came to stay. After watching Bess being breastfed he said, "I want to suck some milk from Mummy."

"There's no milk there any more."

"Mummy put some in."

Just like Nicola he was interested in Oliver and me cuddling, but also like her, not anxious. "What are you doing?" he would ask.

At two years and two months he came to a great conclusion. After lying silently in bed with me for an hour in the early morning he said: "Mummy is not Daddy."

My life was easy. After breakfast I would push Danny up to Hilly Fields with schoolgirl Nicky. At the top of the hilly park she would give us both a hug and walk down down down the other side. At the bottom she would turn and wave to us. How tiny she looked to be doing this herself! Then she crossed a quiet street and went round the corner to where there was a school crossing.

Back home Danny would go to sleep. When he was two he was still keeping up this morning sleep, long after other two-year-olds had given it up. It just always was, and remained, a time when he was drained of energy.

In the afternoons children would come round and Nicky would take them and Danny up to the now empty again playroom (except for Danny's cot in the corner, and two mattresses stacked against the wall). I don't remember any screams or demands. I suppose Nicky organized games because that was later what she became supremely good at. At any rate these playtimes I was ignorant of, glad to be free downstairs and reading a book.

At two, Danny was showing signs of his later dogmatic self. He was convinced that he knew how night and day worked. When I said goodnight to him he said:

"See you a-lunchtime."

"Not lunchtime, breakfast time."

"LUNCHTIME!" he shouted.

"It's night now my poppet. Look outside at the moon and the stars. When the night is finished it will be breakfast time."

He saw the point, but was unwilling to give in completely.

"Breskit time OR lunchtime," he said, gloomily.

What Danny wanted to do he wanted to do with crazy intensity and focus. He was not distractible the way Nicky had been at this age: showing him a flower when he wanted to work the record-player by himself was disdained in a loud, wild rage. As with Nicky we did not hit or punish or call him naughty or say we didn't love him. We believed in "unconditional love". But the child is cleverer than the theories. He knows that a parent is not feeling loving during the frustration of the moment. Screaming to get to Nicky, when it was inappropriate for some reason, he said, "Mummy doesn't love a boy …"

Later, when he was lying quietly with me, I said, "Do you feel very cross with Mummy sometimes?"

"Yes. And I snuggle Kitty."

That was "putting him in touch with his emotions", as recommended.

I read another useful book at this time, which I've never heard of again. It was simply called *Consistency*. It was very convincing and I did try to be absolutely consistent if I had made a clear decision. It requires self-discipline and a toughening of one's too soft heart, but the rewards for family harmony are great. The kids know where they are and stop pushing the boundaries.

But there are always sudden moments where the parent needs control, when the old-fashioned "Because I say so" would be useful. But liberals couldn't use it.

I don't remember Danny just having a tantrum on the floor. That would have been easy! One could just have left him alone. But if he was going after a passionate "want" which I couldn't let him have, I used to wrap my legs and arms around him and let him yell. This could last for half-an-hour. I felt I was at least being supportive of him.

If Oliver was there, I would just hand Danny over to him. Oliver would carry on doing whatever he was doing with screaming Danny on his hip. One day I took him back again, sensing that Oliver had had enough. Now he shouted: "I don't like Daddy. I like Mummy and I don't like Daddy,"—over and over in his obsessive way.

But life was mostly not like that. Mostly I would avoid problems by talking about them ahead of time, or hiding something away that would set him off.

In the car we never had problems. Oliver and I would sit in the front and chat, and Nicky and Danny would sit in the back and sing: in unison, or two different songs at the same time, or some sort of quite musical combination of sounds and tunes. Before we left England, when Danny was not quite three, they were able to sing a round together.

Danny had no fear of the dark or of visitors or anything else at home that I can remember. But he suddenly did have a huge fear. We were going on a slow meandering walk, stopping to look at pipes or to talk about them—a lovely day, and nowhere to rush to.

A man on a motorbike stopped to talk to us. Then he offered Danny a ride. Danny clutched me, screaming, and saying, "No! No! No! Don't want a ride don't want a ride". I picked him up and carried him home. He had been riding his tricycle quite happily in the front space up to now—had said of his tricycle: "not a car, not a motorbike". But now, if a motorbike roared past he would run into the house in a panic.

A few weeks after this incident he saw a man on a motorbike in the newspaper. He asked, "Is that man cross?"

"A bit cross perhaps."

"Cross man goes on motorbike."

The fear faded, and soon he was riding his tricycle again in the front and saying, "Brm, brm, I'm on my motorbike."

He developed a passion for vehicles and had a collection of toy ones. His favourites were "working cars"—cranes and tractors. Oliver had no interest in cars and never talked about them, so Danny's passion was not modelled by his father. In the same way Nicky had a passion for clothes—not modelled by her mother! I would stay all day in my slightly short Marks & Sparks slacks, while she ran upstairs and down, appearing in a new variation every time. I remember her coming down in summer pyjamas with a short tartan winter skirt over them.

I continued to love my life with my two children—except when Danny was teething and Nicky had measles at the same time and Oliver was away. I was awake with one or other of them all night—and then I longed to hand over to someone when the day dawned. But I had no relatives in London, and my friends lived far away and had children of their own. I used to invent more sensible communal living in my head.

LOVE AND LEAVING LONDON (aged two, 1969)

By 1969 we knew about the Hippie communes. My imagined communal place was nothing like that: mine still had separate families in separate houses, but common places for laundry and chat and easy sharing of some of the parenting duties.

I sometimes called myself a "Hippie"—and picked a wild flower at Hilly Fields and put it in my hair. After all I did believe in "make love not war"—but was simply more in touch with reality. We knew, by the end of the sixties, of nursery schools and primary schools where the children did "whatever they wanted to"—but that often meant the more bossy were bullying the others, and the more careless were destroying the careful paintings and block-buildings of the others.

One of the couples we knew well was going in for "couple sex"— where the two couples swapped partners. These friends got divorced a year later.

In the Hippie communes there was Free Love and No Rules. The kids were neglected or indulged—usually both. Into this chaos the drugs were arriving. People took drugs either to experiment or to relieve the pressure of their lives—or both. Oliver was given pot on one of our last nights in England. He smoked it, but said it did nothing for him.

We didn't drink on a daily basis—only if we were giving a dinner or going to a dinner.

There were no McDonald's then, nor any other fast-food outlets—except for the age-old British institution: the fish and chips shop. As soon as we had a little money to spare we would have a weekly treat of fish and chips. I remember once going across the big road and along a side road, and it was winter so already dark, and it was snowing slightly in the lamplight. I ordered rockfish which we had found both the cheapest and the one we liked best—beautifully crunchy, and fresher than anything we had had in Jo'burg in the 1950s. A matey chat while the fish was being wrapped in newspaper, then back through the pretty night.

At Christmas all the houses had Christmas trees lit with real candles in the bay windows for all to see. We did have a Christmas tree—but no bay window. One day Nicky and I found about 50 Christmas card envelopes dumped in our front yard. We went on an enchanted night walk delivering all the cards to the twinkly houses.

In the 1970s, gentle non-conformity became the glorification of nastiness and cynicism and violence, but that we only heard about much later.

In our last year we achieved the unachievable: new people next door who became close friends; although for our passionate two-year-old there was sadness too.

Our previous next-door neighbours had been unfriendly and we hardly noticed that they had left and others had arrived. However, Nicky, now seven, saw three girls around her age who appealed to her: but they kept disappearing. Frustrated, she wrote a letter saying that she would like to meet them. The adults, George and Irene, warmed to her letter and wrote one back, inviting her round. They explained that the girls were George's children from his previous marriage: Sarah (12), Helen (8) and Philippa (6). They only came at weekends. Nicky was soon friends with all five of these wonderful people. We left it like that for a while—it was her triumph; but that didn't last: soon we were all friends.

And Danny fell in love with Sarah. He was two-and-a-half. He had all the symptoms of a teenager or an adult in that state. When Sarah appeared he blushed and ran behind the couch and then took little peeps. I don't think we ever told Sarah about her admirer. All during the week, when Sarah didn't come, Danny would ask, sadly, "Where's Sarah? Where's Sarah? Where's Sarah?"

It was a pity to leave London at this point, but we had already decided to go back to South Africa: Oliver had decided and I had given in. Our parents needed us. That was the main reason; and our relative poverty and the absence of a good school for Nicky were secondary reasons. My dad bribed us with a house. Oliver the artist no longer wanted to paint boats, and craved the South African land and rocks and mountains and trees: he was to paint them all.

Our neighbours George and Irene were high school English teachers at one of the new giant comprehensive schools. They were Labour voters like we were. Irene used to come round and visit me when she got home in the afternoon. I would make coffee and then we would go upstairs to the playroom. We now had a record-player in there and I would put on a record for Danny to dance to. I put the two mattresses on top of each other for a seat, and Irene and I chatted and drank our coffee and watched Danny dance.

Sometimes we stopped talking and drinking coffee because Danny dancing was a feast. He took no notice of us. Unlike Nicky he didn't seem to want our attention or approval. He danced to the music, hopping and turning and flinging out his limbs: a future rock star.

Irene said, "George and I have decided that you are a professional mother."

We thought parenting was easy—as simple as the two lime trees in our front yard, so honest and clear in their obedience to the seasons: new tiny buds in spring, and old fallen leaves to kick around as they lay there wetly in the autumn.

How would we deal with going back into that dastardly system? Keep our beliefs and pass them on to our children was all we could think of.

Nicky said, "Kevin is coming to visit me soon in South Africa." (The boy from Guyana.)

We tried to explain, but she protested, "If people say they are not coloured they don't exist. Even white is a colour. You can be buff, or pink (when you are cold), or blue (when you're cold) or light brown or dark brown."

On the last day our friends lined up on the pavement and we hugged them all goodbye. Then we got into the taxi.

Somehow in my next image (and written-down quote) I am at a station with the children. Perhaps Oliver had gone with the luggage to the airport.

A train poured noisily in, unstoppable. Danny tugged on my hand. I leaned down: "Carry me, would you please Mummy. I'm frightened."

Me too boykie.

Chapter Two

NURSERY SCHOOL AND THE GUITAR
(3 TO 5)

WHICH WAY IS ENGLAND? (Aged three, 1970)

The house we chose in Johannesburg had a large, run-down garden, which the children immediately took to, and there were lots of neighbouring children who could be reached through broken fences. The house itself was single-storey with a flat roof. That they loved too—taking their friends up to see the view and run around—and later sleeping out up there.

Danny missed England and "the girls" (all three) and of course, in particular, Sarah.

He said, with his usual confidence, "Let's go and see the girls now, shall we?"

He didn't believe the grown-ups when they said it was too far, and decided he had better do something about it himself: "Mummy, which way is England? I'm going to visit Sarah now."

I found him standing silently in the driveway.

The big wooden crate which contained all our belongings from England came about three months after we left. We unpacked, and Danny recognized one thing after another, saying joyfully, "That's from England!"

In one of his last references to Sarah he said to me, "I want to eat Sarah."

The Baruch book I had read in London came in useful. It had said, "Allow them to *say* angry things, but not to act them out." So when Nicola, now eight, came to me and said that Danny was hitting her and that she didn't know what to do because she couldn't hit him back, I took him away and held him until he calmed down. He didn't do it again.

He had some notion that he ought to control his angry urges: "Later I'm going to knock down all the things. I'm not well yet."

Both children when little used the word "naughty", even though we never did.

At the garage I said, "That silly man put in too much petrol."

"That man was naughty just like I'm naughty."

At just three he went to Nursery School—a good one, for teaching future nursery school teachers. He was fine there but one night after a couple of weeks he got into bed and said, "Mummy and Danny go to school and all the children stay in their homes. Then I can play with the toys." He knew it was a wish and not a possibility, so I joined in: "We'll have to go in the middle of the night—when the other children are all asleep in bed."

Another day, while putting on his pyjamas, he told me, "When I put on my pyjamas I be a little boy, and when I put on my clothes I be a big, big boy."

He continued to get strong ideas which he didn't want to give up. At three-and-a-half he decided to take his toy gun to school:

"No, you can't take your gun to school."

"Then I'll take my gun and I'll shoot you dead and I'll walk to school and I won't come back because you will be dead."

"Who will look after you then?"

"Another Mummy just like you."

"Do you think you'll find another Mummy like me?"

"No—but you won't be dead, because only a bullet gun can really shoot people dead."

Suddenly reality—South African reality—intruded. Danny came out of the front door of the house next door—alone—and saw a dead man lying on the grass. Soon other people were there, but he had seen it first. The man had jumped over the wall to avoid a pursuer, but the pursuer had already stabbed him and he died.

The morning afterwards, on the way to school, Danny sang:

The man was dead, dead, dead,
He couldn't walk
He couldn't stand

He was dead.
He couldn't mend railways,
Or robots
He was dead.

For weeks he ended all his songs with: "And the man was stabbed."

Then he drew a circle, and put another circle around it. "Now I've buried the circle." Then he drew another line leading away from the circles and said, "No he was only stabbed once, not three times, so the ambulance is coming to take him to hospital to fix him up."

He seemed quite calm about all this—didn't have nightmares or anything like that. He was preoccupied with it, but not anxious.

Nursery School Report
Danny is a thoughtful, even-tempered little boy who delights in making new discoveries and, for his age, has a good sense of understanding and judgement.

He is content to follow the lead of his companions, yet is always ready and willing to offer his ideas and suggestions for their games, accepting the decisions of others with equanimity.

RIGHT AND WRONG (Aged four, 1971)

Now Daniel was four, which seems to be the age for the concepts of fair and unfair, right and wrong. For the grown-ups in that era, only the government was "bad"—not children.

I overheard Danny asking his sister:

"Do you know what love means, Nicky?"

"What?"

"Love means a very good boy."

Next door were two children with Portuguese parents, Nadia (9) and José (8). Nicky and Nadia were good friends. Danny at three became an admirer of José. José had learning difficulties at school, and was always in trouble at home. I thought how nice it was that at least somebody in his world thought he was marvellous! It didn't occur to me that he could influence Danny in a negative way. Now Danny said, "When I was little, José took me to the shops and we stole sweets."

Another time he declared: "If somebody won't let somebody play with another person's guns and that somebody is big like José and has two guns then that somebody is horrid!"

Oliver and Danny got on very well. Oliver was mostly a kind, warm, educating father. He was a spontaneous person and unlike me he never told Danny in advance how to behave, or made up rules—he just sometimes got suddenly angry and shouted at him.

"Dad should have shouted at me because he was cross but he shouldn't have broken my gun."

But he did identify with Oliver and with future fatherhood: "When I am twenty I am going to study to be a daddy."

Nicky was educating Nadia: "I keep telling Nadia about our family's ideas—like not hitting children but rather giving them reasons why they shouldn't do things. And I gave her a brown bread sandwich to eat and she said she liked it!"

I told Danny a made-up story about a monster who was very tiny but got enormous when cross. Later the monster was able to take over Danny's crossness. Danny said, "I wish I really had that monster. I'm a bit sick of getting cross. I'm not going to get cross any more."

Their grandmother, Oliver's mother Sally, came to live with us. Of Danny she said, "I worry that his mind is too active." He did sometimes pour out words very fast, but at that time they always made sense. Mostly I didn't manage to write down his long fast flows, but once I did. He was criticizing the bedtime story I had told him: "I don't like to cry. That story made me want to cry. Tell me a story about a little boy only three who could jump from one house to another without falling off. He jumped all the way round the world and never got tired. Then he went to the army and never got killed. Then he blew up the whole world ... No, don't tell me that one. Tell me about a little boy about four who went in an aeroplane with his mummy and daddy. He went to England and to America but he never got out of the aeroplane. Tell me that one." I kissed him goodnight and went to write down his stories.

At other times he came out with extremely condensed thoughts (like "Un-la"): "Do you remember when my leg was very sore and I cried and cried and never stopped?"

"Yes I do."

"Do you know another way to say I cried and cried and never stopped?"

"No. Tell me."

"Sea."

"See? Oh, the sea—because it's salty?"

"Yes—and it comes through small holes."

We had been to the seaside when he was three, by car, which took nearly a day's driving. At the end of the long drive home, Danny, who had looked out of the window all day, said, "There is more land than sea in the world." We all tried to persuade him that this was not true, but he was certain. Back home he fetched an atlas to prove to us that we were wrong. He stuck to this belief for the next year. When we returned from the seaside the next time he said nothing, but in the car a few weeks later he said to his cousin, "You know something Cathy?" "No, what?" "There is more sea than land in the world."

All his cousins were older than he was, and all the neighbourhood kids were too. So when his younger cousin, Bess, visited us, we thought that was nice for him, and they played well together at first. Bess was the child whose photo Danny had taken to bed with him when she had been recently born. Now she was two and she didn't know the rules. We were playing Bingo at the farm where my parents lived. Danny was the caller of the numbers. Bess was messing up the numbers he had already called. We tried to persuade him that it didn't matter, but he said, "I read in the rules that if a baby comes and takes the finished numbers the caller stops calling and goes away." (Which he then did.)

We were a happy family, each getting on with each of the others. But sometimes at table Danny would be formulating one of his marvellous thoughts. I would see him concentrating and I held my breath for him—and then, before he could get it out, Oliver would interrupt with something else. Was he somewhat jealous? Or just impatient? Or perhaps, being a male, just completely oblivious?

Here are extracts from the three reports on Danny when he was at nursery school at four years old:

First report: Danny is a gregarious little boy who makes contact with children of all ages. However, he is beginning to be more selective in his social contacts and invariably joins boys of his own maturity in active, boisterous, imaginative games.

Second report: Danny is a highly imaginative child and is very often the one to initiate games. Although he has very definite and decisive views he is able to accept the opinions of others and share leadership with them.

Last report: Danny is a happy and even-tempered little boy who has very decisive ideas and is not easily influenced by others. He is independent in his relationships with others and has a well developed sense of what is right and wrong.

He seldom seeks the support of familiar adults. His mind is alert and he finds his surroundings of infinite interest.

Danny is able to express himself very well verbally and is a great conversationalist.

NURSERY SCHOOL DROP-OUT (Aged five, 1972)

Towards the end of his second year at nursery school, Danny had had enough, saying, "I'm so bored of that school!"

Another time he said, "I don't like my life. I only like my life at birthdays and Christmas and sometimes on Sundays when Dad is home."

Children stayed three years at nursery school because the government schools wouldn't take them into Grade 1 until they turned six. I don't think the activities changed much in the third year—or not enough for Danny, who was now at the end of his second year there, in Middle Group. One day he said, "I was sitting at the Older Group's table at lunch but they were all telling lies, so I'm not sitting with them any more."

"What were they saying?"

"That they would chop me up and throw bombs at me and things."

"But why were you sitting at the Older Group's table?"

"Because the teacher said I was more like Older Group."

And another day, driving home from school, he asked, "Mom, why do children have to go to school and daddies have to go to work?"

"Well, children have to learn about everything."

"I know about everything. You can ask me questions if you want to know things."

"How big is the world?"

"The world is as big as a very very big big big gigantic giant's castle. And a cat's world is ten houses."

Back home he said, "Ask me another question."

"How does that light come?"

"That's easy-peasy. By electricity."

"But what is electricity?"

"Well, you see … there are wires … (long pause) … and little fires sparkle along the wires." He went on, "I know about fighting too. If I have a real fire-gun I would have to go in the army, so when I'm a big man I won't buy a gun. I will buy work things."

One day he asked for a day off from school. He didn't pretend to be sick or anything. I, in my flexible way, couldn't see why not. Nursery school was not compulsory.

He did this regularly in the last few months—once a week? I don't remember. What did I tell the school? The only rule I made was that he was not to bother me, since I was doing my own writing work in the morning. There were no other children around. Mostly he stayed in his room. Promptly at 10.30 he turned on the radio—the Springbok radio station—and listened to a women's serial.

The other thing he did was to "read" his favourite book, *What Do People Do All Day?* by Richard Scarry. He couldn't read it himself yet, but the pictures are extremely informative: all the drama and the how and the why and the what of urban life: pipes underground, planes in the sky; how the postal service works, how paper is made—and then on to farms and ships. The child who at 21 months had asked: "Pipe down down down a-water Mummy please show me," could now see the hot water being heated and the pipe taking it up to the bath, and the dirty water going down and out.

This was a big, strong hard-cover book, but Danny wore it out completely. I bought him a second copy, but by then, like nursery school, he was done with it.

He forgot about the boredom of nursery school when I took him to Jabula to swim. Jabula was our local recreation centre. "Jabula" means: "Rejoice, be happy, joyful, delighted". It had a children's pool just the right depth for Danny. The first time I took him there he walked on tip-toe across the pool with the water touching his chin. Then he (a complete non-swimmer) got out of the pool and threw himself in—a shallow, flat, "dive". "Danny!" I shrieked, but too late. He got out and did it again and again. And taught himself to swim by wriggling and kicking—like dancing in water. Other children in our family had been taught to swim by older siblings or parents—held under their tummies while they kicked. But Danny taught himself.

Danny had been missing his dad. One bathtime when Oliver had come home early, Danny said, in a friendly voice, "I would like Dad to come and see me bath because I need a rest from you."

All the above was at the end of 1971, when Danny was four, and still officially at nursery school. Now it was January 1972 and Danny about to turn five and the new school year about to start. But Danny was not going to the third year of nursery school. Our plans had changed dramatically—and this was to lead to both triumph and tragedy in our future lives.

In 1971 Oliver had almost been an absentee father. He was working at Mullers music shop in town—town being the original centre of Jo'burg and still the main shopping area at that time. Mullers sold musical instruments and also hi-fi's. In those days hi-fi's—or "sound systems" as they would now be called—were sold in parts: two speakers, one amplifier, and one turntable. A technical expert had to set all this up for you. Oliver became a well-loved expert at setting up hi-fi's in people's houses—in the part of the house they wanted it in, and with the best possible acoustics—plus their personal tastes in sound.

He did this in the evenings and at weekends. On Saturday mornings he taught guitar in the shop: Mullers offered free guitar lessons to anyone who wanted them. Oliver loved doing this, and it reminded him that his ultimate goal had always been to teach music, and in particular to teach music to Africans—as they then wanted to be called. I had taught music to all races in my youth and now Oliver was doing that at Mullers. (Oliver had taken a huge Zulu dictionary with him to Paris. I don't know whether he had intended to keep up his Zulu there; it seemed to me more of a token from South Africa—and one which was rather heavy for us to shift around. I still have it—it's where I looked up "jabula" just now.)

We now made a decision: we would take a drop in income—no more seaside holidays—and Oliver would find pupils and become a full-time music teacher.

Since at first he would not have many pupils, he would be able to spend a lot of time with Danny; so the other decision was to let Danny off the third year of nursery school.

What happened now in the mornings I don't remember. I had been an over-involved mother and I was backing off. Oliver took him to the zoo and showed him how to use a camera; Oliver drew and painted and Danny watched, and then at other times he tried himself.

How and when and why did the guitar lessons start? Again I don't really know. Oliver had a friend, Tony, who made guitars. Danny often went with his dad to visit Tony. And then all of a sudden Tony was making a small guitar for Danny. But given the expense and time and trouble involved I hardly think Oliver would have set this in motion if he hadn't won Danny's strong interest in the first place.

Soon Danny was having an after-breakfast guitar lesson every morning with Oliver. This continued throughout his year of being five. One of the reasons Oliver was such a good guitar teacher of beginners was perhaps because he had only in very recent times learnt the guitar himself—and with that star guitar player and teacher in London: John Williams.

Danny soared. He became in a few months a child prodigy, able to play short classical pieces most beautifully. He was very poised and still when having his lessons with Oliver; I suppose the music steadied his over-quick brain. We made no fuss about it—did not show him off anywhere. Oliver thought of taking him to play to Tony the guitar-maker, but Tony's brain was deteriorating through dagga-smoking. Whenever Oliver went to visit him he was smoking dagga. Oliver up to then had simply accepted the liberal view that "dagga is less harmful than alcohol", but now he was losing a friend through it. Tony died the following year. (Dagga: cannabis, or pot, or marijuana.)

The terrible twins stormed into our lives towards the end of 1971. We lived back to back with them. They were now seven, and together with five-year-old Danny they made a gang. Harry and Alex were tremendous enthusiasts with uncontrollable curiosity. If no one was in our living room they would touch and examine all the objects, and even open Oliver's instruments and try them. Oliver wanted to ban them from our house.

But I valued them. They were wild, but not mean. The three boys would tear around our house with wild calls, which I simply endured. It was good for Danny to have close friends in his drop-out year. And often he went to them and I had peace. Oliver was soon teaching in the afternoon at a school, so he seldom had to suffer them.

Their parents were Greek. Both parents worked a full day, so they were left with an elderly, immobile grandmother who had no control over them.

These were the most non-identical twins you could imagine: Harry was rough, tough, firmly built; and not interested in chatting to adults or in feminine pursuits. Alex had a softer, gentler face. He loved talking to me; he loved feeling the texture of Nicky's dresses in her wardrobe; and he loved coming to watch the ballet classes.

Nicky was doing ballet very close to us, across two roads. I played the piano for the classes on two afternoons a week. Sometimes I took Danny, who sat cross-legged and silent at the front, watching them. Then one day Alex asked to come too, and he too sat silently watching. Harry had gone off, disgusted.

In the holidays I would drop the three boys off at the edge of the Royal Johannesburg Golf Course—near Jabula—with a picnic. Few people played golf during the week, so the chance of a stray ball hitting them was minimal. At the edge of this golf course were trees and ditches and thorns and debris: a fine place for adventures. They often needed plastering and bandaging on return.

Nicky was doing well at ballet, and that year she took part in an Eisteddfod. Danny and I went along for an endless day, while a large variety of types of dance went on: character, Scottish, Irish, classical—solo and in groups. Danny was fascinated. Nicky won Second Prize in one event and Third Prize in another. She was not the star of her age group. The star was the daughter of the ballet teacher—Wendy. Wendy was ethereal: watching her was a "getting lost" experience.

Danny said to me, "When these children go home their mothers will say, 'You did very well my child,' and they won't know that all the other mothers are saying the same thing."

In the winter holidays Alex and Harry and Danny and Nicky went to a local Baptist Church which was having a Vacation Bible School.

Danny seldom had temper tantrums any more, but one afternoon when they came home he had quite a violent one. I had asked them, "Are we allowed to sing hymns at the Bible School concert?" "No," said Danny, "But you can say the … what's that word Nicky?" She tried "prayer". Danny was frustrated. "No, you know, Nicky. Harry just told you when we were walking home."

Nicky struggled to find the word he wanted but couldn't. He had a temper tantrum thinking she knew but wouldn't tell him.

Later Nicky asked Flora, another neighbourhood child who had been there. Flora suggested "verse". This was the word Danny had been looking for. He was quiet by now and he realized that Nicky really hadn't known.

Alone with him later I said, "At least you didn't hit me while you were in that temper. Last year you would have hit me."

"I didn't hit you because it wasn't your fault."

"But you didn't hit Nicky either."

"It was my fault and I couldn't hit myself."

He could be critical of the twins, who were probably not as articulate as he was and who would therefore sometimes tease him: "Alex and Harry have never learnt to talk properly. They only talk a little bit of sense words. They've just lied and lied and lied and lied."

Little Bess came again, now three years old:

"I don't feel like playing with Bess. You see I've got used to playing with big boys."

"The other morning you played very well with Bess."

"Yes. I didn't seem to have any of my own things to do. I was like a machine."

"Why don't you like it when Bess copies you?"

"Well, you see—those are my words. I don't like Bess taking my words."

He was interested in the voting that was going on, and wanted to know if anyone looked after the whole world.

I told him the story of Sparta and Athens.

"I will tell you about brave/wise," said Danny. "If a child tried to do everything and he got a beating for the naughty things then in the end he would be very wise because he knew all the things not to do. And he would be very brave because he was not afraid to risk the beatings. But he shouldn't ask his mother first because then she would just tell him what was naughty."

On Christmas Day we went to my parents' farm, 20 miles south of town. Sometimes all of us three sisters were there with our families, and sometimes an aunt and uncle would come. Always a good-sized group. And it became a tradition for our family to entertain everyone else before lunch.

That year Oliver and I played a flute and piano Telemann sonata, then Nicky played a Bach prelude, then I sang a folksong with Oliver playing the guitar.

Finally: Oliver on his big guitar and Danny on his little guitar played a classical guitar duet.

Chapter Three

HA JACK SCHOOL (6 TO 9)

SURVIVING THE WICKED WITCH (Aged six, 1973)

In South Africa the school year starts in January, so Danny was exactly the average age for his class. He was keen to catch up to Nicky and to Harry and Alex and to his older cousins. Before Christmas he asked me, "Why has Nicky got so many presents to give people? It's not fair."

"Well she didn't give lots of presents when she was five."

"But when she was five she didn't have a big brother to be jealous of."

He couldn't wait for "big school" to start, so that he would be part of all that "big boy" stuff. He loved buying his uniform and his stationery. He was excited and optimistic and enthusiastic.

School started on January 10. He would be six on January 24. He was going to a school called HA Jack where his sister was starting Standard 4 (Grade 6).

After the first day he said, "It was much, much nicer that I expected."

After three days Harry came round and asked him, "Are you the strongest in your class?"

"I don't know. I haven't fought any of them yet—I mean! I've only been there three days."

After five days: "Today was just like real school. D'you know why?"

"Why?"

"Because the teacher shouted at us."

But after the first week Danny was disgusted and disillusioned. Not because the teacher shouted, but because they were doing play-play work. Danny thought it was like first year nursery school. I thought it was more like pre-nursery school, because what they were doing was matching shapes, and the children at this school would all have been given shape-boxes at about aged two—with a triangle shape for a triangle hole and so on. This was for "reading readiness". After Danny had told me all this he said, gravely, "I don't think we should tell Harry about this."

Danny already knew the sounds the letters made, and when they got on to reading he probably shot ahead. At bedtime one night he asked:

"Mum, do you think I am a genius?"

"Well you know, all mothers think their children are geniuses."

"Well Miss K said today, "I SUPPOSE your mother thinks you are a GENIUS."

I didn't ask him what had caused this remark. I think I was embarrassed and moved on to something else.

There were three Grade 1 classes and he sometimes met the two other teachers. He compared them:

"Teacher A can't control a class of 40. Teacher B is horrid to us. Teacher C CAN control a class of 40 AND she is kind. She NEVER hits visitors."

Yet the children in Grade 1B did not report back to their parents about what Miss K was doing to them, and even Danny was being oblique in that quote. Miss K was not Teacher C—that's all I can be sure of.

Much later, when he was nine, Danny said to me, "I really think Miss K was evil."

"As bad as that?"

"Yes. Do you know that she once took the whole class out of the school to sell us!"

"To sell you?"

"Yes. We had been noisy, and she said if we went on like that she would sell us. We ignored her and went on being noisy. And then, quite suddenly, we were all lined up and walking right out of the school, along those roads near HA Jack."

"But you didn't believe her—I mean you personally?"

"I didn't know what to believe. We all went absolutely silent. And we walked and walked and walked behind Miss K."

He told me about a girl in his class called Sharon. Sharon used to be sitting at her table, quietly, but as soon as Miss K walked in she started weeping—always.

"Miss K even *looked* like a witch. She called Sharon a cry-baby, and then Sharon would stay away from school for a few days. Then she would come back and the whole thing would start again."

At the end of that year, Sharon had a nervous breakdown and Miss K was dismissed. We parents all heard about it and discussed it. Miss K was later brought back—but as a teacher of older children. She never again taught the first-graders.

At the end of that year I wrote in my diary: "He is an enthusiast. When his interest is captured he responds hugely. When his interest has lapsed—that's that. And if forced to go on, as at school, life is very tedious indeed."

That means he did report "school boredom" to me, but he didn't crumble with boredom the way he did later.

At home he seemed a peak confident child, confident that he could survive:

"If you were a child would you rather you died or your mother died?"

"That's a very difficult question! I think I would rather I died. What about you?"

"I would rather live than die. I would go and live with someone else."

He still sucked his thumb at home, but when the dentist told him it was pushing his teeth out, he stopped. But at night his thumb went back in and he was upset when he found it there in the morning.

I told him there was a way to solve the problem: put a horrible-tasting stuff on his nail. He agreed to this. The first night he woke up screaming from the taste. The next evening I asked him what he wanted to do. He decided to have the stuff on again, and from that day on he didn't suck his thumb any more—neither at night nor in the day.

One bedtime I said, "I don't know why the other children have smooth hands. Perhaps their parents bully them more to put cream on."

"Well you should bully me more. But when you say nicely that I must put cream on my hands then I say no, but later I do it. But if you say it crossly then the next time I don't want to do it."

In their News books at school they were allowed to write without worrying about spelling or anything else. Danny wrote:

> *my roof is fLat roof and it has u room on it it has got A Lot of cracs and it is saf on The roof. cum over to my hows we can hav u feste in the dak an pLay sPooKs. I went to bed that nite I had u breme. bfro i went to bed i brusht my teeth Then i went to bed cosie and snug i fell u Slepe i landid in A munchn with golde and SiLvre ono it was all u drem cum ovre to my hous.*

"What a lovely dream you had, Daniel," wrote the wicked witch.

SICK AND WELL (Aged seven, 1974)

In the Christmas holidays after his release from Grade 1, Danny was very merry—he listened to our folksong records and sang them around the house. He made up songs and poems. He read comics and the Asterix and Tintin books.

One day I was in the kitchen sitting at the table, with pen poised to write a shopping-list. Danny came in from outside and said, "If I say you my poem will you write it out for me?" "OK".

REVENGE (BY DANNY, aged 7)

> *There was an old man of Tangeree,*
> *Whenever he met a bee: "Let's dance together—just you and me!"*
> *So one day he went to the town*
> *Got a ten foot ladder, and by mistake, fell down,*
> *And fell down on his head*
> *And HE WAS DEAD.*
>
> *The bee wept with his sting,*
> *Oh poor little thing!*
> *But he said, "Not tears!"*
> *So he went to the army and got some spears,*
> *Threw them at the ladder,*
> *The spears got very bent,*

37

The ladder said his last words,
And down he went.

He liked dressing up, but unlike Nicky didn't then show himself to anyone. It was for his own satisfaction. He showed me his book about pirates: "There are six pirates in this book. I've done three of them and I've got three more to do." (He was dressing up as each pirate in turn.)

I have a photo of him and his cousin Hector, two years older than he was, being pirates together, with strong crayon markings on their faces and bodies.

But after he turned seven in January, there are no more photos and no more writings in my Danny diary until July. Did he say nothing of interest in all that time? He was not so ill that he couldn't talk! But for half-a-year he scarcely attended school.

Danny had gone back to school at the start of his Grade 2 year resigned and prepared to accept his fate. But he didn't like his new teacher at all. She was an elderly, experienced teacher who expected performance. She was the vice-principal of the school and had been there for years and years. My sister had done her teacher training practical under this teacher: "Yes, she can be abrupt and rather humourless, but she has a reputation for getting every single child knowing what they have to know by the end of the year."

These somewhat spoilt northern suburbs kids had not only to learn to read and write and spell and do sums. They also had to learn to sit still and listen and to finish whatever they had started.

Danny hated the whole thing. There was no lightness and warmth. No laughter and imagination. And he simply did not like being talked to crossly. He responded much more to enthusiastic encouragement.

In the third week he woke up white-faced and with a tummy-ache. He had never used sickness to get out of school, so I let him stay home. The next week I took him to the doctor, who said he had swollen groin glands and swollen neck glands, but no clear symptoms. He put him on an antibiotic. It made no difference. Every morning I took his temperature. It was between 99 and 100 (Fahrenheit).

What was going on? What was causing what? Was hatred of school causing his immune system to function badly? Or was a mild chronic illness causing his motivation for school to slip into a donga. Danny was a child who could slip into demotivation rather easily and now he just lay in bed and did nothing.

I gave him a diary to write in, and at mid-morning gave him some tea and read to him a bit, and then left him to write half-a-page in the diary. His writing was dismal and defeated:

> *I was in bed for two weeks. I didn't go to school. I was sick again and I have to do some homework in the morning. Mummy reads me Winter Holiday. I don't want to write and I can't think of anything to say so I'm stopping. Sorry but really I can't write.*
> (I've corrected his spelling.)

In the evening he perked up. This had always been my own metabolic pattern so I recognized it in him. However, Oliver, who was only seeing him in these more lively times, felt I should try harder to get him to go to school. He felt that Danny might, whether consciously or unconsciously, be getting out of school. So I made heroic efforts and got him to school a few times.

Oliver was now leaving the house at 5 am. He had a morning job at a school on the other side of town and liked to avoid rush hour and then do his own practising at that time in his teaching-room. So he never saw Danny being white-faced and as inert and heavy as a corpse.

Our own doctor thought he had a chronic virus which would gradually burn itself out. No more antibiotics.

Eventually I took him to a specialist paediatrician. No one had looked at Danny "all over" for some time. (He bathed alone.) This expert took off all his clothes and studied him all over. Then he called me in.

"This child has Cat Scratch Fever. Look at all these scratches on his chest. Do you see that some of them are septic? It's a virus. There's nothing you can do—except that I'm afraid you do have to get rid of the cat."

This cat had lain on Danny's chest in Danny's sickbed. And no one had thought about it. I don't think any of us had any particular affection for that cat, and Danny both accepted the doctor's verdict and wanted to get well again.

I took Danny home and took the cat to the vet to be put to sleep. Danny was completely well within a week. And then it was the holidays.

Neither Danny nor I even tried to sort out when the original sickness had turned into the cat scratch fever. But Danny did say in my first diary entry afterwards, "I would like to be a doctor—because you make a lot of money, and also because I would like to understand about how the body works."

It was July. We were away from town and winter and sickness. Up in the Zoutpansberg mountains in the Northern Transvaal—east of Louis Trichardt. This was my parents' pine farm, near Venda. My sisters no longer lived in South Africa, so we had this soothing and healing place to ourselves, year after year, for three weeks in the winter holidays. The bright tropical flowers around the house greeted us as we wound up the mountain after our long trek through the dry lowveld. Beyond the flowers were the deep green pine forests.

It was warmer up there, but not so warm that we didn't have a wood fire every evening. I lit the fire and watched it growing from tiny twig flames to large palaces with deep orange caves. From the kitchen came the aroma of Oliver's herbal or spicy meals. He did all the cooking up here, and the catering too—driving with the kids to Louis Trichardt for supplies. So what did I do? Nothing! The Venda caretaker did the washing-up. This year I had ambitiously brought *War and Peace* which I had never attempted before. I read it in front of the fire, or in bed, or in the indigenous forest where I found a comfortable 1000-year-old jungle tree to lean against. I lost myself in this book and finished it before we returned home.

We all walked. After ten minutes along a farm road we entered the jungle, where a boss Samango monkey barked his echoing orders across the vast gorge; or sometimes the whole troop of them swung across the road for us to watch. We saw pale green leaves turn into butterflies; the children collected porcupine quills; and we heard indecipherable flutterings and trillings.

After supper we sat watching the ever-changing fire and Oliver and I took turns to read a book which suited us all. This year it was Jules Verne's *Around the World in Eighty Days*. We were all hooked. We wanted Phineas Fogg to get there in time, but we also didn't want the book to end. And then the day came when the book would end. Oliver and Nicky and I knew of course that he would make it back to London in time to win his bet. But Danny did not. Because of time changes and clocks, Phineas Fogg has apparently got back to London too late. Danny burst into tears of disappointment and rage and ran to his room. We finished the last few pages. Danny's shouting had stopped. I went into his room and sat next to his bed and told him the real end of the story. He smiled—reluctantly.

We were on our way back to town. Oliver was driving. Danny leant forward, "Dad, can we stop for milkshakes?" Oliver said, "Maybe." Danny said, "Well what does that 'Maybe' mean? More to the yes side or more to the no side?"

When we got back to town he accepted that he had to go back to school. There was no "Maybe" about it. He went every day, but he still hated it.

A great joy for me at that time was that he was now reading books to himself. I had read him *The Wizard of Oz* six times! He seemed to want to swallow it whole, like he had done with *What Do People Do All Day?* When he asked for it a seventh time I said he would have to read it to himself. Which he did. I then started getting books from the library which I knew would absorb him, then reading the book halfway and stopping. That did it.

He also read Nicky's Standard 5 History books. The pupils stuck photocopied stories in their exercise books and then answered questions. Danny always loved history.

I began to dream of a different school for him. I knew that in other places there were primary schools where children's curiosity and imagination thrived. But I knew of none in Jo'burg.

That's why I went to see Sonia Machanik. She was a renowned educational psychologist and I thought that if there were any interesting little schools hiding away somewhere in our town—she would know about it.

She wanted to test Danny's abilities. I said I was dubious about IQs, but she said that this was not a pen and paper IQ but a more comprehensive type of test that would show where his strengths were. We spent the whole morning there. I read a book in the waiting room. Then Danny came out, smiling. "It was fun," he said.

I went in. Dr Machanik seemed almost angry with me. In an indignant voice she said: "No wonder this boy is bored! He is age seven and his reading ability is age eleven. His reasoning ability is age thirteen."

"So where should he go to school?"

"St John's."

But St John's just wasn't in our ideological world. It was High Anglican and wealthy children went there. I also thought it would be completely conservative as far as teaching methods went.

In Dr Machanik's report she stated:

> *Danny was alert and co-operative during the test. He is socially mature and very independent for his age. Verbal reasoning ability— good at 13-year level. Comprehension—good at 13-year level. Arithmetical reasoning ability—good at 11-year level. Auditory memory—superior. Visual memory and visual integration—above average, but not as mature as his other intellectual abilities.*
>
> *Recommendations: This is an extremely able little boy whose intellectual interests are currently not being satisfied. He could be moved up a class.*

But stern Mrs van N was insulted. "Absolutely not!" she said, "Just look at his handwriting!" He had missed half a year of learning to join up letters, and now his writing just looked messy.

In her report at the end of the year Mrs van N stated: "Danny has adjusted well to the classroom situation."

For the moment there was no answer.

When Danny was six-and-a-half, the year before, he had, all by himself, entered a talent contest at the Jabula Recreation Centre. He and Oliver chose a piece and he practised it diligently.

On the Saturday afternoon we all went along. The hall was crowded with mothers and fathers and sisters and brothers. Danny sat there nervously with his little guitar. When it was his turn he walked up on to the stage, sat down, and played—perfectly—a serene Spanish guitar piece. The crowd clapped politely.

After Danny came a little girl, glittering with bangles and dressed in pink frills and a swirling skirt. She danced and sang to a well-known popular tune—and the crowd roared.

We had been so proud of Danny's playing—and our extended family too, so I think that Danny had clearly expected to win. In fact he didn't even come second or third.

In a few years time the crowds would roar for Danny.

Danny didn't touch his guitar during his illness. When he started playing again he had lost ground. He found it very difficult and got discouraged. He had not gone far enough to slip easily back to the level he had reached before.

Then came Nicky's bombshell. She was 12 going on 13 and very much a young adolescent. She announced: "Classical music is YOUR music, and Pop music is MY music."

And she gave up learning the piano. She had learnt for six years. She had done reasonably well but had not had an inspired teacher. Oliver had liked this teacher because her technique was good. I used to call Nicky to practise at 5 o'clock every day for half-an-hour, and this she had never questioned.

Nicky was Danny's role model. What she did he would do too.

The next thing that happened was that the twins, Alex and Harry, came over with a plan to form a pop band. Neither of them learnt music, but they could bang drums and sing riotously. Danny soon learnt to strum chords. He listened to records and the radio: anything they could do he could soon do himself.

He took his guitar to school and the kids crowded round.

Oliver was devastated. This was the end of classical music for both our children. We lived in the wrong place at the wrong time.

WORTHWHILE? (Aged eight, 1975)

This was a good year. Neither Danny nor I can remember anything about his Standard 1 teacher at HA Jack. Nor is anything written down about school in the Danny Diaries. Plenty of other chat, but not school. I think he had a pleasant-enough teacher, got good-enough marks, and the kids had settled down. Danny made friends and went visiting and went to raucous birthday parties. He got into the swimming team, and I motored groups of excited boys to galas at other schools.

One thing did happen at school right at the beginning of the year: the whole school were given pen-and-paper IQ tests. Danny again scored higher than high. The headmaster phoned me and told me to take him to the Gifted Child Association at Wits University on Saturday mornings.

Dutifully we went along. I left Danny there and wandered around the grounds of Wits and then settled with a book. At the end of the morning I fetched him and we walked silently to the car. In the car I said, "And so?"

"This is not a 'have-to' thing is it?"

"I suppose not."

"I registered for Music and Astronomy. The Music was completely below my level. Astronomy was OK, but the thing is—I'm just not THAT interested in astronomy. And it's a nuisance for you, isn't it?"

"Ja well ..."

So that was that.

At home Danny said, "I would not like to go to a school just for gifted children because they would make us work too hard."

"Well they might have a different approach."

"We would think things out for ourselves."

Another time he said, "I would not like to be top of the class."

"Why not?"

"Everyone would think I was a snob."

About books Danny was "over-decisive", judging books by their covers. "No I won't like that one," he would pronounce, putting it aside. The idea that he would only put his energy into truly worthwhile activities was an important part of his personality. In contrast Nicky read everything; if she had nothing new to read she would read her own books over again.

About the books he did read Danny could be very critical: "This is a very soppy girl's book. So what if she found the baby's hand! Anyone could have done that—it didn't require any skill."

"I may be a scientist," he said one day. He always got full marks in Science at school. He did it without having to "work hard".

"Why a scientist?"

"Well science is complicated and I like complications. Working things out."

Movies too were either worthwhile or not. Returning from *Zorro* he said, "I'll never see a film like that again!"

"How was the walk home?"

"I didn't even notice it. I was thinking about the film all the time."

He then created a Zorro outfit and was so absorbed in it that he couldn't eat any supper.

Oliver read him the Greek myths and he particularly liked Hercules. Later, Oliver, who had a rich, warm, expressive, compelling voice, read to both children: the Tolkien books, and later the Sherlock Holmes books.

Danny was still great friends with the twins, and together they did daring deeds. One which paled me when he told me about it consisted of climbing to a high point on a warehouse building near us, and then working their way round the building on a narrow ledge. At some points there was a window ledge to hold on to, at other points nothing for their hands at all. If I had looked up I would have seen these three boys plastered against the wall like cut-outs.

I took him skating. Danny was both a know-all and a risk-taker. He had done roller-skating on our flat, cracked roof. Realizing that he might be over-confident I talked to him in the lift going up to the Carlton Centre rink. I told him it was quite different from roller-skating and that he should hold on to the side at first. I don't think he heard me. We hired skates, he put them on—and skated to the middle and fell down. And that's how he learnt. No lessons—just experience. Sometimes he skated even in his darkest years and it always lifted his mood.

Danny decided to do karate. There was a centre a few bus stops away. I took him the first time and then he went on his own. He started on 7 May 1975, and achieved his Yellow Belt on 7 August the same year. Then he stopped. Later on karate was to play a big part in his healing. He asked me why I had allowed him to stop at eight. But it was not a question of "allow". It was his idea: he started and he stopped. I had no idea at the time that karate "built character". Character! What a word.

We were still flower people at heart: this word would have sounded hard and cold and Victorian.

The first maxim of karate was: "I will constantly train my body and mind for perfection of character."

The reason he stopped then might have been simply because the swimming season started again, with training and galas.

A holiday drama course showed up Danny's motivation system very strikingly. It was a daily course, which both children attended. The play they were putting on was Robert Bolt's *A Man for all Seasons*. Nicky, at thirteen, was already known to have acting talent: she was given the lead female role. Danny, as the baby of the course, was given a minor role. But even this role did require him to learn a few pages.

Nicky, Oliver and I all nagged him: "Come on Danny! Learn your part! We can test you on it."

"Nah!" said Danny.

On the day before the performance the second male lead fell ill—too ill to do the part. Danny was given the role. I don't know why—perhaps he had tried it that day. That evening he locked himself in his room with his part. We heard him reciting it to himself into the night.

Oliver and I went nervously to the performance. At interval Oliver said to me, "He's as good as Nicky!"

He had swallowed the play whole and understood both the play and his role in it. We had never seen him acting before and we watched in almost shocked amazement.

So that was "worthwhile".

Chapter Four

SAHETI SCHOOL (9 TO 11)

TWICE RESCUED (Aged nine, 1976)

At the end of every year Danny went to the Happy Acres Holiday Camp in the Magaliesberg. He loved everything about it—walking and climbing, playing games, putting on entertainments. He would return in a state of collapse. Luckily this didn't matter because the camps were at the beginning of December so he had the rest of the holiday to recover in.

Nicky had been to these same camps but under different owners. Nicky was never ill afterwards. She of course was not the one who got ill, but also I think that there was more supervision in those days. As children felt entitled to more freedom, so adults became more helpless in dealing with them.

At the end of 1975 when Danny was at camp we got a phone call saying he had fallen down the mountain. They had all been out on a hike and a climb. Suddenly the horrified children saw Danny flying off a ledge and landing far below. They hurried down, and found he was conscious but unable to move. The older campers made a stretcher with branches and clothes and carried him back to Happy Acres; then a car took him to Krugersdorp Hospital. By the time we were phoned he was having X-rays to see if his spine was damaged.

Oliver and I drove in total silence to Krugersdorp, imagining what it would be like to have a child with a damaged spine. By the time we got there the X-rays were finished: nothing broken, no spinal injuries; Danny cheerful in his hospital bed. So it had been shock and bruises.

"I'm not going to tell anyone at school about going to hospital because they will make too much fuss about it. Like they did with my burnt finger and my ankle."

We were not expecting school to go wrong, Standard 1 having been perfectly OK. But school went wrong. Other teachers had criticized him, but this Standard 2 teacher seemed to dislike him. Perhaps she saw any lapse in his application, given his "giftedness", as some sort of personal insult. She sent him to the headmaster to be beaten. He didn't tell me at the time, so I don't know how often this happened.

Later, in summing up HA Jack School, he said, "You know I had absolutely no idea why those beatings happened. I just didn't know what I had done wrong."

He was not disruptive or cheeky. I think he probably went into a dream when it got too boring. Or he was in one of his sluggish states, when good handwriting required more effort than he could manage— or perhaps more effort than we had trained him to exert.

He came home one day very excited and asked me to help him research material for his Churchill speech the next day. In a way the success of this speech made his life worse.

Danny started missing school again. He was never at his best in the morning, and given the negative school experiences he often flaked out before he could get up. I don't think he did it consciously. I was helpless. I was not strong enough or bossy enough to force the issue. In other situations I could "say no" and be consistent about it, but this task was like trying to get an unwilling child to eat: a no-win situation; and Oliver was still going early to work.

I made an appointment to see his teacher. I recognized her as one of Nicola's teachers. "I just can't get through to him," she said. "And his Churchill speech was brilliant. If he can do it sometimes, why not all the time?"

Well that is his nature, I thought. Sometimes he is highly motivated to do something spectacular, and sometimes he is half-dead. But I don't suppose I tried to explain this to her. I thought that for Danny life was so dreary and this teacher so antagonistic that his brain simply withdrew.

Danny later said: "You know the worst thing she did?"
"What?"
"Compared me all the time with Nicky."
"Teachers should never do that! What did you feel then?"
"I just wanted to kick her."

Nicky had had a huge start at HA Jack. When we came from England she was far ahead in reading, writing and arithmetic. She was put into

Standard One with her age group. She learnt nothing new that year, except Afrikaans. This enabled her to concentrate on handwriting and presentation. At the end of the year she came top of the class. She enjoyed that so much that she went on working diligently for the full five years she was there—and always came top.

By the end of that term Danny had internalized the teacher's view of him. He watched "Longstreet", in which a blind man doesn't try to help himself. Afterwards he said, "He isn't trying at all! Am I as bad as that Mum?"

He listened to the tape of himself when he was 18 months' old. It was the tape where he recites nursery rhymes when alone in his cot. Then he said, "I was good then. I was a different person then."

Of my writing things down he now said, "I don't want you to put me in your book because you would put in all the bad things about me."

So we were in a dungeon. No light.

The holidays came. We relaxed. We left Danny alone to play with his friends and experience joy again. It was late autumn. The many-coloured autumn leaves had not been blown off by wild wind and rain as sometimes happened. I sat outside on a windless April afternoon, reading the paper. I read an article; I experienced shock and hope.

It was about Saheti School. I had never heard of it before. A new school. A ten minutes drive from us. George Bizos, the unglamourous, much-admired defender of Mandela in the Rivonia trial, had helped found the school and was on the board.

It was a project school, educationally experimental. Although primarily for the Greek community the education was in English and as the school was not yet full they were taking some English children.

Off I went the next day to see the headmaster. The school was all light and space— more like a guest lodge, with a circular mini-Greek theatre on the outside.

The head said that Danny would have their best teacher, Miss Terry Walsh, who had an MA in Education.

My father was easily persuaded to help us with the finance. I only told Oliver, the pessimist, when all the research was done. And then I told Danny, who was wide-eyed and instantly optimistic. On the night before he was to start he looked at his new clothes and said, "I can't wait to go to school!"

But the next morning he was nervous as we drove there, muttering, "hut-cha but-cha hut-cha but-cha."

When I fetched him he got into the car and I didn't need to question him. He just couldn't stop!

"That is the most brilliant school! Twenty times better than HA Jack. We did Art and Greek Dancing. I gave a talk on snakes. Miss Walsh asked me all sorts of questions about snakes and I found I knew the answers! Basti and me are going to do a project on snakes. It was so easy! I made friends with everyone straight away. They were all so friendly! No bullies. Basti is so strong. If there were bullies they would be Basti and me. I am much taller than anyone else. Miss Walsh is wonderful. She's quite strict and she makes us laugh. The Afrikaans teacher is very sweet. The Greek dancing teacher is horrible. It wasn't boring at all. They wanted me to be captain, but Miss Walsh said I wouldn't know where everything was ..."

A few days later Miss Walsh said to me, "I love having him in the class. He is so sensitive and imaginative and perceptive."

Miss Walsh handed back Danny's piece on "The Cyclops". She didn't say, "What a mess!" she said, "I like this—would you write it out in neat for the board." In the foyer of the school there were display boards. Within two weeks of being at the school Danny had his neatly written piece there on a board in the foyer:

The Cyclops

A luring shadow loomed over a dusty pathway. Me and my men felt like ants next to a teddybear. His one eye bulging out it reminded me of a frog I had once seen. His long golden but dirty hair hung down, and it was not exactley what you could call beautiful.
He, as you now probably know, was the Cyclops.

Miss Walsh knew that you couldn't concentrate on every aspect of writing at once. In their dinosaur book there is a page of information on the dinosaur which the children simply had to copy, in the cursive style in which it had been written.

In the holidays before Saheti I had taken Danny for a few cursive writing lessons in a beautiful home in Oaklands. Looking out on trees and flowers he looped the loop to music, and his handwriting started to flow.

Danny, in Standard 2, made friends with Harrigan in Standard 4: "You know what, Mum? Harrigan lives on the same plot as Miss Walsh. She says I can go home with them tomorrow afternoon if that's OK with you."

Miss Walsh lived with, and at some point married, John Oakley Smith, who was a well-known rock/pop/folk guitar player and teacher. On his very first visit to Harrigan, Danny met John, and arranged guitar lessons for himself. We of course agreed, and from then on the weekly visit to Harrigan and the weekly lesson with John took place.

"Now I won't be the worst in the family any more," said Danny as I drove him home.

After his first lesson the next week he came home and practised obsessionally for two hours or more. Then he came to play his piece to me and Oliver—but couldn't do it. He was very upset. He wanted to succeed instantly at a high level.

How easy it is to despair if your sister seems to succeed so effortlessly. Nicky had learnt folk guitar for about six months with Edi Nederlander. She sang simple songs with simple accompaniments—and people gathered round her.

Luckily no one at Saheti had even heard of Nicky at this time.

With Greek, where there was no pressure to succeed, Danny soared. The Greek teacher wrote on his report: *Very good. He is one of the best. He tries very hard.*

The balance between trying too hard, trying just hard enough, and not trying at all, was achieved.

When the holidays came he couldn't wait to go back to school. He never missed school any more unless he was seriously ill.

Going to and from school was our talking time. But I used to give lifts, and this Danny resented.

"It destroys our privacy."

"Well I think it's mean not to given these Africans lifts."

"Well you can give one man a lift, but not three women who sit there chattering away."

So I gave lifts on the way to fetch him, and let him talk on the way back.

A friend visited from England. At table Danny explained our family: "Dad and Nicky and I are the artists. Mom just runs the house."

Yet I had the biggest room in the house!

"Why do you have this huge room? Dad should have this room."

"Why?"

"Because."

"But why?"

"He's the boss of the house."

"He is?"

"Well he earns all the money. You don't earn any money. Do you earn money for doing *The Rationalist?*"

"No."

"You do it for nothing? I would never work for nothing."

I edited the newsletter of the South African Rationalist Association, started by Eddie Roux at Wits (University of the Witswatersrand).

I couldn't draw at all.

"Da, please will you show me how you draw a head."

"Well—let's start with something simple."

"I don't want to draw one myself. I just want to see exactly how you do it, because I've never seen anyone drawing a head."

Later he drew a head on the same sheet as Oliver's, and was furious with my genuine inability to see which was his.

The school put on a memorable performance of *Midsummer Night's Dream*. Danny only had a small part, but he loved helping Terry (no longer Miss Walsh nor Mrs Oakley Smith) to produce the play.

Terry told Oliver that he was tremendously aware. She said that during rehearsals he was full of suggestions.

For me a shivery moment came when Puck (played by the son of Myra Kamstra who had partly designed the school) leapt out saying, "Oh what fools these mortals are."

At the end of the year Danny got A's for everything except Afrikaans. Terry wrote: *Danny is a delightfully responsive pupil. His work is imaginative and mature. Spelling is occasionally eccentric.*

He got prizes for English and Greek (i.e. Greek for the English-speaking children), but when he ran to the car he didn't tell me about these prizes because he was more excited about his friend Harrigan being made Head Boy.

"I wonder if I will be Head Boy. I don't suppose so, because Nicky wasn't."

He was very pleased about taking a hamper to old people on Xmas Eve, which his class collected instead of having a class party.

A LUCKY, IF OPINIONATED, BOY (Aged ten, 1977)

When Danny was ten I thought of him as "the luckiest boy in the world". One extraordinary bit of luck was that the best teacher he ever had—and one who was so right for him personally—moved up with his class. So he had Terry Oakley Smith for nearly two years.

Other things went well too. He played in the soccer team and sang in the choir. At the Springs Eisteddfod he won first prize in "Verse Speaking 10-11" and brought home a Gold Diploma and a report which said: *Very good indeed. I felt that you had thought hard about the poem, and about the snail herself.*

And, best of all, he had good friends at his own level of intelligence. One thing the Gifted Children Association was aiming at was to get these bright children to meet each other, so that they would not have to bluff and "dumb down" to be accepted. At Saheti he met two boys, Sebastian Ahrens, and Paul le Cock, who were at least as clever as he was, and immediately became friends with them. Sebastian ("Basti") had a well-structured mind. Terry put Danny and Basti together for projects—Danny had all the bright ideas, and Basti could organize the project.

Basti came to my parents' farm with me and Danny. In the car they discussed what they were going to do. I heard Danny telling Basti:

"Well if she disagrees that will be that. My mother will never give in. However much I nag and beg and plead she will never give in."

I was surprised! We often argued, but I tried not to argue when there was something he had to do since he could go on and on. But I was not a dominant or a bossy person. Danny knew this. He said to Oliver of us three sisters:

"Of the three of them, Mum is the least bossy and Jenny the most. G (Jenny's husband) is the most irresponsible of them all—but I like him very much."

And Jenny said of Danny, "He's alarmingly dogmatic!"

Peddie Masango, who now worked for us once a week, asked Danny:

"Can you tell me what love is, Daniel?"

"Love is when you can say no to someone and have your own opinion." (A different definition from his "Love is a very good boy," when he was four!)

Basti came for the weekend and we spent it at the farm where my parents lived. On our return I wrote:

> *Things reached a crisis at the farm this weekend. Granddad kept going on and on about what Basti and Danny had done in his office last time, until Danny exploded, saying something like, "You've told me that a hundred times already."*
>
> *Granddad became paranoiac after that, saying that Danny was totally undisciplined etc. We had a row about it at breakfast. Danny and Basti just listened. When the grandparents had left the room Danny said: "Mum, I just couldn't help shouting at Granddad because he went on and on and I got so frustrated."*
>
> *Basti and I tried to persuade him to apologize, but he refused. "I can't do it straight away. Maybe tomorrow if this is still going on I will."*
>
> *Basti told us how his father (nearly 70) used to send him to bed for the day when he cheeked him, but that now they had discussed it.*
>
> *Basti said: "Now he understands that if I cheek him it's not my fault because I'm one of these modern children who haven't been brought up not to cheek parents. You should apologize, Danny, so that Granddad will like you again".*
>
> *Danny said: "But I don't want him to like me."*

Finally he apologized, then came to me very worried saying: "Now Granddad will be all nice to me—and I don't actually want that."

I told Danny about his grandfather's achievements as a preventive health guru. He said, "Granddad had everything—high IQ, very organized and good application."

Later that year Daniel gave a speech on his granddad. Afterwards Basti said, "You know, Danny, when you grow up you are going to be *exactly* like your grandfather."

Decisive and dogmatic. But Danny had more empathy than Granddad, and more understanding of human interactions.

A friend who had gone to England when we did, now sent her son back to visit relatives. Few of my exiled friends would come themselves during this apartheid regime.

I took Danny and this boy, Paul E, exactly his age, to the farm and left them there for three days. This time the grandparents had no complaints—I think these two just talked all the time!

The next day Danny and I had this conversation:

"Now I have two brilliant friends called Paul. But this Paul drove me a bit mad—I would say 'about seven' and he would have to say, '6.873'. I tried him on all different sorts of jokes, but he didn't appreciate any of them."

"His father, David," I said, "used to sit in a tree and read maths books and he didn't have any friends."

"I would hate that. It would be like being in a dungeon. I would rather be less brilliant and have a social life. With Paul I found myself using all sorts of words I didn't know I knew the meaning of. He is more brilliant than Paul le Cock because he is brilliant in words and maths. I asked him whether he had any burning ambitions, but he didn't answer."

Danny was still good friends with Oliver and me. He and I had arguments, but good-natured. He didn't like me watching "his" TV programmes, so I didn't.

Terry Oakley Smith became a friend of ours as well. Basti's parents were also friends with Terry. Terry let Basti and Danny call her "Terry" at school. Just them. Was this appropriate?

Terry often left her class to do administration work for the school, and had taught her class to get on with their work alone.

"There's such a shortage of teachers at the moment," said Danny, "that we're left alone a lot of the time and we just get on with our work."

"It's lucky for them that your class has learnt to work on its own."

"And you know Terry was so pleased with us! Because when she expected us to be all wild and fighting I was reading the class a story in the quiet corner."

He was worried about wars: "I'm glad I don't have to go into the army. I don't want to die young." (He was British—we had kept his British passport.)

"But you used to want to go."

"Well I thought it was all cops and robbers and bang-bang. Now I know it is shaving off your hair and having generals shouting at you and working hard all day. I wish there was no fighting. A country could have an air-pressure wall all around so that no one could get in."

"What would you do about Idi Amin killing people inside his own country?"

"I would put him to sleep, whisk him away to a mental home, cure him and then send him back again. But what about his army? They would have to be killed."

"Well if he was a good leader then they would follow him. Soldiers follow leaders."

"Maybe I will be a leader then. A leader of all the pop groups. We would fight wars with pop music—so loud that it would kill people."

"Then you would kill off all the mothers first and there would be no one left to look after the children."

Terry introduced them to the Greek gods. She had been "Terry Walsh"—and she came from Wales. But now she was teaching in a Greek school. She put Danny and Paul le Cock together for a project on the gods.

Paul and Danny's project was 12 blue cardboard pages. On the cover, Zeus rises out of pointed peaks with his square heavy face and his broad shoulders—holding up four prongs of lightning to symbolise his power. Drawn by Danny.

Paul and Danny took it in turn to tell the stories. Of Zeus. Apollo, Athena, Dionysus, Pan, Hera, Hercules, Perseus, Theseus, Poseidon, Aphodite, Hades and others.

Terry wrote, "I am very pleased with the work you have done, particularly in such a short time. I am also pleased with the way the work has been evenly balanced between you. I particularly like the cover. Well done both of you."

At the government schools this age group was learning about the Great Trek.

Terry loved Danny's enthusiasm for everything she taught them about. However she was sometimes shocked by the contrast between his best and worst work. Those slumps still happened.

Danny never seemed to have any homework. When I asked him about it he said he always finished it at school. Terry didn't complain about his homework so I accepted that.

"We had to describe one of our parents today. I did Dad—because you are not the sort of person one can write about."

When the last term of Standard 3 (Grade 5) started, Danny said, "I've decided to work hard this term. Alex and I have been talking about it. I'm doing my science swotting like English at school: first in rough, then in this old English book you gave me, then on the wall."

Terry said that he really was putting more effort into his work this term and realizing his potential.

"It's nice really putting an effort into something and then it turns out well. Like this skateboard."

John Oakley Smith was not his guitar teacher any more. I don't think John was a real teacher—he simply showed Danny a few things. Danny remembers *The Maple Leaf Rag*. And now he had no teacher, but was hooked on jazz.

"Pop songs are all about love," he told me. "Jazz songs aren't. That's better."

"What's wrong with love?"

"Oh nothing's wrong with love—I like love. You just don't understand."

"What are jazz songs about?"

"They can be about anything at all—about the universe, space—anything!"

A hero now came into his life who was to remain one right through his breakdown and beyond: Robbie Robb: band leader, composer, guitar-player, famous in young Johannesburg—and Nicky's first real boyfriend. (She was 15.)

Robbie had a bright red, huge Afro hairstyle. Granddad called him "the golliwog". Robbie's family came from Ireland.

Robbie would visit with his musician friend Georgie and sometimes they would allow Danny to play his guitar with them—on our flat roof.

And now the two years with Terry were over. On December 4, Danny wrote her a spontaneous letter:

> *Dear Terry,*
> *You took all the gloom out of learning, you gave me two years of learning fantasy.*
> *A million thanks for all you have taught me.*
> *Best of thanks,*
> *Daniel*

Terry, when she heard about his breakdown, many years later, said, sadly: "I can't believe it. He was the most delightful child I ever taught."

A BOY'S LIFE (Aged eleven, 1978)

Danny, still at Saheti and now in Standard Four, had another good teacher—Kevin Barnes. Mr Barnes gave the class empty exercise books and told them to keep diaries. There are no ticks or initials or comments, so I'm not sure what kept them going, but Danny seems to have enjoyed writing his, and kept it up from January to May. He invented a friend called Engelbert. I have quoted from his diary in this chapter.

24 January 1978

Hi Engelbert,

Today is my birthday; it's been pretty lousy because I gave up all my Xmas and birthday presents for a racing bike. But at night my dad said I could have this quite advanced camera and trade in my two small ones when I knew a lot more about cameras. I said, "That's great," and asked if I could have a look at it. He said yes and we found out it had a bust shutter. My dad said it costed R40 to fix a shutter, so I fiddled around with it and saw a green lever that was on X. I asked what it was for and my dad said it was an automatic flash timer, so I shifted it to V, and the shutter clicked into place! And just for fixing it he gave me the camera. I'm reading a book on photography now so I can get a bit more knowledge before I use the thing.

    That's all,

    Daniel

I wrote: "He is growing rapidly taller, but there are no signs yet of adolescent behaviour. There are no reports of negativity and rudeness. He loves to talk and discuss all sorts of things, but hates me to pin him down on a logical point. Terry, however, insists that he is very logical. He has definite opinions on everything. He is happy to talk about people and feelings. He is happy to be hugged, and tolerates, perhaps even likes, being kissed goodnight—unlike last year."

22 February 1978

Dear Engelbert,

<u>*News RHODESIA*</u>

Last time I said I would write to you about Rhodesia, well I am: every Rhodesian whatever colour is allowed to vote for the government. This means that the blacks will rule because there are more of them and I wonder why the terrorists are still fighting?

<u>*Relationships*</u>

I have just phoned Paul Buck, because Sebastian wanted him to come to his party but didn't want to ask him himself. Anyway I phoned him and we had a chat about his school and other things, (including girls!)

    Yours

    Daniel

11 March 1978
Dear Engelbert,
Last Sunday we had the gala. I had to swim against High School boys because there weren't many in our team. I swam the Under 14 Butterfly and came 3rd, the Junior Open Breast Stroke where I came second and the Medley where I almost came second but Harrigan beat me by a smidgen of an inch. My biggest achievement this week is Riding to School on my Bike; it's about 4 k's and it's pretty tiring but it will save money because the petrol price is going up on April Fools Day so that means that the bus fares will go up as well
    Yours
    Daniel

He rode his bike to school through the quiet suburb of Sydenham and then along Club Road, Linksfield, where cars go fast. It frightens me to think about it now.

… Last week I went to see Mike S (husband of my mom's best friend) and he said I needed new gears for my bike because they are not ideal for hill climbing. I went into the kitchen of Jo S (my mom's best friend) and she asked me why I was annoying her, and I said, "because you're the easiest person to aggravate," and she said, "But that still doesn't answer my question." and I said, "I'm not aggravating you it just seems like I am," and she looked at me very erratically and then we started a new argument about her buying white bread!
    Till next time,
    Daniel

My friend Jo thought him amazingly confrontational for a child. She was herself a very dominant person and not used to being challenged. Danny said, when he saw her using white flour, "Don't you ever take any notice of anything my mother tells you?" And on another occasion he told her, "My mother never ever eats white bread."

When he and I were visiting the farm I said to him, "Danny, Do you see me eating this white roll?" "I see it, but I don't believe it!"

He now knew hundreds of jokes, but was dissatisfied by our response to them: "Why do you two always laugh at each other's jokes and never at mine?"

He was sensitive to my moods, especially if I was tense. One day when I was getting things ready for a party he asked me, "Why are you talking in that irritable way all the time?"

"I'm sorry. I'll relax now."

He still craved "time to talk"—and still valued me as a talking companion. I asked him, "Have you discussed the danger of cars in your travel project?"

"No. That's the trouble with school—with any school. We don't do the important things. That's why I want to go to Durban with you in the car, so that we can discuss everything."

So he and I drove to Durban—quite a long drive for me to do alone. The evenings at the International Fun Hotel, where we spent three nights, showed him at his entertaining best. After supper every night there was a comic in the main lounge, and the guests gradually drifted in. The comic demanded responses from his audience, but the people when we were there were quite dumb. Except for Danny. To everyone's delight, and I imagine especially that of the comic himself, eleven-year-old Danny began giving him appropriate and confident feedback. This time his humour was not unappreciated.

He didn't ask for alcohol in the evenings, nor to go out in the evenings. He stayed within the lifesavers' boundaries when swimming. The next visit to Natal was a little different.

On a freezing Highveld day I was standing on the Johannesburg platform waiting for the Krugersdorp train to come in. I would whisk him into the car and in no time would be home and I would be hearing all about this particular Happy Acres holiday.

This time he had gone as a "senior"—much like he had been put with the "Older Group" at nursery school—for the seniors were 12 to 14, and he was still eleven.

This time I had to wait at the station for a new happening: all the girl counsellors lined up to hug Daniel goodbye! I watched in awe, and forgot to be cold.

In the car Danny told me, "I don't go to Happy Acres for the games any more. I go for pillow-fights, cook-outs, party-nights and girls."

A few days later there was a phone call. I answered. A woman was raging into my baffled ear. The gist of it was that my son had slept with her thirteen-year-old daughter at Happy Acres. When she stopped I said, "But he's a child. He's eleven years old. A boy." That silenced her. "Anyway," I said, "I'll ask him about it and get back to you."

"Danny, um, Mary's mother says you slept together!"

"Yes we did! It was a game—she came to my bed and we lay in bed for five minutes and pretended to sleep. It was in the afternoon."

Mary's mother was contrite, and invited Danny to go to Kyalami to see the car racing with her family. Which he did.

But in this second half year of being eleven, Danny, now almost his full height, started to be spotty and croaky. Was there any connection between his general "fast-tracking" and his early sexual maturation? His urge to go upward, ever upward, faster and faster? Urban children and modern children mature faster; but in Danny's school groups for the next two years he was the only boy who was no longer a boy. It seems sad to me: he could have done with more time for other maturation to take place.

Danny said to me, "I think I will get married at about 23. I don't want to hang around for too long after school waiting to start my life."

Two years before, when he was nine, I had written in my own diary: "I know that this stage Daniel is at must end, so I appreciate it all the more. He is so intelligent and yet has the naiveté and gentleness of a pre-adolescent. I'm inclined to let him keep this terrible cat just so that he can have a way to express his gentleness." (This was a cat we had failed to train not to mess in the house.)

Back to this year: he went to Happy Acres again in the October break, simply because he loved it so much:

"Flip! That was the best camp I've ever been to! I made proper friends with girls—not shy with them—like a best buddy. My first girlfriend was there—but my tastes have changed since then. This other girl—she started off like a kugel, but I had a very good influence on her. Then she went off to try someone else. But on party-night they brought her back to me. She had such guts! She's only eleven, but so mature!" (Kugels: frivolous, materialistic, complaining.)

By the Christmas holidays Daniel had become restless and careless. I told him to take responsibility for his knockings-over and messes. He protested: "Not a single child my age would! At Saheti no one owned up and took the blame—yes, one: Sebastian. But they will all turn out all right in the end." (Sebastian was the boy with the elderly father—the one who got Danny to apologize to his grandfather.)

Other Danny thoughts at this time: "I would like to be a movie director—I've got lots of ideas for movies. But it's very difficult to get a job—so I may do law. I would rather prosecute than defend."

He was absolutely furious because in a film which he was enjoying to the hilt the gangster turns into a goody at the end. "That doesn't ever happen on telly. A romance must be a romance and a gangster movie must be a gangster movie."

Books he had loved were: *When Hitler Stole Pink Rabbit; The Diary of Anne Frank;* and *Animal Farm.*

"You should read every good book three times—once have it read to you when you are about five, just for the story. Then when you are about ten you can understand the plot. Then at 19 you can understand about communism and so on. Like *Animal Farm.* Come to think of it, the camp in *Watership Down* is like communism. I wish we could go to Molozi to read *Animal Farm* aloud again." (We had read it up at the pine farm when he was eight.)

A last thought on "hurrying ahead":

"I don't feel like eleven. I feel more like thirteen. I think at the end of Standard 5, I should go into Standard 7. I want work to be difficult. Work isn't work if it's too easy."

"But you could be a leader of your own age-group and have time for other things."

"I don't want to be a leader. I want to get on. And I wouldn't mind being in the middle of the class."

Chapter Five

ST JOHN'S SCHOOL
(AGED TWELVE, 1979)

What happened in the middle of his Standard 4 year at Saheti was that we learnt that his close circle of friends were all leaving at the end of the year. All the English boys were leaving. Why? There seemed to be a feeling that although they had had great fun with their projects, they were lagging behind the equivalent boys who had gone to the all-English boys' private schools which had a high reputation for excellence. This didn't apply to Basti. He was emigrating to Spain with his family.

Daniel was definitely going to Woodmead for High School. It was a project school like Saheti, and we believed he would thrive there. But they didn't have a Standard 5 class.

He could have course have stayed at Saheti, but in the end Daniel himself decided on St John's—the school we had earlier rejected for ideological reasons. It was only for one year, and he would certainly experience a different culture. Danny's reason was that he was losing all his Saheti friends and that he already knew boys at St John's.

Daniel had known Pippin all his life in South Africa. Pippin's mother was a lifelong friend of mine. They lived near St John's and Pippin went to school there—in Daniel's year. Danny often got on the bus along Louis Botha Avenue and walked to Pippin's house, and often spent the night there. I had not realized until now that he had met Pippin's St John's friends there. And liked them.

He did a test for St John's. At the school I watched him going off glowing and being social and light-hearted with the young teacher. He was in a "fast-brain" state and I knew he wouldn't be accurate. He seemed more interested in making a social impression than an academic one. Afterwards he said that he and Mr H had joked their way through the whole thing.

"He's so nice! You'd think he'd known me all his life. Now here are some of the difficult questions I was asked:

'What is the difference between laziness and idleness?'

'There is an exception to every rule even this one. Explain this.'"

There were two Standard 5 classes at St John's. The A class had mostly been there all along, were very bright, and were used to working very hard. Daniel was relieved to be put into the B class. The reality of it was getting to him—and Pippin was in the B class. For French he was put into the A class, because they were all starting from scratch.

Coming home on the first day, Danny said, "It was nice. I know all the boys in my class. It was formal my foot! The only formal thing was chapel and that was brilliant! We sang the tune and the choir sang against us. Such a good choir! Better than the Drakensberg."

The next week he said, "It's so hard! I'm going to have to work my arse off this year. I wouldn't like to go to the College because you have to work so hard. It's only now that I realize how easy the work was at Saheti. If I had to choose now I'd choose Saheti because the work is so easy—but St John's is nice. I'll probably be bottom until I catch up a bit. History was the best—it was so interesting."

History remained fascinating all year: the First World War; the Second World War; and Communist Russia.

"At least there's one thing I'm ahead in—or at least not behind, and that's swimming. I'm in the top swimming group and I'm a 'specialist swimmer', so I don't have to play cricket. I did better today. He explained something new in Maths and I understood perfectly. Even Paul le Cock wouldn't be in the A class at St John's. I'm only average in the B class."

He had to go to school on Saturday mornings until 10.30. Having chosen this school himself he accepted this without any argument or indignation.

Socially there were no problems. I asked him, "Do you go with Pippin in breaks?"

"Sometimes I do, sometimes I don't."

"So you don't think it's a snobby school?"

"Are you kidding! If St John's is a formal school I'm Mickey Mouse!"

He called the masters "sir" as if he had been doing it all his life. Quite a jump from calling Terry by her first name.

"School was great. I enjoy it more every day. Our Geography teacher knows all about Saheti. He said: 'Hey, Daniel, how do you like being in an old-fashioned classroom?' I said: 'Well sir, I don't want to hurt your feelings!'

"But I like having my own desk," he continued. "We don't talk to each other much—both because of the desks and because we have so much work to get through. It's a good school for work—but I miss the leisured life."

Within a formal, consistent structure you can still have fun:

"School was tit today. I joined in all the backchat and the general mischief. I tried that posture thing and it worked fine. Pippin is quiet in class. He doesn't pass smart comments or dance around or go for jacks and that. Saheti was so slack and slow. There's no messing around at St John's. People who get over 80% wear a special tie. Even if I work my very hardest I'll never get that."

Oliver thought that Danny was better able to work when he was a calm child. Now he didn't always think before giving an answer. He would jump to conclusions and then defend what he had said.

Danny (grinning) said, "Now I know what it's like not being at the top of the class."

"What's it like," asked Oliver.

"Nice! I like being around the middle. At Saheti they always gave me extra work—but I still lazed around."

Being very much taller than everyone else didn't seem to be noticed or commented on.

His voice had completely broken by halfway through this year and he was his adult height: six foot, two inches.

After going out socially twice with a boy called Beezle, this boy said, in my hearing:

"Oh Danny! You always *know* don't you?"

My bossy sister Jenny from Canada came again, and again she said of Danny, "He's alarmingly dogmatic!"

He and my dominant friend Jo S went on battling with each other. At breakfast I said to Oliver, "Jo says Daniel is a cool customer."

"Why does she say that?" asked Oliver, himself also rather a dominant person.

"Oh I know why," said Danny. "It's because she says, 'Oh Danny you *know* I've got this *marvellous* job at Wits'—and I just say: 'mmmm'."

Jo said to me that Danny was the only child she knew who couldn't be talked into a response.

In the holidays Danny and Pippin flew to Durban without adults and then they both went to Umhlanga Rocks to stay with my sister Hilary's family. Danny was already this lanky adolescent with a deep voice. And Pippin was not. They were quite amiable with each other, but Pippin, who matured more slowly, was no longer where Danny's social thoughts were.

At the hotel was a Happy Acres counsellor, a Matric boy at St John's. He invited Danny to have drinks with him and his mates, and no doubt Danny was delighted. When they came home Hilary reported to me: "He disappeared after dinner every night—and then I noticed him with those boys. I didn't feel I could do anything about it."

And in fact nothing went wrong. It was just that a pattern had started. Danny was still twelve, but he looked much older. He became a sort of mascot for older boys, who would pay for his drinks and later for his drugs.

WORK ETHIC

Danny went and came home by bus now, so we didn't have car chats, but he still enjoyed talking to me. We were sitting in the garden having tea. I said to him, "Mr Gruber said a surprising thing—he said you were conscientious."

"What's that?"

"Well, that you care about your work."

"How do you mean, care?"

"The opposite of being slapdash and just doing it any old how."

That my very verbal child should not know the meaning of "conscientious" was that this word, like the word "character", from the karate document, was not in general use at that time.

The year before, on a Saheti report, alongside "sensitive, aware, articulate etc." came this remark from a maths teacher: "Daniel does not always work with diligence—I feel he enjoys being entertained, and a non-entertaining lesson is not acceptable to him."

These children of liberal/therapeutic parents were at a disadvantage in the school situation. We had friends whose children were dropping out or failing simply because they had not learnt diligence.

Pippin's mother, who was in fact a therapist, said: "We must love our children for what they are, not for what they do. These children who want so much to succeed have been loved for what they do."

In the end of course the much loved children grow up—and then they have to learn to get up in the morning and to go to work even when they don't want to work, and to do the more difficult and tiresome things before the more agreeable things.

Oliver had the example of himself. He was the elder of two children of passive parents. His father had been sent away to school in Germany when he was seven: he stayed there in a boarding-house for years without his parents. He became a very good student, but had no idea of how to be a good father. Faced with his young son Oliver, a delightfully jubilant, extremely attractive child, his father just gave up. In adolescence as soon as work got difficult Oliver would bunk school and visit the house of a schoolfriend's mother and play jazz on the piano.

Oliver, as a young adult, suffered from low self-esteem and depression. At university he passed one subject in three years. Then he discovered the flute, and was highly motivated to work at it. But he didn't know how to work! In Paris he trekked across miles of winter snow to his flute teacher, for his third lesson with him. As soon as he began to play, the teacher stopped him and said, "I am not teaching you today. You have not practised. You will be charged for this lesson." So Oliver learnt, more or less, to be diligent enough to survive.

What Oliver thought now was that Danny was an absolute marvel compared with himself at the same age. Danny admired Oliver for his art, humour, cooking—and generally laid-back personality. Nicky wasn't in South Africa this year, but she had the stamina to go out until midnight, come home and write an essay and then get an A for it. So he didn't observe much diligent work at home. (I worked at my writing when he was at school.)

My father, at twelve, started to work for an incentive: the Rhodes Scholarship.

Now there was Daniel. He had a mind that formulated his own thoughts about other people and the world. Simply to learn textbook facts was often neither interesting nor worthwhile. School was something to get out of the way. He worked well in class I think, but at home he played soccer and swam at a neighbour's house; or he fooled around with paper darts; or he watched television. He was phoned regularly by a girl he had met at Happy Acres, and also by one of his old Saheti friends who still lived in Jo'burg.

If he couldn't solve a problem instantly he tended to give up on it.

One day after official "homework time" (5 pm) he said he was going to have a bath "because we beat this team that has never been beaten before and I pulled a muscle." After his bath he flopped on my bed and told me about a literary competition in which he wrote a narrative poem about "Rembrandt Park". He was pleased with it, told me some and then said, "I'll go and write it out for you."

"Shouldn't you do your homework?"

"Yes I better."

He did Geography for about 20 minutes, then came to me and said: "I've got a proposition. If you let me watch *Chips* now I will do French for as long as you like afterwards—because I've got a test and I want you to help me."

Today, with hindsight, I would simply chuck out the television. I don't know why we ever bought it.

There were other slightly dreary and boring things he "couldn't do".

"Why don't you get into the habit of winding your watch?"

"I can't. I've tried, but I can't. You don't know me."

"If I gave you R100 a week you *could*!"

"Oh, for R100 a week I could do anything!"

"It would save a lot of frustration, both for me and for you."

"Yes, I know. That's why I should get a digital watch."

His intentions were often way ahead of his actual carrying-out of them:

"I'm going to limit myself to two hours tonight."

"Two hours of programmes or two hours of work?"

"Work."

"I bet you fifty cents you can't work for two hours. Your intentions are good but you run out of steam."

"I *have* to work for two hours. I've got Maths and I've got an Afrikaans speech. So I *have* to. You can take your bet back if you like."

"No, the bet stands."

In fact he worked for two half-hours with a ten-minute supper break. He asked me to look up words for his Afrikaans speech and then became perseverative about not getting it done. That was his other problem: not being able to stop. But in the end on that occasion he accepted quite reasonably that he would have to tell the teacher he was not ready.

He got a letter addressed to him from Woodmead. This pleased him very much.

"I don't know about my behaviour, but my work will be OK—nah, my behaviour will be OK too."

The next evening he again worked for two hours on the Afrikaans speech.

"I've *enjoyed* working on this speech. This is preparing me for Woodmead. We'll do a lot of this at Woodmead, won't we?"

Sometimes I just left him alone and hoped for the best, but halfway through the year his report was not good. I was at my parents' farm when the report came. Oliver reported to me that he had said to Danny: "Your report is a little disappointing," and that Danny had then spent the whole of lunch defending himself. Oliver asked him, "What have the A-stream guys got that you haven't?"

"They've got the personality to work hard."

Pippin's mother was shocked at how much work the St John's A class was getting. She said they would spend the entire weekend on their projects. She felt this was very wrong and that adolescents needed time to think and dream and be themselves.

On Sunday night, when I came back from the farm, Danny asked me, "Oh, by the way, have you seen my report?"

"Yes."

"What do you think of it?"

"I'm wondering what makes you do so well in History and Science."

"It's the teacher—he's just so nice. Everyone likes him."

"But everyone doesn't do especially well. Why do you think you are below average in Geography?"

"I suppose I don't learn. I should learn more. You'll have to give Woodmead my Saheti report. Otherwise they may not accept me."

Oliver and I discussed the whole issue: "Well just tell him that his report is not good enough and if his marks don't improve you'll cut out telly altogether."

But I sensed the arguments that would meet this approach.

Instead of having an incentive to do schoolwork, like the Rhodes Scholarship, Danny had incentives to play his guitar. He had kept his early technique from learning classical with Oliver, and now he could pick up anything he heard on the radio. Any young people who heard him play were full of admiration. Nicola later admitted that she had brought friends home "to hear her genius brother".

Daniel learnt the guitar for a while with a jazz guitarist named Lucky. This worked very well. Lucky taught him to play scales, and Danny got faster and faster at doing this, and loved practising. But something had happened to Lucky, so those lessons had fallen away.

I felt he needed a teacher—not so much for technique but to have a mentor. I contacted Edi Nederlander, who had been so successful in teaching Nicky folk guitar. Danny went for a lesson. Edi said to me afterwards: "But he's better than I am! You would be wasting your money. He should be a jazz guitarist."

But jazz was no longer inspiring to the youth of that time. Electronic rock/pop bands were now what it was all about. A pupil of Oliver's had a brother named Ross, and Danny made a fatal visit to their home. There, in the family living-room, was an entire rock band set of equipment—all for Ross. Danny was stunned. He felt Ross had been very spoilt just to be given all this, but at the same time Ross needed a lead guitarist for his band, and if Danny had his own electric guitar ...

This was all in the middle of the year, when his report had not been good. This was also when we heard about the Merit Certificate. This he could get within his B class, for final results of 75% or above. We said, OK—get that certificate and we'll buy you an electric guitar.

"It would work at first, but then I'd slip back into my old ways."

In the end I established a "guitar fund" in which money was put in for eight hours work a week. That worked very well indeed, although he still feared boredom if he got too far ahead.

"Mr Muir is very pleased with my project. I've done more than anyone else. But I can't do any more of it at home, because then I'd have nothing to do at school."

He got 90% for this history project on the Wooden Horse and came top. A combination of interest and number of hours worked. Since he was studying the Second World War at the time, I think his project must have been on the story where the prisoners used a gym horse to dig a tunnel and escape.

Danny always worked steadily when he started: he was not a dawdler or a ditherer. But he didn't always check. His worst mental fault was still his over-quickness and over-simplification. Perhaps his assertive drive together with wanting to get things done quickly combined to make him think things were easier than they were.

He also still easily got chronic infections from late nights. From now on we did not let him go out at weekends during term time and he did not have one day's absence. But in the short October break he went to a friend for four days—and got acute tonsillitis.

He sold his electric train to a boy at school: "David will pay me the R50 for the train tomorrow and pay the other R25 off in 25 cents etc. from his pocket money."

"Oh no, Danny! He'll never do it—and you'll have to keep records."

"You don't know him! He's in the A class!"

That was what happened: Danny got his money and I found it interesting: the A class were not just swots. They had self-discipline which would help them in the next world. The adult world.

Near the exams I said, "I haven't helped at all with these exams."

"All the better. If I get a Certificate of Merit it will be all my own doing."

On the last day of term I fetched him from school. He gave me his self-conscious teenager's look and got in the car without saying anything. At Pippin's house where we went for tea, he said, carelessly, "Oh, by the way, I got a Merit Certificate."

DEFIANCE (Christmas Holidays, Aged 12/13)

Nicky came home from England, where she had been studying for O-Levels at a tutorial college in Oxford, financed by my dad. She had thought she might stay in England, but now wanted to come home.

A month before the holidays started Oliver came home sheepish but glowing, "I sold a bassoon and bought an air ticket for London!" It was his turn to go. I had visited Nicky during the year. He had looked after Danny, but it was term-time and there were no issues. So none were expected now.

We went out for a family dinner at a very good restaurant down the road from us: the Hacienda. Nicky leant over to me and whispered, of Danny, "He's beautiful!" We hadn't noticed this. It had happened gradually while our minds were on other things.

Outside the restaurant Oliver and I were waiting for the two of them and having a hug. Danny watched us and said, "Really, you two behave as if you weren't married sometimes!"

Later that week Nicky left for Cape Town, where she was spending the holiday with friends. Then on the Friday night Daniel and I took Oliver to the airport. On the way there we all chatted happily. But after we said goodbye to Oliver, Danny turned teenager, walking behind me to the car and not saying a word coming home.

On the Saturday night I came in to watch *Starsky and Hutch*—into the living room, which did after all belong to all of us. I didn't think of it as one of his special programmes. Danny said, "You won't like this. It's not your sort of thing at all. All violence and 4-letter jokes."

But I was soon absorbed in the story.

Danny wouldn't give in: "Are you sure you still want to watch this? You can't be enjoying it."

"Yes I was, but I am not any more. Good-night!"

Another time I went to watch the pop group ABBA. Danny started up again. "Why are you watching this?"

"I thought I'd see what they're like."

"Give me one good reason why you are watching it."

"I like to see who they are, to compare them."

"To compare them with what?"

A few minutes later he said, "Are you enjoying this?"

"I don't mind it. They are surprisingly gentle."

"All pop music is gentle. It's rock that's not."

The house was empty. And all Danny's band members, whom he had been playing with every Sunday morning, had gone away. Danny told me, "Ross and I must be the two best guitar players of our age in this country."

I wrote in my diary, "He is good. I enjoy listening to him, finding him tasteful and musical. Between skating and electric guitar he has two good hobbies."

My birthday. Danny came in to wake me. Stood at the door. "Wakey, wakey," he said, then went away. In the kitchen I found Oliver's present, and Danny's lovely cardboard cut-out with its coloured pattern. I took him tea. He looked very embarrassed and anxious and mumbled, "Happy Birthday".

A supervised party for young teenagers was arranged by someone.

"They want you to bring a girl to the disco party."

"Yes, but they will all be quite young—not more than about 14. So an 18-year-old would feel out of it." (The Happy Acres girl who had been phoning him.)

He was brought back at 11.20. I was awake but didn't emerge, because he had a key and I knew how important "being late" was. The next morning he said proudly: "I came back *so late*! There was a chick there who lives at Midrand. Max is going to get her number for me ... Why am I telling you this?"

That was the only supervised teenage party that was ever arranged in his growing-up years that I knew about. In the extended village of northern Johannesburg, no one was doing this. I looked and looked for clubs and groups. I could only find youth groups through the church—and Danny wouldn't consider that.

Us being alone at home meant more jobs for him, but he got his pocket-money that way so he didn't mind or argue.

"You're doing your jobs so well."

"I need the money."

He used the money for playing pinball at local cafés, or for going skating.

One day we went shopping together. He bought his clothes entirely alone, while I bought groceries and a braai. I told him I wasn't much good at clothes and this made him feel good. At home he put on his new clothes and looked marvellous.

Hector, his 15-year-old cousin, phoned up and I invited him and his brother Martin (18) to come over to try the new braai, and to spend the night, since they lived far away. The three boys talked and listened to music all afternoon. I gave Martin five rand for his birthday present. It was a lovely evening and we had the braai outside. Martin and Hector and I talked about their dad's job. Daniel didn't want to associate with such "adult" conversation and simply put in the odd wisecrack now and then.

After supper they went to the garage—the old garage which Danny had fixed up as his den.

At 10 I called them in to fix up their beds. They did this and I went for my bath. After that I was puzzled, and said to Danny: "The garage is still open."

He said, sneering, "Martin is there."

I left them to it and went to bed and to sleep.

In the morning I was in the kitchen when Martin and Hector slouched past the window on their way out. They looked gloomy, and left without saying goodbye. I realized they must have slept in the garage.

Later I took Danny to an old Saheti friend, Little Stevie, who lived too far for walking or cycling. He was going to a party and to spend the night. In the car he said, "I may become a professional guitarist." This was the first time he had said this.

"But you wouldn't like being poor."

"Some guitarists are millionaires!"

"I think you have to have an abnormal amount of stamina for that sort of life."

"Then I will do law."

When I got back from taking him I went to clear up the garage—and found evidence of debauchery—a pillow which had been vomited on and then scent poured over to disguise the vomit—and an alcoholic smell in the garage. I felt upset, and resentful towards Martin.

Daniel was dropped off the next day.

"There is much evidence of goings-on here the other night."

He agreed soberly, "Ja."

"You'd better tell me what happened."

"Well I was sick."

"But why were you sick?"

"I don't know—I was just sick."

The day dragged on heavily. In the end I said to him, "We must talk about what happened."

"I don't see what you are fussing about."

"Well I know that you had so much to drink that it made you sick."

"It wasn't a lot! It was Cinzano and I just hadn't tried it before."

"You mustn't drink unless you are with us."

"I learnt something didn't I? You just don't want me to have any fun ... Let me tell you, I can hold more beer than most people."

"Oh Danny that's not the point. The point is that alcohol is a poison. It has an effect on you even if you don't appear drunk."

"Well I know that!"

"What do you think it does?"

He mumbled, "You can't do things so well."

This conversation was tense, but it was still communication. But then it got a bit frantic:

Danny (shouting): Anyway you can't ring up my friends and find out if adults are at the party. What would my Happy Acres friends think? You always exaggerate. I knew it would end like this. Everything has been going all right hasn't it? So why?

Lucy: But there hasn't been an issue up to now.
Danny: Anyway they were all offering me drinks last night. They all think I'm sixteen.
Lucy (astonished): Stevie's parents!
Danny: Oh they went out.
Lucy: But there were other adults?

Danny: I suppose you *could* call them adult. (They were older teenagers.)
Anyway I've had enough of all this. If I'm ever in any trouble I
would go to Nicky. Or perhaps Dad, because he's a guy.

Lucy: But the idea is to prevent trouble.

Danny (getting frantic): Well perhaps there won't *be* any trouble.

Suddenly he screamed at me and I screamed at him. He came right
next to me and put his face up against mine. His six foot two size next
to my five foot nine size. Now he was crying and very aggressive. He
shouted, "You better be careful when I get like this." I walked away,
shouting, "Oh that's just blackmail."

He shouted back, "All these years of humiliation and now I'm
getting my own back."

I was very upset all evening and the next morning. I felt quite
desperately that I needed some person to talk to him—a counsellor, a
priest, an elder. I felt that I had failed and that I didn't want anything
more to do with him.

The next morning I still felt angry and weepy and not like doing
his laundry. I left him a note saying he should do the washing-up and
then I could do the laundry (same tap).

I went shopping and had coffee and bought a new skirt and top
that looked good.

When I came back the washing-up was done. He said cheerfully,
"That was blackmail! You knew I had to have my laundry done." I
replied pleasantly, "Anyway, thanks."

We had a peaceful day. I did the laundry and he ironed.

The next day he told me with pleased approval about an ad in which
you think the tramp is asking for whiskey and he ends up drinking
milk.

He went to Happy Acres for a week, and came back exhausted as usual.
We had a contented week. No friends, no phone calls. He played his
guitar and listened to his records and did jobs for me. He walked
around without a shirt, proud. Great mirth over my discovering his
moustache:

"Are you SURE I'm not really 16 or something? You don't think
you might have made a mistake?"

On his thirteenth birthday he jogged to the Hacienda and I walked. When I got there the Frenchman said, "Your beautiful son is sitting over there."

"You can have a beer," I said, warmly.

"You won't let me have a beer when I want one, so now I won't have one just to spite you."

So he had two coffees instead: "I must be allowed my dose of toxification."

Peddie returned. I told her everything. She said, "Daniel is doing too much thinking. I saw him walking around thinking last week and I said to him, 'Daniel you must stop all this thinking or I am going to punch you.' He told me about the drinking and I said, 'Daniel we must keep Mummy happy. If Mummy is not happy then nothing will go right.'"

Chapter Six

WOODMEAD SCHOOL
(AGED THIRTEEN, 1980)

I asked Daniel yesterday (2009) what his thoughts were about Woodmead before he went there.

"I simply thought it was the family plan for me and Nicky."

"In fact it was too loose, too open …"

"And puzzling. I found Woodmead very very puzzling."

"And if you had stayed at St John's?"

"I would not have had a breakdown."

His breakdown didn't directly follow Woodmead. But Woodmead led to Damelin, and Damelin led to drugs.

At the time, Oliver and I discussed leaving him at St John's. And in retrospect I think St John's had long experience with teenage boys. The adults had no uncertainties. Adults need to be in charge, even if "wrong" by some other criteria. But when we suggested it to Daniel he went completely rigid: he was outraged. If we had known for certain, then we could have won, but we were not sure. When you are not sure against a dominant, dogmatic, young human male—you don't stand a chance.

Before he went to school there, Woodmead for Danny was a dream place. He had been there often—to speech days and Open Days and to see Nicky as Bottom in *Midsummer Night's Dream*. All in the open. There was no hall—only sheds and rondavels. If Saheti was a well-designed guest-house, Woodmead was a deserted farm or game lodge. Danny once made a twig house while the speeches were going on, and then the children stampeded over it and it was crushed to randomness. There was a beautiful river to dream by and walk along, alone or with friends.

We had heard the headmaster, Mr Krige, speak about his educational ideas and we had read his articles. Woodmead parents had mostly done the final school "Matric" exam themselves and had found it stifling. But the Woodmead method simply used the first three years of high school for general studies and then did the Matric syllabus only for the last two years. This had worked. These young people had passed their Matric. "Adolescents should enjoy their schooldays," said Krige."Let them do topics which excite them."

But what was now going on in Krige's head was unknown to us. It turned out to be the worst year ever to have gone to Woodmead.

Woodmead was out of town—an hour each way by car or bus. Danny was going as a weekly boarder partly because of this distance, and partly because he wanted to get away from us. But when the day came he was white-faced and in a panic. He knew no one at Woodmead. In the drive there we didn't talk, except for one unpleasant exchange:

"If you need anything from the shops just phone me."

"Nah, what for—I'm going there to get away from your voice."

His class and some of the Matric students went a few days before school started—for orientation.

There was a Woodmead bus. On the Friday I fetched him at the bus-stop, near Waverley Girls' School—not far from where we lived.

In the car he mostly just made explosive sounds; then suddenly he burst out with words: "The orientation was so stupid! Silly games, long lectures. The standard is so low because of the plurals. The Standard Sixes are such turds! I go around with the Matrics. I haven't smoked yet—I've been offered enough times! But it's good because if I run I can't smoke. I don't see what's so special about this method of education. The dormitory is like a barracks."

Oliver couldn't bear his son referring to black people as "plurals". From now on, every Friday afternoon when Danny got home, he and his father sat at the kitchen table and argued about the "plurals". (I don't know where this word came from. I think it started off being a euphemism for black people, but sounded derogatory when Danny used it. The word didn't last long.)

Mr Krige's idea, which he explained only after term had started, was that it was morally wrong to select well-qualified black pupils, as had been done up to now. They had been selected on the basis of their perceived ability to cope with the Woodmead method of education. But Mr Krige had had a revelation—or perhaps the school needed money: all children whose parents could pay were now welcome to come to

Woodmead. The many black children who now came were those with rich parents. Their fathers were businessmen. Black academics and professionals and intellectuals were mostly out of the country—or in jail—or perhaps the parents preferred Waterford, a multi-racial school in Swaziland, away from trauma and civil war.

Taking black pupils was against the law, but from the 1970s first Catholic schools, and then Woodmead, started taking them, and the law did not interfere.

It was the third week. I was doing the washing-up and listening to these two having their desperate Friday argument:

"I know we are an experiment," shouted Danny, "but I don't want to be part of an experiment. I would rather be at a school without them. They bring the standard down."

"But that's not all you go to school for," said Oliver, agonized. "It's also to learn to get on with other people—and especially all the people in this country."

In fact Danny didn't like the white Standard Sixes either. From his point of view they were all "twerps"—especially the boarders with whom he shared a dormitory. However, they became his slaves—and made his bed for him!

His one friend in Standard 6 was a serious Indian day boy, Cass. Danny said, "Cass thinks the praying six times a day that the other Indian boys do is ridiculous. Cass says he has tried to give the black kids a chance but that they are immature, especially the older black girls who giggle all the time."

The big problem for Danny this year was that the teachers were so overwhelmed with helping the black children that they had no time for helping Danny, who simply didn't know what he was supposed to do. The black children not only did not speak English as their home language, but had come from the very inferior "Bantu Education" schools.

Woodmead nearly collapsed that year, because the teachers became so disillusioned and exhausted. It did collapse a few years later.

At the end of the year most of the black children left the school. One or two were put up to Standard 7, and one or two were allowed to repeat Standard 6.

It was a sad year for everyone.

In those early weeks, Danny wrote about himself and his schools:

... My father is a music teacher and musician and started me on classical early, but I have now turned to jazz-rock ... My dislikes are commercial pop-groups that play bad music; and cigar smoke.

I would rate myself as a fairly responsible person and, at times, dedicated to my work. However, I'm fairly lazy and will not always willingly help around the home etc., but I won't disobey orders.

I do not have a short temper, but not a long one either. I will tolerate people's negative actions to a certain extent.

I have a fairly small family: my parents ... and my sister, Nicola, whom I get on unusually well with. This is probably because there is a five-year gap between us, she being the elder.

I have been to a number of schools in the past, all very different from each other. This is perhaps to my advantage but I don't quite know.

The first school I went to was HA Jack, where I stayed until the first term of Standard 2. I then went to what I think is the junior equivalent of Woodmead, Saheti (South African Hellenic Educational Technical Institute). It is a Greek School, situated in Senderwood. The standard was not very high because at least 45% of pupils there were Greek (but fortunately not the teachers). Greek as a subject was compulsory, and by the time I left I could almost speak it fluently. It is one of the most modern schools in South Africa (the designer, Mrs Kampstra, having won a prize for its design), and placed in beautiful surroundings. It's not so good on the "facts" side, and as I said, the standard is fairly low, but it does put stress on projects and creative writing, and has a wide range of encyclopaedias in the library. I stayed there for three years.

The third and last school I went to was St John's, perhaps the opposite of Saheti. It is one of the most highly organized private schools in South Africa; it is incredibly strict in uniform, behaviour and work. It is excellent in the field of fact learning and technical work in general, but keeps you in an inner world of being told what to do, how, where and when—but it does discipline you tremendously. I stayed there for a year.

BEING BIG

Nicola was home from England. Ironically she was at St John's! They had a sixth form class there for doing the English A-level exams, and this class took girls. Nicola was loving it, and very involved in its activities.

We were sitting chatting outside one late summer evening. Danny said with longing to Nicola, "What I really want is your old crowd to come around again—sitting around talking and playing music."

"You should give your Woodmead class a try Danny."

"But none of them have even kissed a girl!"

He said that his only real friend at Woodmead is a Matric guy who has a rondavel to himself. Danny visits him in the evenings. He loves talking to him.

He is going on a school camp to the Drakensberg. I asked him if he was looking forward to it. He replied, "Oh yes, I suppose so. Oh yes—it will be wonderful!" He grinned and said, "I'm a bit scornful of everything these days—like last night. It will wear off." (His band had played the night before for a Wits Rag disco.)

The next day he said quietly, while washing his camping plates, "You see, I am completely independent. I have organized everything myself, even the tent."

Home from the camp he walked in and came straight to find me. "It was much better than I expected. Mr Q is a great guy!" His ban on telling me things was completely obliterated because he had so much to talk about and there was no one else here to tell. He told me how he and a couple of other boys had walked away from the camp and found Basuto ponies and ridden them bareback.

At supper we were all there. Danny said, "I am going to compose songs with Chantal this week." (The band now had a girl singer.)

Oliver asked, "Haven't you got a project to do?"

Danny replied, "I can organize my own life!"

Nicky said, "If you don't do that project I'm not going to take your side against Mr Q." And she left the room. Danny was most indignant. "How can Nicky say that? What a thing to say. It's like saying 'I won't speak to you ever again if you don't do your homework.' Have I ever not handed in a project in time?"

I thought about it: "No, that's true. I don't think you ever have." The problem was not about handing in his projects but about "not doing enough". Not researching enough and not writing enough.

Nicky admitted that most of her long Woodmead essays were just thumbsuck. She got A's for them all, but I now read some of them, and realized that no teacher had actually read them through and criticized her on consistency or working through an argument. They were just eloquent waffle.

Danny summed up his opinions: "I like being at Woodmead more than being at St John's. But I enjoyed the St John's work much more. I don't agree with Woodmead's system. There are a lot of things not good about that school, but I love being there and the surroundings and the opportunity for lots of different friends. I agree very much with the council system. That works well. But not with the tutor system. They keep talking about building up a good relationship with your tutor—but half the time you can't find your tutor—they are busy with other things. And we don't have English—that's one of the things I don't agree with."

The first report came. Mr Q wrote: "Daniel's general direction is somewhat confused at present and as a result he is not being faithful to himself and his talents. He does not have to 'behave big' or underachieve to prove himself to others. He simply has to be himself, namely warm, intelligent and friendly. At present he is in danger of placing himself on 'the other side of the fence' which certainly will have adverse results."

Danny could make no sense of this: "I don't understand it. I think we should all go and talk to Mr Q about it. I try to be original. I use long words. I try to do what he tells us. Some of the others copy pages out of encyclopaedias and then get 90%."

I went to see Mr Q. He said that Danny seemed not to want to be *seen* to be co-operative. He said that Danny's group at the Drakensberg (school trip) cut themselves off from everyone else. I asked him what he meant by "the other side of the fence"—but he didn't really know. I had thought to myself, "well it's not *evil* for adolescents to have an adventure like riding those horses,"—but it seemed that Mr Q didn't know anything about that, so I kept quiet about it.

I reported back to Danny: "In order to *be* big you'll have to stop *acting* big."

"Argh! Mr Q doesn't know what he's talking about. How can I not act as big as I am?"

"Well I think it means not putting people down, not groaning when someone in your class does something stupid. Rather realize they haven't had your opportunities and try and explain to them."

"I'm not *that* mature! I have to be at the stage I am at."

Mr Krige gave a talk, in his usual inspired way, about his visit to Atlantic College. This was an international college for "young people". These students were all very helpful and co-operative. He went on and on saying that this was his aim for Woodmead, and I thought, "But he is talking about 18-year-olds!"

In my diary I wrote, "Danny is out on a limb—will it *ever* work out for him?"

And then, suddenly, magically, there was Adrian.

As awkward as this term of being wrong for his age had been, so the Easter holidays which followed were entirely appropriate for his age. He came home glowing one weekend, with 14-year-old Adrian, who was in Standard 7. When Nicola was thirteen I had tried to liaise with the parents of her best friend, but the mother had just shrugged and said, "But what can one do?" Adrian's parents were different. We talked things through with them. Limits were set. But in these holidays limits were scarcely necessary, since the boys were not doing anything seriously bad—not drinking, drugging, or driving.

Danny spent most of the time at Adrian's house, teaching him the guitar. Adrian's parents and younger sisters were there, so it was all very safe. Danny was extraordinarily nice these holidays. He said it was because we weren't restricting him. Certainly the deprivation he felt until he met Adrian seemed to have come to an end.

Adrian was gentle and quiet. Danny organized the purchase of a guitar and an amp for him. At first he said, "Adrian is brilliant—he's picked it up so fast." Now he says to Oliver, "Da—don't you think I'm a brilliant teacher?"

Danny is somewhat megalomaniac, expressing things in extremes, lording it over Adrian: "I can look after him. His mother trusts him with me—even hitching back late at night." But it turned out that the Adrian's parents weren't quite up to allowing this hitching. We didn't mind Danny hitching, partly because Jo'burg transport was so impossible, and partly because it was a not-too-risky adventure.

"It isn't the wild drunks who give us lifts," said Danny. "It's the quiet lonely people who want a bit of company. You think you know everything about people from your psychology books, but we know from experience."

In my diary I wrote that I was proud of him for:

> organizing his pop group
> hitching home alone
> organizing himself for the Drakensberg camp
> teaching Adrian the guitar and helping him to buy equipment
> admitting faults.

As much as he felt unrecognized by teachers—his efforts scorned—that much was he appreciated in the pop-music world.

Adrian's report had attacked his character even more than Danny's had. His parents were disgusted with Woodmead, and took Adrian away. He was sent to Eden College, a no-fuss school which prepared pupils for Matric. Adrian passed his Matric. He joined a band called "The Elementals", which was written about in our papers, and which toured Britain. Adrian played bass guitar in this band—a simple plucking part, which required steadiness and rhythm rather than a wild creative style. Danny would not have done that, but he was nevertheless proud of Adrian for doing it.

THE PLAY, THE POEM AND THE PROJECTS

Science was taught separately by a teacher who had nothing to do with the confusions of Integrated Studies. Danny always did well and had good comments in his report for his clarity and accuracy and for his responsibility with equipment. Science was a holiday from everything else.

I asked him if he missed Adrian on the bus and he said, "No, not at all. I need that time to think."

In my diary I wrote, "Last week his Standard 6 play, written by him, came first overall: first for the writing, second for acting, first for production. It was a modern version of Theseus and the Minotaur, with Danny as the minotaur."

At supper, Danny gloated, "Ours was the only play with originality and humour. Even Mr Q laughed!"

Oliver said, "All you need is something that you really enjoy and then you work well."

"Oh I didn't really enjoy doing it!"

Oliver got him interested in Berk Lee, a music college in Boston which catered for all types of musicians. Oliver also helped him with his projects at the weekend.

Danny was working much harder now. I asked him how he thought he was doing. He replied, "I just don't *know*. That's the trouble. I have *no* idea how I am getting on."

I drove out to Woodmead. Outside, under the trees by the river, Danny and I talked to Mr Q, who said that yes, he was doing better but that he still wasn't believing in his power—for example he was writing rather humdrum language in his Creative Writing book. (He couldn't win!) Mr Q said, "Come on Daniel! With all that vocabulary at your disposal you can do something more lively."

Danny walked off with his pen and pad into the bushes and came back with this:

> *This handicapped monstrosity*
> *That's standing here in front of me,*
> *Has no kind of memory,*
> *Which is not a catastrophe,*
> *It could live for a century!*
> *Its childhood is momentary*
> *It grows with high velocity!*
> *It could have flexibility,*
> *But has no portability,*
> *Sunshine is its ecstasy,*
> *Gales are its misery,*
> *Anyone can see,*
> *It could only be ...*
>
> *A TREE!*

At home Danny at meals often had us quite out of control with laughter, hugging ourselves to prevent falling off the chairs. He would carry on a non-stop conversation in which he was both people himself—often himself and me; or Mr Q and a girl student. He still talked very fast, but entirely sensibly.

I overheard a lot of argument when he was working with Oliver.

After one session I said, "All this point-winning that you do with Dad actually hampers your intelligence."

Danny looked amazed. "Hey!? What's that supposed to mean? Put it in my language."

"Well say Dad is trying to help with your project and you keep arguing and coming back with quick replies—you don't actually learn anything."

"Oh I can't not do that! Other people's mothers don't talk to them like this."

After working much harder on his project he came home in a rage because of getting the *same* marks for his recent project as he was getting last term for work he had hardly tried for: 64%. He had a new enemy, his tutor Mr Henry, who gave the girls marks in the nineties. "For what!" said Danny and went on, "I *hate* that guy. I swear I'll leave Woodmead if he stays. When they give us marks they are not:

    1) comparing the work with earlier work we have done

    2) marking us for the effort we put in

    3) comparing us with each other."

In his next two projects he went from 64% to 66%. He felt that all his effort had not been worthwhile. Both Mr Q and Mr Henry complained that he had left things out, whereas he was able to show me that he had not left them out at all.

Like me he had a problem of condensed thought. It bored him to be discursive. I think he even saw it as dishonest. His mind had come to certain conclusions and he wasn't going to waffle.

End of term report:
Science: Another good term with good marks achieved by consistent work.
Well done.

Tutor's comment (Mr Henry): Daniel is making good progress at Woodmead. He is an intelligent boy who uses his creativity and initiative to good advantage. He works well. On the debit side he occasionally brings to the class a brand of cynicism which is out of place here—possibly the result of trying to be older than he really is.

POP-STAR DANNY

Danny's band, Streetkids, had started the year before. Four boys—Mark, Howard, Ross and Danny—had practised every Sunday morning at Mark's home. Mark had a large family who took a great interest in what was going on. Oliver too used to pop in and listen to the band and give advice. He was most impressed and said that Danny definitely had leadership capabilities in this situation.

There were no drugs. It was part of a family home and adults were around. Mark was three years older than Danny, and very keen on sport.

In May Danny wrote in his Woodmead diary:

Last weekend I played at a fashion show in Rosebank with my band. We went for two rehearsals and a sound check the day before the show. But the acoustics were terrible because it was an extremely large hall, and seeing that at the rehearsals there weren't any people to make up for it, the sound carried all over the hall and we could only put out about 250 watts—about 80 decibels in a large hall. So anyway we went that night and approached the manager to confirm that we were getting paid. He made out that he knew nothing about it, and when we insisted that we were, he told us to get out. We couldn't do this as we had no form of transport, but the lady whose fashion show it was told us that we were definitely playing, so we did. There were 800 people or so there, so the acoustics were good and we played well. There were also some press photographers there so we should have got quite a good write-up in the newspaper. The way we got home was incredible. We fitted:
1) a 10-piece drum-set
2) 9 drum stands,
3) 6 cymbals,
4) 4 guitars,

5) a Peavey speaker about the size of two large school desks,

6) a Peavey amp-top,

7) a fender guitar amplifier,

8) and our "Streetkids" sign about half the size of a car, plus 6 people, into a station-wagon. But when we got back we remembered that we had left one small amp for the singer's P.A. at the hall! So we went back in another car; and when we got back the manager rushed out to meet us and apologised for the inconvenience and told us we were brilliant!

I was not allowed to talk to him about his music. There was a taboo on this just as there had been on my watching his TV programmes the year before. (This year there is no mention of television in the diary at all.)

The others were allowed to talk about music: new releases, soloists, bands, styles. Nicola, Daniel and Oliver would have cheerful shouting arguments in the living-room standing there with the television full on. I would retreat, putting three closed doors between myself and the din.

He was no longer a boarder. This meant two long daily bus rides, but again he said, "I've got buddies on the bus, but I don't want to talk. I *need* that time for sorting out my thoughts."

He now walked home from the bus stop every day (about two miles—three kilometres) without any complaining. He no longer complained about cold, pain or tiredness.

He was in touch with his former guitar teacher, Lucky, a jazz musician. Lucky lived not far from us and Danny went over there to have sessions of playing scales. Because he had to take his guitar and Lucky was not on a bus route I used to take him and we would chat like in olden times. He said to me of his guitar, "You know what Ma? It's not the sound so much as the feel of my fingers on the neck. The guitar neck is like my own neck." And another time, "Lucky is such a nice guy. He said I can come any time without paying. And do you know that Lucky's group don't smoke or drink or anything? It must be unique."

We also found a point of contact in driving. He asked me for help on a car project he was working on for school: "Ma, can I just go over how a car works with you. I have to write it up. I'm not sure Nicky's got it right. Will you teach me to drive? It's the one thing I'll be better at than Nicky. She was always so good at everything. Just think—I'd be able to drive in emergencies, and if you're feeling tired or sick."

In my diary I wrote, "I have been thinking lately that he often feels put down—by Oliver's sarcasm, by my impatience and irritability, and by Mr Henry."

I said to Danny, "Dad is often sarcastic to you."

"But I'm sarcastic *back* now. We understand each other. He respects me more these days."

"Does Mr Henry put people down?"

"Does he! But only the boys. He can be so nasty to boys. I tried to be friendly the first day, but from the first moment he didn't like me."

Nicola was having a glorious year in the Sixth Form at St John's. She was ahead of the others because of the one-on-one coaching she had had in Oxford. Now she knew so well how to write a critical essay that she often had to read it out in class. They could wear ordinary clothes and were treated as adults. They became a close group—about fifteen of them I think.

But Nicky thought that Danny was a genius at the guitar and that she would never reach his level in music. She also thought that his creative writing was better than hers had been at thirteen. Woodmead often told Danny how well Nicky had done. They seemed to have completely forgotten what a bratty nuisance she had been at thirteen!

Luckily the Battle of the Bands happened in the Woodmead August holidays, so there was no conflict with work. Danny's band, the Streetkids, entered for this competition between the schools, and survived the early stages. Now they were in the finals, which were to be held on 13 August in King David's school hall (Linksfield). I don't remember any discussion about whether I should be "allowed" to go. I was going. The only thing I recorded in the Danny Diaries was supper on that evening. I don't know where Oliver was. The three of us sat silently in the kitchen. Possibly Nicky and I were a little worried that the outcome might not be what Danny thought his band deserved. Danny said, "From all this silence you wouldn't think we were the most amazing family in Jo'burg!"

The school hall was full of shouting and gum-chewing teenagers. Tuning-up was happening on the stage. I was worried about the sound level and my ears.

I think there were five bands which had made it to the finals. Danny's band played about third. He was in front, singing and pointing his guitar up to all the corners of the ceiling, something like the Rolling Stones guy. He was compellingly expressive both in his face and in his movements. "Danny! Danny!" shouted the girls.

The results were announced: The best band was "Streetkids"; the best composer was Daniel; and the best lead guitarist was also Daniel.

No one disagreed. From then and for ever onwards people of his generation would say, "Oh you mean Daniel the guitarist?"

Oliver said, "I don't know whether he is the *best* young guitarist in South Africa—but he is certainly the *fastest!*"

Danny, in his thirties, said, "I think it kinda went to my head."

In the middle of his last term at Woodmead, Danny got a surprising report. For Integrated Studies, where Mr Q and Mr Henry had moaned about him, came this:

Daniel works to a consistently high standard. He is a positive and useful leader. I am certain he will get even better.

He had a new, younger tutor, who was entirely enthusiastic about him. Mr Moonda appreciated Daniel and Daniel appreciated Mr Moonda. I went to see him, amazed. He said, "Daniel is so intelligent he probably doesn't need to do much work. No, I don't find him at all inaccurate in my subject. He is the class scriptwriter. An excellent student."

But his overall teacher was still Mr Q.

Danny said, "They are trying to turn us into such perfect citizens. Mr Q is always going on about human power and good human relations. He's just a word-happy philosopher. Some of the people in our class are suited to Woodmead. But me and my buddies aren't into being such perfect citizens—and Moonda agrees with us. Mr Q just doesn't know how much we can take."

Mr Q gave them an essay to do on saving the world. But he kept giving them different ideas, and Danny refused to tackle this essay until Mr Q stopped talking about it.

From Danny's "Utopia" essay. Introduction: If you think about it a bit there could never really be an ideal society. In the following essay I have tried to make it as ideal as possible, but only from the point of view of one type of person, this person being the responsible adult—the adult who has forgotten what it is like to be a mischief-happy child or a reckless teenager.

Towards the end of the year the headmaster, Mr Krige, called Danny in for a chat. He said that perhaps Woodmead wasn't the school for him, because the work would get harder next year. Danny was not exactly being expelled—had done nothing to warrant that. But he did feel rejected.

"But where could I go?"

The next day, when Danny told Moonda, Moonda said, "If you go I go," and Danny said to me, "If Moonda goes, I go."

The school had had a depressing year—too many unrealistic expectations, and the tutors tied up with helping the children who had come with too little good schooling behind them. I rather felt that Woodmead was falling apart, and Krige's rejection of Daniel was the final blow.

The term finally ended for both children. Nicola had got into UCT Drama School, and Danny was going to his dad's old school: Damelin College. The stresses were over.

All in the kitchen on Sunday night. Oliver on form telling a good story, Danny joking about my having read that "thirteen-year-old boys despise their mothers".

Oliver said, "Never mind my boy, when you're married you'll be saying to your wife: "My *mother* always did this and that.""

Danny (to me), "So you're responsible for my wife trouble as *well*!"

In my diary I wrote: "Danny keeps telling me how wicked he is—how late he comes home, what he drinks. Conventional wisdom would have it that he is 'asking for limits'. But Nicky, who has seen him at these jazz clubs, says that his behaviour is not at all out of bounds and that he simply listens to the music. I think he is basically law-abiding but feels a need to prove that he is not too tame."

Nicky told me that he was most perceptive—and socially very good.

At table Nicky asked me, "Is this a recipe or did you make it up?"

"Well ... I ... er ... um ..." I mumbled. Danny said, "All those ers and ums mean she got it from a recipe book but she would like you to think she made it up herself."

"Yes, you are quite right!" I admitted, laughing.

Chapter Seven

DAMELIN COLLEGE
(AGED FOURTEEN, 1981)

Oliver himself had been to Damelin. He had been a drop-out teenager in Standard 8 who despised learning and culture. But by the time he had been at Damelin for two years he had discovered Western Civilization under Dr Isaac Kriel. Kriel took Oliver for History, English and Afrikaans. Now, in 1981, Kriel was still the headmaster of Damelin, but he no longer taught individual subjects.

People went to Damelin for all sorts of reasons—some to get better Matrics so that they could enter Medicine, some came from other countries and didn't fit into the South African school system, some were for some reason older—through illness perhaps. And then there were all the rest of them: those who weren't succeeding at ordinary schools.

The school was there to get people through Matric. It offered no extras and no sport. We felt it would suit Danny so that he could use his extra time for his music. I took him to a gym club three days a week after school.

In one way Damelin suited Danny very well: he was never criticized either for his character or for his work. The rules were clear. If you broke them you got detentions, but no moralizing. Work was clearly set and clearly marked. Danny didn't feel out of place because there were so many fully-grown boys there. On the whole the boys his age who were still children did not go to Damelin.

Danny phoned Adrian and said excitedly, "You should see my class. There are three *ou's* (guys) taller than me!" To us he said, "Damelin's *lekker*! They make you work hard, but it's OK."

I think Eden, where Adrian was, probably took the younger ones, and also had strict rules about no one leaving the building during school hours. Damelin students could wander around Jo'burg City during break—as long as they were back in time for the next lesson.

There was a bus almost door-to-door from our house to Damelin, so that was another problem solved.

In my diary I wrote, "This evening he was high on Damelin—rushing around in an excited mood collecting pencil crayons etc. for Geography—just like Standard 2 or something!"

A week later he said to us at supper, "This history teacher he comes in and calls us all shithouses and shows us these giant hands of his. And then he gives us this brilliant lecture on the French Revolution and the Congress of Vienna—I would never have understood it from a book. They say you hate him after a while because of all the work he gives you, but in the end you love him because he gets you through."

From the diary: This morning he got up and worked. He has done long periods of work on Wednesday night, Thursday night and this morning (Saturday). Then we had our meeting, but it didn't go well. He again didn't want to accept the going-out rules. Later however we talked about pocket-money and associated it with room-tidying and teeth-brushing and he accepted this like a lamb.

Striding up and down the passage he said, intensely, "You just don't understand me—I have to get out. You'll see—I'm very stubborn. I'll accept your rules for three weeks and that's all."

The rule was that he could only go out at night once a week in term time—realistic to keep him rested and well.

He was very happy about the teaching. "I really understand the Afrikaans for the first time in my life. We do this difficult book very slowly—only about two pages a day, but I really understand it." And, "Our English teacher is on an ego trip. I just laughed, and he referred to me as 'that grandfather'. He didn't realize I wasn't one of the older ones!"

One supper he said, "Oh Nicky, you know what I did … oh no, I better not tell you in front of Mum—she'll get upset."

I was peak curious, "I promise I won't!"

He looked dubiously at me. "We played this game and no one chickened out." (He showed Nicky a cigarette burn on his arm.)

I thought: So his inability to stand any pain when he was younger is one thing I needn't have worried about!

The only dry subject was Accountancy. At first he didn't understand it at all, and then he did, but found it impossibly boring. He was allowed to give it up halfway through the year.

In English he could fly free:

A Bird in Flight. 19th February 1981
It self-admiringly strutted up to position itself on the sun-bleached rock, proudly flapped its wings once or twice and gracefully threw itself into the cloud-studded atmosphere and boastfully showed off its two-metre wingspan. It sailed over the multitude of farmhouses and winced for a second as it caught the sun in its eyes, and then, letting the wind carry it, torpedoed away into the romantic firelit sunset, making its exit like a king from his parlour ...

What was he doing at weekends? His successful "boys' band" of the year before—Streetkids—had broken up by now. All his friends, including Mark, at whose house the boys had rehearsed, were now smoking dope (as they called cannabis), but we didn't know this at the time. Danny, who for so long had had glowing feelings for the musicians who didn't smoke dope, was perhaps trying to avoid it himself by staying home at weekends.

All this year neither Oliver nor I, nor Nicky when she was at home, knew that Danny ever smoked it.

From the diary: Danny came home totally exhausted after tests and a detention on Friday afternoon and went to sleep at 8.30 pm. Now he is cheerful, sings and chats and since the last no-Happy Acres-next-weekend argument at Friday supper, has been completely calm. Nicky and Danny both enjoy the Saturday morning vacuuming of their rooms. (The vacuum cleaner was a new thing for us.) Danny has played his electronic game in the cafe, worked on some music in the garage, played the piano, and watched "Conduct Unbecoming" on telly last night, when we were all out. And now he's out skating at the Carlton.

Since his tests on Friday he has been worried: "This is the only year I'm likely to fail—and it's all because of that nursery school Woodmead. I should have stayed at St John's."

All the work that I have seen has been done perfectly—nothing careless at all.

"Hey, you know what? I got the top mark for my Afrikaans essay!"

Nicky quoted Danny as saying, "I met this smashing chick—she looks just like you!" He also told her that all the guys at Damelin talk about girls all the time but that he isn't interested.

Yesterday afternoon—Nicky's last day before Cape Town—she explained a list of art concepts to him which he had to learn. He will benefit from Damelin simply because he will never "just learn by heart" even if told to do so.

Damelin, before the drug scene exploded all around it, was a good school to go to.

JOYFULNESS

In March Danny passed his first term's exams—with an A (80%) in History, and a B (77%) for English. In his free periods leading up to the exams he spent all his time swotting Geography, which he had done badly in before, and brought it up to a B.

In April he went with a new Damelin friend, Pierre, to a big game farm. They went game viewing at night and Danny came back exhilarated and well. While he was away, Oliver and I celebrated our 21st wedding anniversary. I wrote in my own personal diary, which I still kept from time to time.

> I am reading *Isn't Today the Day?* by William Saroyan. He is a life-liver and I love him. Also because he was 55, had a ringing ear, didn't blame people and told it how it is.
>
> I have absolutely no worries at the moment. I can hardly believe how contented Oliver and I are with each other after 21 years of marriage. The children are away, and here we are, good companions, always plenty to talk about if we feel like talking. We freed ourselves from the niggling things that go on in most marriages by having our weekly meeting on Friday evenings.
>
> Danny's preoccupation with the guitar has been like this too: anything else he simply wants to get over and done with as quickly

as possible. The exception is grown-up work and earning money. He so wanted that job with Adrian's dad last Xmas. Now he works in Magnets music shop after school. He doesn't get paid—just free strings when he needs them. But he enjoys all the music talk and is allowed to try out the equipment if he plays very quietly.

Oliver responds strongly to the outside world. Danny responds to the world in his head. But neither of them finds it natural to sit back and work things out. That they leave to me.

It is June. We are at supper. I ask Danny, "What do you do in English?" He gives me a scornful look.

Oliver helps out: "What setbooks do you have?"

"*The 39 Steps*—the new version."

"Do you read it in class?"

"Ja. He reads it until he gets tired and then he says, 'Take over, Daniel'—it's always me."

I said, "Perhaps he likes the way you read?"

"Nah—it's just that ever since that first day when he nearly got me expelled I'm the teacher's pet."

The next week he told me, "At school today the teacher said to me: 'We had a meeting and out of the 50 Standard 7s we chose four who would definitely pass Matric. And you were the first of them.' I had forgotten a book and she still gave me some extra work to avoid the 'teacher's pet' idea. But she really likes me." He added, "I didn't mind doing well at Saheti—because I was bigger than all of them!"

Sheer size was a big factor. Danny later said that two of the teachers— English and History—were *huge* men. "And the Afrikaans teacher was tall and wore high heels and was able to cut us down to size."

By July he had a new friend, whom I will call Jan K. A large guy with a calm manner, whom I thought I could trust. He was in Matric at Damelin. It was holidays. Jan K would fetch Danny and bring him home again. Danny said, "You wouldn't know your own son! Me and Jan K we go around helping people. I've been a child psychologist, a drug counsellor—we're so nice!"

Mark from his old Streetkids band was still a good friend but he was not driving yet. He lived about three miles away in Houghton. Danny liked him for short visits. One night he and I had this discussion:

"Can you give me a lift?"

"No, I've got a programme."

"If I walk to Mark can you fetch me after your programme?"

"No, that's too late."

"You don't know what you're doing to me!"

In the end Oliver gave him a lift to Mark's house and he walked the three miles back in the middle of the freezing night.

Another day he said, "Dad is coming to the jazz club." He smiled. "But it would be better if he didn't and then you could see whether I'm responsible or not." This meant whether he could get back at a reasonable time, and also whether he had drinks there.

In September it snowed heavily. This was the first time Danny had ever seen snow. Damelin sensibly didn't react when the students ran out and didn't come back to school all day. They built snow sculptures all around Jo'burg city.

Danny's snow diary (a school essay):
Thursday 6am: It was a strange eerie atmosphere. It was dark, humid, superior, malevolent. I felt at home, strangely enough. I would say the feeling of that particular morning was not unlike that of a windy crag—dark, desolate, untouched and—again—superior. The morning appealed to me. I like variety, and something different was in the air.

9am: Looking out of the canteen window. Something happens. Everyone looks.

10.30am: The College was abandoned. The streets were strewn with insane, different-coloured people. The steel blanket of the city has been ripped beyond repair. People stop cars. People want more snow.

1pm: A quieter atmosphere; but still special. People start to use the surprise intelligently and to their advantage. The blind childlike delight has now diminished considerably.

5pm: The finishing touches are added to glorious masterpieces. People abandon the blanket in the hope of a nip, or a cuppa.

Friday morning: A much plainer atmosphere. But somehow a sense of freshness and renewal is just caught. Threads of the blanket are seen. Only threads.

Friday evening: I am finishing the last words of this conveyance of natural senselessness. I have now finished my essay.

"EVERYONE DID IT"

The received wisdom among "intelligent people" was that pot/dagga was no worse than alcohol, and in many ways better.

In the 1970s we knew it was around, because of Oliver's guitar-making friend; and then Nicola smoked it in a mild way. We followed the advice given in those days not to over-react.

But by 1981 we were more definitely against it—had seen or heard about its damaging effects. Danny's cousin, Hector, about seventeen at this time, had been having problems at home; his parents were about to get divorced. Suddenly he left both home and school and drifted around for three months. One Saturday afternoon Oliver went to Danny's garage and found Hector smoking a joint (a stick of dagga, like a cigarette). Oliver knew the smell of it by that time. He was enraged, and shouted at Hector: "If you *ever* smoke pot here again I will forbid you from coming to this house."

Hector stayed with us for a few days and he and I talked through his situation. In the end I offered him a loan, provided he gave up dagga and went back to school.

When Danny and I were alone, he said, "Hector got such a shock when you told him he'd have to give up pot."

"Well, with *his* ambitions!"

"Ja, he'll probably end up with his brain all turned to cottonwool, as a roadie (someone who lugs band equipment around). He'll sit in one corner and we'll all have to say in chorus: HECTOR GET MOVING!!!"

Hector moved in with a friend who went to Sandringham High School, got his Matric from there, and much later paid back everything he owed me.

Grant, a much older musician friend of Danny's, said to me recently, "But everyone did it you know? We would have a jam and then a joint would be passed around from one person to the next. Danny was so much younger than we were. How could he have refused?" (The dictionary defines a "jam session" as "an unrehearsed or improvised performance by jazz or rock musicians".)

As the year went on Danny was more and more in demand as a musician who could raise the musical level of these older boys who met in different groups.

Grant said, "Danny was five years ahead of us in his musicianship—and five years behind us in development. In general conversation he wouldn't know how to contribute and would look uncomfortable. But we all loved him you know; he was a very delightful person."

So Danny must have smoked pot by the middle of the year—but not at home and not in great quantities. His mind still held together. In August he asked two questions which should have alarmed me, but didn't. I never dreamt he would smoke pot. He was outspoken, but came across as eminently sane. He asked, "Does a persistent twitch under your eye mean you are going mad?" "Not at all," I answered. I often have twitches. It's from tiredness I think."

Another time he asked, "Is there any madness in our family?" I told him about my dad's cousin who had gone mad while a student in Hitler's Germany—and never recovered. The next day he said, "I hope you don't mind. I used that story you told me for my English essay." "That's fine." "It was a very good story. Only I changed it and I was the one who went mad."

When he did go mad I blamed myself most of all for the weekends at Midrand. I felt bad about moving him from one school to another, but there were thought-out reasons for doing that. Whereas I didn't think enough about Jan K and the Midrand weekends. And Oliver was used to leaving such things to me, and didn't check that I had checked.

In the second half of the year Jan K was forming a band, and wanted Danny to be a part of it. Danny had had friends to jam in the garage—the old garage which he had turned into a den. (We didn't have a real garage so we went on saying "the garage".) The problem now was that Oliver had started an Early Music group, which rehearsed every Saturday afternoon in his studio—near the garage. This was an impossible clash. So when it was decided that the band would rehearse on Saturday afternoons at Jan K's place, I drove Danny out there, and Jan K brought him back in the early evening. I met Jan K's parents—an elderly German couple. Very formal. We had tea and made polite conversation. Danny said that Jan's father was very strict and that Jan was afraid of him.

One day Jan K came to see me with a plan: he would take Danny home to his place on a Friday afternoon, and then bring him back after lunch on Sundays. At the time this seemed practical. But what was I thinking about! What did I think they were doing in the evenings? To me Midrand was in the country—far away from the wicked city. They rehearsed in a barn, which I suppose the parents never came near.

Danny says now that in 1981 they drove around looking for places to play—clubs or friends. "We all squashed into his little orange Volksie with all the equipment! Like fitting 100 people into a telephone box."

I thought these weekends at Midrand would give him the freedom he yearned for, but he often came back irritable and frustrated, so it was not the release I had thought it would be. Of course I blamed "tiredness" and didn't suspect pot.

One day Danny said to me, "I think I'll tell you something if you promise not to tell anyone."

"Not even Dad?"

"No. I don't know why—I just feel like telling you these things."

He then told me about drugs and drug-peddling in the city, and finished by saying, "The drug scene is sad—very, very sad." Nothing in his manner or behaviour or speech suggested that this had anything to do with him personally. He looked so young and fresh and healthy.

In the second half of the Damelin year, work became revision and repetition. Danny hated it, and probably didn't need it. But it was Damelin's way of ensuring that non-workers passed exams.

Sometimes Danny was extreme about school, sometimes resigned. Here's Danny being extreme: "You don't know how much I hate schoolwork—what agony it is to have to do schoolwork when I could be working on my music. I don't know how I can stand another three years of it. Every time I pick up my pen to do Maths or History homework and I think I could be doing something like composing it's a terrible feeling. I've got something I can achieve at and there's no point at all in sitting there in school. I *hate* it. Damelin does its best—they have better methods than other schools, but any school would be a waste of time for me. I could work all day at Magnets standing at a counter because I knew I was going to be paid for it—but to think that you even have to *pay* for me to go to school! Being forced to do it makes me hate that sort of work more and more."

I now think that this outburst came from his heavy weekend pot smoking as much as from Damelin revision. The after-effect of pot is poor concentration—so it was becoming more and more of an effort to study.

Damelin's rules could irk him too. At supper: "Can you guys do something to get me out of detention for going up in the lift last term? Tell me one single reason why I should not go up in the lift."

I said, "The penalty probably reflects the amount of disruption which would be caused if everyone went up in the lift."

"But everyone *doesn't* go in the lift."

"Oh, they've probably learnt not to from dire experience. The staff have to be able to get up and down quickly."

"Ja, that's true."

Oliver said, "Perhaps it would be worth phoning up and finding out just what they give detentions for."

Danny was startled! "No, don't do that! They'd probably give me *another* detention! I'll just stick it out. It's only for a few more days."

On the issue of being more organized at home he had a good reply, good that is for a disorganized teenager. He made this speech:

I'm not mature enough yet. I'm not advanced enough to become a really disciplined, organized person. I'm happy with myself. If I changed, my personality would change and I don't want that to happen.

I've got my life
I've got my goals
I've got my ideas.

People will stop respecting me for what I am. You don't know the other side of me—the conversations I have, the way of life that I lead, the people that I help.

I understand me as I am.

COUNSELLING MANDY

Danny had been interested in girls since he was eleven, and since he was now nearly fifteen, there had, I suppose, been some sort of development from smiling at them to wanting to go the whole way. The pattern was always older women taking an interest in him, so when Mandy, a Matric student (but not at Damelin), started phoning him up in the second half of the year, we thought it was life as usual. But Mandy phoned very regularly, and Daniel took the phone to his bedroom and they had long conversations. "I'm counselling her," he said.

One day he was about to go for a run when the phone rang. As he ran out he called back, "Just tell her I was cut off."

He did running now instead of gym. We had worked out a click system—a small clicking gadget which you banged on the top to change the number. Clicks were for running and for work times and so on. It was so easy for Danny to put off things he had to do that some parental shaping seemed necessary. His pocket money was related to these clicks. This worked much better than lecturing him about self-discipline and arguing about how long he had actually worked or what time he had actually started and so on.

He said in a good-humoured, glowing mood, "After supper is the loveliest time of all—so I'm glad I don't have to rush back to work at the time I used to."

In this last term of the year he was accepting school better. There was a lot of discussion both at school and at home about what subjects he should take for Matric:

"I think I'll do Geography. I like it so much more now because it's become human. We discuss the difference in house prices between Harlem and Houghton!"

I asked him, "Which do you prefer out of Physical Science and Biology?"

"Physical Science. It's more challenging. I mean biology is more my sort of thing—but not *all* biology. I want to do Physical Science and Geography and Art and English. I know it's a strange sort of Matric."

"Not History?"

"No. It's pretty dry really—and we'll never get another Riley to liven it up. I am interested in history—but it's more, well, you know, historical sociology—if there is such a thing."

"Very hi-falutin'."

"What's that mean?"

"Well it's a very sophisticated concept."

"But is it a real one?"

"I don't know."

One evening after running the bath he came to me in great excitement, like a young child: "Hey Ma, an incredible thing just happened to me. When I was running the bath I was just wondering about how the water came from the Vaal Dam and how they got the chemicals in and all that. And when I turned the cold water on, *muddy* water ran out!"

He was starting to read newspapers and asked us why the SA army had gone into Angola in the first place. Mostly he tuned out Oliver's and my adult conversation at supper, interrupting suddenly to put some musical point to Oliver. Oliver continued to get at him a lot of the time, but on music they got on well. Oliver was interested in the new records which were coming out, which were different from pop and rock and jazz. Sophisticated fusion: Queen (rock and classical); Weather Report (rock and jazz); Dixie Dregs (rock and country); and Shakti (classical Indian and experimental jazz).

Just as Oliver and I had our Friday night meetings, so Danny and I, with Oliver if he was there, had a Wednesday meeting—to discuss home chores and work times and so on. It avoided unnecessary confrontations. Quiet discussions. If I brought up some issue outside a meeting, Danny would remind me to keep it for Wednesdays.

In the diary I wrote, "He was working in the lounge—ordinarily I would think not a good idea, but I went in and read the paper there and he read me passages he had liked from both his English and his Afrikaans setbooks."

The phone calls from Mandy continued.

In the diary: "He feels he can help this mixed-up girl Mandy better than any psychiatrist could, because he knows what she is like and what she likes."

I asked him, "How would you counsel someone who had no good feelings at all?"

"No one could be that bad. I would find out all about their personalities ..."

"But what if they didn't have personalities?"

"Oh, Ma! They must have some of the time or they wouldn't be alive. Even if for only five minutes of the day they were OK, I would *use* those five minutes."

In later years Danny didn't talk about Mandy as if she was "mixed up". He said she was intelligent—had won literary prizes: "I missed an opportunity there." We never met her—they had met through his weekends away with Jan K.

It was spring. Mid-September. I wrote in my diary: "He is caught up in some personal drama which cannot be revealed. I am a little worried that he will be over-confident about his counselling ability."

He told me that he had gone for a long walk the night before, intending to visit "the girl", but had thought the better of it and now "felt a better person". This was the first hint that he might be talking about a girlfriend, rather than "a girl he was counselling".

I said, "Being human is not the easiest thing in the world."

"No, it isn't. But it's fun."

From the diary: "My laborious building-up of his habits is working now—he is following the schedule, remembering his key, and noting the day he takes cigarettes—and all this in spite of his personal preoccupations."

And then suddenly he went off with Jan K after school on a Thursday, not at all part of his orderly life—because "we don't have school tomorrow". On the Sunday he was due to rehearse with two other friends who had organized a place where they could play and get paid in Orange Grove—twice a week. Danny had expressed great eagerness for this, so his not remembering the rehearsal was puzzling. When I phoned Jan K, Danny was not there. When he finally came back on the Sunday he said he had been counselling Mandy. It only becomes clear to me now that this was when he and Mandy made love. Danny later said the first time was at a party, when they were encouraged by everyone at the party to get on with it, so off they went to a bedroom. We were still in the era of celebrating sex. Girls were on the pill. It was the end of 1981: AIDS was first isolated in 1982.

He came in beaming from a phone-call to Nicky in Cape Town: "I haven't been in such a good mood for weeks. We are both having the same hassles. We can really talk to each other."

But then Mandy disappeared. No one who knew her understood this and it has never been clarified. Daniel went on expecting her to turn up or to phone, but something had gone wrong. We had not been told at the time that it was a love affair, so now we didn't know that it had ended.

Danny came home late from school: "I had to stay in town to get over my depression. It's nothing to do with school. It's to do with social matters."

Danny, in spite of a failed love affair, in spite of adulation by older Jo'burg youth, in spite of school resistance and pressure from me to study—and in spite of dagga smoking—ended the Damelin year perfectly sane and well. He passed all his Standard 7 exams and was promoted to Standard 8.

It was November 1981. He was still 14. The school year had ended. He felt fine about himself, so we felt fine about him.

CHRISTMAS HOLIDAYS (1981/1982)

We had a swimming-pool, for the first time in our lives. My father had been worried about his grandson's sportless school, so he had financed this pool. I had designed it and I watched it being made from my bedroom window:

> I look out of my window and see the full swimming-pool with my mosaic patterns in place round the top and the red earth surrounding the pool. When the green grass replaces the red earth it will be good in a different way—but I will miss the red earth.

I had made the pool long and straight for good swimming, but at the side had designed a paddling part on two levels: one for my toddler grandchildren, and one for when they were older and learning to swim. Well, that was thinking ahead.

But Danny in these holidays seemed less organized than he had become during his Damelin year. He got scattier and more forgetful. Even ordinary unpaid jobs which he had done since he was a child were forgotten.

> Danny is furious because his room hasn't been done. Peddie comes once a week and I say she will clean the kids' rooms if they have cleared up in time. But at the moment he is so incapable of thinking ahead and tackling a job that his only solution is to live with the mess—and also to live with no pocket-money.

The next week however he did clear his room. He really couldn't stand Peddie not cleaning it. He also did it two days in advance!

On my birthday he slept until lunchtime. At 2 o'clock he barged into my bedroom when I was resting—napping with my eyes shut. Danny said, puzzled, "Why are you sleeping now?"

"It's resting-time. It's 2 o'clock."

"Oh, I didn't know. Well, when you wake up you'll get your present."

The present was a birthday card which said:

A very sincere Happy Boifday to a real live 50-year-old Mother. You now have at your disposal: My services until 6pm today for less 50%. I will do it for nothing when you are 100!

I hadn't the heart to point out that he would only be able to give me a half-day. I was just delighted that he was offering me something at all. I took my tea and book and sat under the huge Australian Chestnut tree with its flaming orange blossoms, looking up from time to time to watch my son vacuuming the swimming-pool. When he had finished I went up to it to look. I said, "You did an excellent job my love. I've never got it that clean."

"Well you have to use more pressure. If you use light pressure you only pick up the loose dirt."

It was very difficult now to say that he had to be home by a certain time, because his present friends were all 20 or more. I remember earlier in the year when a young man came to fetch him at 8 pm to go to a jazz concert at Wits.

"He has to be home by 10 pm," I said—which was true then.

"But the concert only *starts* at 10 pm! Never mind, he can sleep over at my place and I'll bring him home tomorrow morning." Which he did. This was Toby, aged 21, with his delicate, pretty face. He was the older brother of a friend of Nicola's, and I had met their parents. I trusted him completely. He had often come over to play music in Danny's garage.

One day Oliver came back all smiles: "Guess what! I saw Daniel coming out of a shop on the arm of this beautiful, tall model." I was horrified. I didn't say a thing, but I phoned Nicky to see what she would think. She was still in Cape Town. She was as horrified as I had been.

Danny, getting such a positive response from Oliver, told him other things too: "This morning I was sitting on her bed eating chocolates when her ex-boyfriend walked in!"

Nicky phoned her Jo'burg friends to see if she could find out more. It turned out that this woman, Daphne, had been living for a long time with a forty-year-old man. Now they were breaking up, and she was enchanted with Danny's youthfulness. But she did not know at first exactly how young he was. She was 26. "A woman older than I am," said Nicky, disapprovingly.

All through these holidays, Danny slept at home. That was a relief. Jan K's band had not worked out, so those weekends were over.

Another thing Danny was doing these holidays was going to Hillbrow where the Johnny Fourie band rehearsed. Danny had been introduced to them and had played to Johnny and now he was allowed to go any time to their rehearsals. We thought this was a harmless and interesting thing for him to do. Oliver and I both loved that band, which was jazz, not rock. I had the idea that jazz musicians were more stable than rock musicians. Since Danny only went there during the day, and since Johnny himself was a 40-year-old adult, what harm could there be?

On Christmas Day I gave Danny a lift to the Fourie studio. As we drove there, Danny said that he was now "counselling" Johnny Fourie. I asked him what on earth he meant. He said he was encouraging him not to lose heart, and he was telling the band what to play and criticizing them afterwards. I said nothing.

Toby's friend Max came to see me. He was also 21, and he idealized Danny. He said to me, "You really should understand Danny better. He's an adult! You should hear the conversations he has with Johnny Fourie! Deep philosophy. It would be better if you just let Danny go his own way. You can't tell Danny what to do."

But Nicola was fed up with Danny. He had not been at home when she came back from Cape Town, which was unheard-of in the past. She had been looking forward to one of their intense conversations into the night. She didn't like his adolescent mannerisms or his older girlfriend, and she felt he had become completely unreliable and also too full of himself. She said, disgustedly, "I saw Danny on the opposite pavement in Hillbrow today. He is walking around like the King of Hillbrow!"

Johnny Fourie told Danny that he could be South Africa's next great young guitarist and that he should leave school immediately. (Later we learnt that Johnny had also fed Danny non-stop pot/dagga while the band rehearsed.)

I thought that all this unreality would stop as soon as school started again and we were back to ordinary family rules.

On New Year's Eve, Daniel was fetched by Max, the young man who so approved of him. On this one night of the year we didn't stipulate when he should be home.

Oliver and I did not go out. Oliver watched television and I reflected on my year in my diary:

Now that I have turned fifty I don't expect anything dramatic still to happen to me. I shall just go on living quietly, and thinking and hoping about the world.

It has been a good year in spite of the problems with Danny. He did in the end stop saying negative things about himself—all those disparaging sentences!

I enjoy everything about the pool—its changeability, and analysing the reasons why it changes; the efficiency of the engine— that it works; and the simple joy of the water.

Well now I am going to join Oliver and see the New Year in with him and the television.

What are my resolutions for 1982?
I shall look for elegant solutions,
I shall fly down the foofy slide,
I shall breathe to the slow baroque music,
I shall let the sun penetrate every cell of my body,
I shall never surrender.

At this stage of our lives, neither Oliver nor I knew that Danny at fourteen had ever:
1. Slept with a woman.
2. Smoked dagga.

We kissed each other a Happy New Year—and slept soundly.

Chapter Eight

BREAKDOWN PART I
(AGED FIFTEEN, 1982)

It was January. Nicola was leaving for Cape Town on the 5th. Oliver's teaching term was starting on the 6th. Danny had another week before Damelin started on the 12th. I was looking forward to getting back to the book I was writing.

Before Nicky left, she and Oliver had a conversation—which Oliver reported to me. Nicky told him that she had been talking to her friends and she now knew that Danny was often stoned. She asked Oliver if she should tell me. He said, "Why not?"

"But she'll worry!"

"I don't think she will."

I of course was immediately worried. "Being stoned" sounded like "being drunk"—not like just having a puff now and then.

Then Danny had a conversation with Oliver in which he said, "Daphne and I are completely honest with each other. She knows how old I am." I hoped this meant that the relationship was dying a natural death.

On the Wednesday I told him we would be starting our meetings again. Oliver had to stay late at school, so it was just Danny and me.

"So what's this meeting about?"

"Just things for school."

"Oh—books and that?"

"Ja. I wondered if a jacket mightn't be a good idea?"

"You've really got something there! A person could really do things with a jacket. Walk around crammed with notebooks …"

"A sort of walking office?"

"That's right!"

I gave him money and a list of things to get—bus tickets, shirts, books … These were all things he had managed perfectly well on his own the year before. But now he seemed a bit switched off. He went to

Damelin to get his books, but it was the wrong day. He was in such a vague state that I decided to help him. We went to Hepworths clothes store. We did the shopping and then I said, "That's R21 off—it was really worthwhile coming here."

Outside the shop Danny said, "You shouldn't say things like that in a shop."

I was bewildered. I protested, "But I said it very quietly."

"Yes, but people can hear very well in shops—it's only a small point, but you shouldn't do it." I thought his imagination was running wild.

On the day before school started he still had made no attempt to get his books, so I took him to town and waited while he got his Standard 8 books. In the evening he practised the guitar for the first time since before the holidays. During the holidays he had only played the piano and drums. I was relieved. We were getting back to normal at last.

He went to school on the Tuesday. When he returned he said, "I'm enjoying the work. But I'm quite confused about the class discussions because they don't find me OK, so I just sit quiet."

"It will take a little time to get back into the swing of school life I guess."

"Ja."

He had five school days and there seemed to be no problems. On the Tuesday, a week after term had started, I decided that I had been a bit heavy and tense with him and that I would switch to my friendly/loving/cheerful motherly self. It was a beautiful evening and Oliver was home, so the three of us had turkey casserole outside. The meal went fine, but then Danny said, "What would you guys say if I was to have a few friends round in the evening, after 10 o'clock—in the garage. Very quiet. We wouldn't worry you at all."

"On a school night?" I asked.

Oliver said, crossly, "The answer's NO. I'm surprised you even ask."

"But now that I've got myself so together and I'm working so well, and if I had done all my work. I would sign a contract."

Oliver said, "The answer is still NO. We've let you do things before delivering the goods. Now we know better."

"But you guys don't know how difficult it's been for me."

I didn't think we were being unreasonable. He was allowed almost complete freedom at the weekends, and as far as we were concerned he could continue his social life then. Later that evening he was still coming back to us with new proposals—all part of a game now, I decided. We were reading the paper and not taking much notice.

The next night, Wednesday 20 January, Oliver was out. Danny came to me and asked if he could watch early TV. I said no. He got into one of his persistent states. I had nowhere to escape to because I was sitting in my bedroom. I exploded and shouted at him to get out. He left the room and the house, and didn't come back all night.

I didn't see Danny the next morning, but I found out later that he had come back and fetched his school-bag—and he had left a note:

Dear Extremely Concerned Parents,
I can handle the shouting, but I cannot handle the exaggeration of the whole petty episode. I will handle my life accordingly until I feel the time to be right. Do not look for me. I will be back in a few days.
Love ya both,
Tarra,
Danny

His intention may have been to go to school, but in fact he did not go. The Damelin teacher we spoke to, Mr Hall, was concerned, but said they would wait and see. He felt it was something more than simple truancy.

Later that day I found Danny's diary and saw that he had written in it that Toby and Debbie were going to Shaka's Rock at the weekend—a seaside place in Natal where Toby's parents had a cottage. It was now Thursday. Toby and Debbie were a young married couple who were friends with Daphne, Danny's girlfriend.

By the Friday we knew that Danny was staying in Toby's Hillbrow flat with his friend Max. Toby himself was not there. Oliver went round there in a rage. He knocked and rang the bell and shouted, but they were not there, or not answering. He left a note saying that we would charge Max with harbouring a minor and get the truant officer to fetch Daniel.

They were in fact there, but as soon as Daniel saw the note he left, telling Max he was not ready to come home. He wanted to live on his own and go out to work. He wanted to prove himself.

On Sunday it was Danny's fifteenth birthday. I expected him to phone, but we heard nothing from him or about him. I was miserable and confused.

On Tuesday Jan K phoned me. Jan K was his Midrand friend in whose parents' barn he had often stayed at the weekends the year before. Jan K said he would look for Danny. He said, "Daniel hasn't phoned me because he knows I will tell him to go straight back home and he listens to me." I felt relief at this support—the first strong-minded person who felt he could handle Danny. I didn't yet know about the heavy pot smoking at weekends in the barn.

I wrote a letter to Danny in my diary:

Dear Danny,
I didn't think it was possible to be as unhappy about a child as I am now about you.

In the last few months you have been becoming an absolutely marvellous person, and you seemed all set to have an excellent year.

I know that you have been trying to overcome your past indiscipline, and we were being unnecessarily fussy. But you had been living in a very adult world and we just felt it would make it easier for you if we insisted on a few broad outlines, to prevent the temptations becoming overpowering.

This has been a nightmare, Danny. That shout of mine will haunt me for the rest of my life if you don't come back soon.
I love you,
Mom

It was now the second week of his running away, and no one knew where he was. Then his adult girlfriend, Daphne, phoned me and said that the two of them had gone with Toby and Debbie to Shaka's Rock at the weekend. The four of them were there alone—without Toby's parents. Daphne said, "He was very withdrawn on Sunday—on his birthday. He was showing none of his usual exuberance. He lay silently on the grass. I thought he was against me. I had been trying to persuade him to go back home and to school and to give up the pot smoking."

Toby and Debbie, and Daphne, and Max, and Jan K, were all now in touch with us—but none of them had any idea where he could be.

Mr Hall of Damelin phoned me and said they would now have to phone the truant officer.

I lay on my bed and sobbed.

On Thursday a young man we had not met before, Jonathan, came to see us. He said that Daniel was staying with Shaun Fourie and his uncles in Hillbrow. Shaun was Johnny Fourie's son. Jonathan said that Daniel was bathing and resting and eating, and that Shaun's uncles had given him some clean clothes.

On the Friday Danny phoned us to say he was coming back the next day, which is what he did.

He arrived home on Saturday afternoon at 3.30. His hair was very short. He looked good. He looked different. We hugged. I made tea and we took it out to the front, under the Australian Chestnut tree. Oliver was having his medieval music rehearsal in his studio at the back.

Danny said, "How have you been?"

"Oh fine since your call yesterday. I worked properly for the first time this morning."

"My first plan was to hang around for three days, then go to Cape Town, make it up with Nicky and spend six months away from home. I could have done it. How has Dad been?"

"He got into an ancient mood of hopelessness. He did realize that he over-reacted with that note about the police."

"Yes. I was just about to phone you, and then when that note came I just wanted to escape further."

"Jo S was intensely loyal to me, and angry with you for making me unhappy."

"Well, what did she think—that I was just having a jol or something? I wasn't worried about the truant officer or the police—only about making you unhappy."

Danny had an amiable supper with me and Oliver and went early to bed. The next morning he and I visited Jo, who lived very close to us. She was the one who had had such feisty arguments with Danny when he was a child. She said to him:

"Look here Danny, I know it sounds boring, but I have got a 40-year lead over you. That is *all* I have got, but I have got it. That means 40 years more of looking at life and people, or reading novels which portray life, or reading books which study life in various ways."

"Well let me ask you this: have you ever heard *everything* anybody says as having a double meaning?"

"What's that supposed to mean?"

"You hear what people say and you hear another meaning as well."

"It sounds like madness to me."

"Yes, I sometimes think so too."

But he had said this with such relish and confidence that neither Jo nor I thought about drugs or insanity.

KINGSWOOD IN GRAHAMSTOWN

While Danny had been away I had phoned Terry Oakley Smith. She had been Danny's miracle teacher at Saheti. Now she was a lecturer at Wits University. We had stayed friends, but I had not seen her during this time when things had started to go wrong.

"It's so sad. I can't really believe it. It just doesn't sound like Danny. But I knew about drugs in the music scene. I should have warned you. The fantasy about 'a few months away from school' might mean he is more into drugs than we realize."

"What do you think we should do?"

"Well, you could try boarding-school—if he would accept it at this stage. Boris Kamstra, who went through a very rebellious stage, is now head boy at Kingswood College."

"Boris who was such a marvellous Puck in your production of *Midsummer Night's Dream*?"

"That's the one!"

Terry gave me Myra Kamstra's phone number. Myra invited me round to visit her. She gave me glowing accounts of what Kingswood had done for both her sons.

"It is strict, but it's small and everyone knows everyone. My boys have turned into fantastic human beings."

For the moment we were sticking to Damelin. Daniel went willingly on Monday morning. But he came home at lunchtime. He looked pale and ill. He said he was having problems with elimination and that there was something wrong with his foot. He had forgotten to take his glasses.

I put him to bed, brought him tea and gave him a while to rest. Then I came in for a chat. He said College was so formal—like a rock, pinning him down. He wanted "real life"—going hungry for a week and not paying the rent.

"How would you feel about going to school in another town—to boarding-school, if we could find a school with a good vital atmosphere and lots going on?"

"Possibly, possibly. Ja, I'd like to get right away from these people."

"Well, I'll see what I can do. The good schools are probably all full, but I'll make enquiries."

He smiled with interest and hope: "Thanks!"

I made an appointment with the doctor for the next day. In the doctor's waiting-room we talked about child-upbringing.

I asked Danny, "What would you do with a self-willed toddler who didn't want to go to bed?"

"Oh I would just leave him entirely alone and then talk to him about it the next morning. When you are a child and you want to do something very much, it possesses you and you can't think of anything else."

Our own friendly doctor was on leave. I went in with Danny. We didn't know this Dr G, who looked at Danny with disgust. He examined his foot and took a blood sample. Then he told him he was a wreck and should give up smoking cigarettes.

On the way home I said, "He wasn't very nice!"

"How could smoking affect my foot?"

"It affects the oxygen supply."

Danny had started smoking at Woodmead when he was a boarder. One evening when they were unsupervised and strolling along the river, he had accepted a cigarette, and then another. Since then he had been constantly trying to give it up.

I phoned the headmaster of Kingswood, Mr Todd. He told me that the atmosphere was disciplined, but within that structure they do consider the boy's needs, and they try to maintain a relaxed atmosphere.

I sat on Danny's bed:

"What do you want first—the good news or the bad?"

"The bad—as always!" He grinned nervously.

"Well, it's very structured."

"What do you mean?"

"Fixed times for everything."

"Oh I see. Ja. Well that might do me good."

"The good news is that you can do Music as a seventh subject on standard grade.

"That would be wonderful!"

"You would go to Rhodes University for guitar lessons."

"I can't believe it!"

"But Danny, listen. He is reluctant to take you, because he feels you have had a lot of freedom and might not settle down."

"I'm not basically a rebel."

"No, I don't think you are. All right then. I will convince him that you have accepted the conditions."

"It will be so interesting!"

I suggested he take a five-day anti-smoking course, but he felt it was not necessary.

"You will feel strange and under stress and then someone will offer you a cigarette. I want you to have some resistance."

"No—I'm not like I was at Woodmead. If I've decided to stop I will—I will gradually give up over the next few days. Anyway I don't think it will be that stressful—they are bound to be nice to somebody new."

He was keen to start sport again and sorry that his foot would prevent him doing so. Of the music he said, "It will be so great! I will learn to read music and then I can do session work in the holidays and earn good money."

It was a Methodist School, but Myra told me that the school drew on a very wide range of people. I asked Danny, "Do you know anything about Methodists?"

"Not really."

"Well it's the same type of religion as St John's but less fancy—more down to earth. No incense or anything like that."

"Well, that sounds practical."

"Yes, it kept people going there on the Eastern Cape border, where some of your ancestors came from."

The two people we knew who had gone to Kingswood were both people Danny liked a lot—his great-uncle Hal, and his good friend Mike S (husband of my friend Jo) who had taken him to cycle races and helped him fix up his bike.

Danny said, "It's a bit impetuous isn't it? Turning up there with no uniform or anything?"

Oh it's been done before. People send children to boarding school because of some sudden emergency. They're used to it."

Oliver came back from work and to my bedroom. He lay down with me and I told him the news. He said, "Well, if Danny is enthusiastic then I think he should do it and I wish him luck."

At supper Oliver said, "It's better to give up cigs suddenly—like I did."

Danny said, "Well if I really need one I can have it on my way to Rhodes each day."

Oliver was shocked: "In your school uniform! You'd be expelled." I added, "And you won't have guitar lessons more than once, or at most twice a week."

The next day, Wednesday, Danny was depressed. He hadn't realized that boarding meant weekends as well. He came to find me. "I'm sure I could discuss it with the headmaster and he'd allow me out one night a week to go to clubs and things."

"No, I'm afraid you just have to accept their system. Make what you can of it."

"I'm prepared to put 90% of myself into the school and their clubs and so on. But I think I ought to have 10% to myself … Oh well, I suppose I'll just have to accept it. I'll start psyching myself up for it."

Kingswood phoned to say he had been accepted. I booked a return train ticket to Grahamstown. He was leaving on Friday.

I phoned Myra. She said, "Tell him to lie low the first term. He can be as much of an individual as he likes later on."

On Thursday at 8:30 am I phoned Dr G for the results of Danny's blood tests. He said, "The bile pigment in his blood suggests hard drugs. As did his defensive manner."

I sat stunned for about half-an-hour. Then I realized that I had to fetch Terry and her young son, Lucien, at 9:30 am. This gave me a focus. I woke Danny with tea, and then again with coffee. The four of us were going to the farm, so that Danny could say goodbye to his grandparents.

On the journey, Danny called out from a noticeboard, "Hey! Kingswood!" (not the school, just the word). "I never noticed that before."

"It's what happens. And you are wearing your glasses!"

"I'm reformed! I'll probably be a teacher's pet. I'm a person of extremes."

At the farm we had coffee and talked about child-upbringing. Granddad said, "I *had* to finish my food." I asked him, "Why did you feel you *had* to?

Danny answered, "If the child is shown that the parent has absolute authority the child just obeys."

Danny showed his foot to his grandfather, a doctor, but Granddad had no theories about it.

At lunch I prodded Danny about his birthday present. Danny said, "Oh, by the way, Grandma, thank you very much for my birthday present. It will be put to good use I assure you. I'm sorry I didn't thank you before—but I've been, well, busy ..."

Grandma said, "Don't be funny Daniel!"

"Ja, well ..."

When he said goodbye his grandmother said, "Well I hope you'll be happy Daniel—and I don't mean just happy living there. I mean enjoying learning and enjoying your music."

"Oh I intend to! And don't worry, I won't be changing schools again, even if ..."

"You don't have to make any promises."

On Thursday evening his old friend, Mark G of Streetkids, phoned. After the call Danny came to me and we had this chat:

"Mark's been giving me all sorts of ideas on how to get fit. Basically I am quite fit.

"Except for your blood."

"Well, let's have it."

"Your blood shows signs of having taken hard drugs."

Danny, astonished, said, "Hey?!"

"That's what it shows."

"Well I did once on New Year's Eve. That's why I was so odd the next day."

"How did that happen?"

"I gave Grandma's Christmas money—that R50—to Max and he bought a cap of acid, and we took it to a park."

I was silent for a while, trying to take this in. Then I said, "We can't protect you if you are found with drugs."

"Well obviously."

"It's not obvious. Max's dad bribed the police and got him off."

"Well I wouldn't expect you and Dad to. I would go to Boys' Town."

Oliver had said goodbye to Daniel because both of them were going out—Oliver to a pupils' concert and Danny to say goodbye to his friends.

When Oliver came home I told him about the blood test and Daniel admitting to hard drugs—just once. Oliver was shaken. He said he would definitely kill Max if he ever came here again.

We knew that "acid" was LSD. We looked it up in Hutchinson's Encyclopedia. We read: "A hallucinogen. One of the most powerful mind-changing drugs known, a derivative of ergot (a parasitic fungus). Colourless, odourless, and easily synthesized. It is non-addictive, but its effects are unpredictable and may be disastrous."

On the Friday morning, his day for leaving, we were rushed. I waited and waited at the doctor's to get the test results and the X-ray. We were going to a neurologist in Sandton to diagnose Danny's foot.

"I don't want to be late, since he is doing us such a special favour by fitting you in."

We got there just in time. I ran from the car to the clinic. Danny limped after me. I was drained by now. I sat in the waiting-room with my head in my hands. When I looked up Danny was looking at me in a concerned way. I noticed that his pupils were still small. I had noticed this the day before and thought it was related to pot smoking.

Dr Maxwell called us in, looked at the X-rays and test results and spoke to Danny for a while. Then he took him next door for a very thorough neurological test—eyes, ears, hands, feet, every part of him. He kept coming back to his desk to fill in marks on a body shape, not saying anything. I was just sitting there waiting. Then he said he was going to do some more tests. I could sit patiently by no longer.

"Is there nothing you can tell me at this point?"

"He has a compressed nerve in his knee, which will take a little time to heal. That's what's causing the problem with his foot."

I sighed with relief and said, "Oh well then it's all right. Nothing permanent."

"I'd just like him to have an EEG."

Danny and I went downstairs together. The nurse who did the EEG told Danny not to clench his jaws because that distorted the results. He had to do a session of deep breathing. While the EEG was being recorded she suddenly gave Danny a quick alarmed look. We went back to the consulting-room holding the results.

Dr Maxwell said, "There are a certain proportion of people—two in five—who cannot smoke pot. Your brain has deteriorated and your reactions have slowed down. This is still reversible. But if you go on smoking pot it will become irreversible. Lethal. You are at a turning-point." He showed Danny the EEG of a normal person and how it compared with Danny's.

We rushed out. We were late for the train. I don't remember it even occurring to me to change the Grahamstown plan.

Danny said, "I knew my mind was slowing down." He said this in the tone of "there is nothing you can tell me that I don't know already."

Then he said, with supreme adolescent omnipotence: "I could have made normal loops on the EEG if I had wanted to."

We drove to Johannesburg Station, numb and dumb.

I said, "The holidays might be a problem—when you come back to this pot-smoking environment."

"Not at all. *I'm* the one who smokes."

At the station Shaun Fourie and his uncle Denzil were there—from Danny's last refuge. Danny wanted to go off with Shaun to get a coke. I said absolutely not.

Denzil said to me, "The only way to get through to Danny is with quiet intelligence."

"Is that how you persuaded him to come home?"

"Yes."

"Thank you." I shook his hand.

Finally Danny was on the train. I kissed him goodbye, and off he went.

But what Danny didn't know, nor I, nor Denzil and Shaun, was that he was taking his voices with him.

THE VOICES

At home that evening Oliver said, "Danny always enters into the spirit of the situation he is in—so don't worry. The danger of his flouting the rules is not *now*, but later, when he becomes more familiar and confident." But I thought that Danny was not the cheerful child he had once been. He was physically in poor shape, mentally slowed down and feeling strange.

Danny was to be met by Boris Kamstra—the memorable Puck of Saheti. A new type of role model for Danny, but from an artistic family like ours.

At home my sense of relief was tempered by terror. Every time the gate clicked I imagined that Danny was home again and that the whole nightmare had started up again. At night I dreamt of schools and schoolboys. In one of them I was in London, and I came upon a group of schoolboys talking to each other in quotes from Shakespeare.

From Friday night to Tuesday night I don't think I was ever far from the phone. But it did not ring. Could our lives now be normal again?

On Tuesday evening I had bathed and was quietly reading in bed, relaxed at last. At 10 pm the phone rang. It was Mr Gardener from

Kingswood. He said, "He's at Alicedale—at the station. He had the return ticket and he got there through the fields. Don't worry about it—it's happened before. I'll drive over there and talk him out of it."

Mr Gardener got there and suggested that Danny phone me, which he did, in an unsteady voice: "Mom, I'm feeling very confused and I want to come home ... I'm in such trouble. I don't know how I got into this."

Mr Gardener said his behaviour had been fine and that the other boys liked him. But I knew Danny was talking about his inner drug-induced world. The school had not been told about the tests.

"Danny, if you come home are you prepared to see a psychologist?"

"Yes yes yes."

There was no way I could not let him come home. It was not a discipline issue. He was panic-stricken and needed healing. So he came on a slow train home: all through Wednesday the train stopped at little stations; then on Thursday morning at 6 am I fetched him at the large Johannesburg station.

I took him straight to the farm—away from all drugs.

The farm was a 40-minute drive away. He cried in the car—and was glad he had. "I was heading for a nervous breakdown. If I had stayed at Grahamstown I think that is what would have happened."

He didn't talk about Grahamstown, but went back to when he had stayed with Sean Fourie and his uncles, in the second week of running away. "Denzil and co speak a special language. At first I didn't understand it and I just used to sit there playing my guitar and feeling inferior. But then I started to pick up some of it. It's so complex! Ordinary things like, 'Shut the door' mean something quite different. Often they were talking about me."

During the morning he seemed normal. Then he started again about double meanings. Grandma told him to get some figs, but he found the wrong fig trees. He feels his problems are unique and no one can help him; it's how he sees the world; everything links up. He wants to see his EEG.

On the Wednesday when he was coming home in the train, I had told his story to our own family doctor, Dr van Niftrik. He had been our doctor since we came to South Africa—was warm and supportive, unlike his locum who had seen Danny the week before. He gave me some pills which would help Danny with withdrawal symptoms.

Danny didn't at first want Dr van N's pill, saying he didn't want any more drugs of any sort. The pill, Surmontil, was an anti-depressant which would also be a sedative at night.

We sat outside. Danny said, "If I could be by *myself* it would be better. If only I didn't have to socialize at Damelin. I don't know what will happen when I go back."

"How do you mean? That you might accept pot?"

"No, it's not that."

I spoke to Oliver on the phone. He said, "He is just using this double-image thing to get him off the hook. He can't just be allowed to get away with it. There must be sanctions."

It was evening. He had reached a low ebb, but went to bath and said he would accept a pill. I brought it to him with some hot milk. I said, "Wouldn't the social situation at Damelin be easier to handle if you didn't go to the canteen."

"No, because a lot of people stay in the classroom; and any group of people is a social situation and I can't handle it. As soon as they start talking I freak out."

I thought: This does not sound like "using" it to get out of something. It was said in a very quiet way, and not to "prove" anything.

The next day he was dopey from the pill, but very relieved at the picture I had given him: go back home, but under strict supervision; no school for next week; see the doctor at Tara.

It was Friday now so he would have ten days free of pressures.

He said, "I think you people are handling it right."

In the car coming home I said, "Perhaps you should invite friends home instead of going out."

"You are still worried about the pot aren't you?"

"No. I told you I believed you would stop it altogether. Even Dad felt better when I said you were to have another EEG in April."

"Sometimes I talk far out. I say: 'I am going to give up smoking,' and I say it so convincingly that I convince everyone, but not myself."

"And about pot?"

"I think I have even convinced myself. It's so wonderful to be straight! Instead of concentrating on just one single thing you can see the whole picture."

At home we phoned Nicky in Cape Town. We were talking to her on two phones so I could hear what she said.

Danny said, "You start off trying to make things interesting and then it takes over. In the end you start taking everything metaphorically. It's quite unnerving."

Nicky said, "Well, you sound quite normal!"

Danny said, "Yes, I am—on the outside."

Mrs Gardener phoned from Kingswood, concerned and upset. She had taken Daniel shopping for school clothes on the Monday. She saw herself in him—something of a loner. She was an only child. She thought him sensitive, friendly and relaxed.

We did not think he was mad—Oliver and I. It did not even occur to us. Oliver thought he was imagining the voices to get out of facing up to things. I thought the voices were real, but caused by stress and drugs. I had hallucinated a few times myself in my twenties—from stress alone. I had three separate visual hallucinations. They were frightening, but I knew what they were, and they lasted only for a few minutes at a time.

Danny had a strong imagination, and sometimes believed what he told himself. When he was about eight years old he had come to me with his left elbow stuck up in the air. He said he couldn't move it. I left it for a while, knowing that it could be a hysterical thing, but later phoned Dr van N, who came round. We were all in the living-room. Dr van N said something cheerful to Oliver and at the same time tweaked Danny's elbow back into order!

So it was this sort of "unconscious imagining" that Oliver thought Danny was doing.

Danny now told Oliver that Terry (his Saheti teacher) and I were talking the second language in the car going to the farm (ten days before), when he and the child Lucien were sitting in the back and Terry and I were nattering away to each other in the front—but of course not about him.

Danny said, "I can turn it off though."

Oliver said, "Well maybe they really were trying to say something to you."

"Ja they were."

I said to Oliver, "Danny is having verbal hallucinations which he believes are real. I don't think he can just turn it off at will.

It was autumn—our loveliest month. Oliver and Danny and I had supper outside on the porch, and talked and talked. Danny defended dope (another word for cannabis/pot), saying we had no idea how many marvellous, creative, productive people smoked it.

At one stage Oliver said how one needs less and less pot to get high. Danny, genuinely amazed, said, "How did you know that? Dope can do nothing for me any more. I don't *need* it any more."

The next morning he walked to Toby and Debbie's place. They were married now and lived in a house in Orange Grove, about a mile from us. They smoked pot themselves but now knew they should not give Danny any. He was to stay only for one hour.

An hour later he phoned: "Could I perhaps come back at 5?"

"No, you have to come back for lunch and your pill. I'll come and fetch you."

"I'll meet you at the corner."

"No I want to come in and say hullo to Toby and Debbie."

"They are not here."

"So who is?"

"Lots of people. Well, Max."

"Then I'm definitely coming to fetch you. "

And I put the phone down and fetched him. It was Max who had kept him out all night without letting us know, when Danny was thirteen. It was Max with whom he had taken LSD on New Year's Eve. He was a tall, lanky, goofy-looking lad—and the only one of Danny's friends not to have talked to us in a worried, responsible, realistic way.

That evening Danny said, "Ma, listen. Max and I have had a good talk and he says he's going to cut down—and that maybe smoking too much *is* bad."

"But with you it's not a question of too much. It has to be none at all."

Danny said, (with absolute conviction): "No I *know* that. I was able to refuse quite easily this morning."

"We've been grossly irresponsible as parents. I just do have to check up. But you did phone and I am beginning to trust you."

"I'm beginning to trust myself!"

Mark G, his Streetkids friend, phoned me up: "Danny told me about the brain scan and how he could handle cutting out pot and how he wasn't even going to take the sedative for withdrawal symptoms." (This was the Surmontil, which I think I gave him daily and he took without fuss.)

The next day Danny and I had lunch at the Doll's House. I asked him, "Is Jan K still smoking pot so heavily?"

"Well the doctor says to him: 'If you smoke no more and no less for the rest of your life you will live to 108.'"

"No doctor would say that."

"It's ridiculous anyway, because no one lives to 108."

"I'm very glad to hear you say that. Do you think Jan K is living in a bit of a fantasy?"

"I think so." (Then bursting out): "But he's so ENTHUSIASTIC! ... I don't want to talk about Jan K."

It was Jan K at whose barn he had "rehearsed" for the second half of the year before.

Danny said, "The reason I went on to hard drugs is that I was irresponsible and I wanted to get more and more fucked. I don't know why you are pursuing this drug thing—it's finished, it's past, it's over. I don't know why I told you if you are going to get so worried. Last year we used to smoke *far* more. Those weekends when I went away on Fridays and came back on Sunday nights with Jan K—we used to smoke 50 joints a weekend. We used to have competitions to see who could smoke more. Our team used to win."

One evening Danny and I talked about the three methods of child-upbringing: strict and authoritarian; democratic and firm; permissive and laissez-faire. I said, "I don't know about the laissez-faire children. I suppose they either end up as drug-addicts or else ..."

Danny interrupted: "I don't like that word, 'drug-addict'. You haven't smoked pot for months and months so you don't know what the hell you are talking about. There's no such thing as 'addiction'. You go from one drug to another and you decide to live out your life in this way, even if you die at 20."

"Danny you are either profoundly ignorant, or on a complete fantasy trip."

"You just think that because you have read a lot of books you know all about it. The doctors know nothing!"

We were tense and shouting.

Oliver came in: "What's going on?"

Danny said, "Oh we were just having a good argument."

I said, "We gave you too much freedom."

"I wouldn't say so, no."

"You couldn't handle it. It led to bad things."

"What bad things? Other than smoking pot?"

"And running away twice from school."

"That's because I was schizophrenic."

"You were schizophrenic because you couldn't handle your own strong drives, and society didn't protect you from them."

"Well yes I do have strong drives, I'll admit that!"

We had calmed down by now—we were almost enjoying ourselves—and we were both using this word, "schizophrenic", in a popular way. I was very much aware that he wasn't arguing like a mad person!

TRYING DAMELIN AGAIN

Danny, buoyant with all these confessions, seemed on the mend. But there was a problem: Damelin did not want him back.

"Damelin might not take you back."

"Oh really?" said Danny, very alarmed.

"Do you *want* to go back to Damelin?"

"Yes I do."

I went to see Dr Kriel, the head of Damelin. He was the man who had made Damelin famous, and who had introduced Oliver to culture and civilization, through teaching him English and History for Matric. He said, "We are not a small college any more. We are not in a position to handle problem children. We simply offer consistency of teaching and high standards."

I told him about Danny's relationship with Neville Riley (his history teacher), and Kriel agreed to put it to Riley.

When I came home tired from Damelin, Danny asked if he could make me anything, and brought me tea and toast.

He plays the clarinet a lot—Oliver has given him a lesson or two—and he makes up compositions. He thinks the clarinet "difficult" and so feels he is "being disciplined", but in fact it is all very immediate and highly pleasurable.

Neville Riley phoned me and said he'd like to come and see Daniel.

Danny flopped down in my relaxator—a canvas-on-metal chair on which one could tilt far back: immensely comfortable.

"So what's Mr Riley want to talk to me about?"

"I don't know. I've got to cook now—do you want to listen to one of my relaxation tapes?"

"Ja—OK."

So he did. When I came back he looked very calm.

"How did you get on with the tape?"

"Fine. What's Mr Riley want to talk to me about?"

"I don't know—life I suppose."

"There's so little I can say in half-an-hour."

"Perhaps you can arrange to talk another time as well."

"There's really nothing I can say. I can't tell anyone what's in my mind."

The next day he and Riley talked for about an hour in the kitchen. Riley left and Danny came in to me. "Phew! He's such a fantastic person! We are exactly alike! He's not only been an alcoholic, he's smoked pot and popped pills. We talked about everything! Socialism, religion. We kept going off at tangents—and then he'd say, 'But we must get back to you.' We were talking like two totally berserk humbled talented people. He says if I come back to Damelin I will have to behave like a normal 15-year-old."

"Does he think you've got a chance?"

"He's going there right now to talk to them."

The nicest thing about the last four weeks has been so many people phoning up and coming round. Jo S phones almost daily.

The next day Damelin said he could come back. Daniel immediately got into a panic. I thought he had developed a phobia. I said to him, "If you feel the slightest panic, just imagine your teacher upside down. Or do deep breathing—that's another way."

"Ja—in,2,3,4, hold,2,3,4, out,2,3,4. That tape's really quite good."

He says he is "fucking worried" about going back to school but that he is "getting near a solution". He of course doesn't want to see it as a simple phobia. Ten minutes after I told him about Damelin he asked for the Surmontil. "It's not just in my head—it's out there too. Three months of humiliation with people downgrading my anatomy."

"Riley says to come to him at 8 am on Monday: he who is in with Riley is OK."

On Sunday I took Danny and his Jewish cousins, Martin and Hector, to the Zoo (our family's peak calming place to go). When I was alone with Martin I said: "He's scared stiff."

"Do you think it's too soon to go back?"

"No, no, the sooner the better."

"What's he afraid of?"

"Social humiliation, real or imagined."

Martin was astonished: "Daniel! But he's always the *centre* of any social group."

In the evening he was "psyching himself up"—sitting upright on his bed in the dark with his guitar. He came in to us in the living room, strong and confident, having talked to Nicky on the phone.

"It's going to be very strange for a while because I am working things out. It's going to be difficult working on ordinary Standard 8 work while I'm handling everything else.

I asked him, "Couldn't you just postpone the higher matters?"

"Impossible! I can't suddenly not catch up with what people are saying. But I'm nearly there. I've almost mastered it."

Later I went to his room and in a very matter-of-fact way refused to respond to his elated smile. "Look Danny, I want you to remember what Mr Riley said about being an ordinary 15-year-old."

"I can't just undo all the work I've done in the last few weeks."

"Well please just try and just be ordinary tomorrow—as if you are making scrambled eggs like you did tonight."

"Well I will try. It's just that there might be too much ..."

I left him then, but later I couldn't stand it any longer. I barged into his room where he was still playing the guitar with an inane grin on his face.

I shouted, "That playing the guitar is real, but this double-voices business is not real."

"How can you come in here and say it is not real?"

"Because it's not. It's simply something your mind has made up to boost your self-esteem."

"Well I'm just seeing how far it can go, exploring religion."

"But you need pot to do that, don't you, and pot is destroying your mind."

"I don't need pot. Can't you see I am high without pot?"

"Look you are to go to school tomorrow and just be humiliated and stop this nonsense."

On Monday I drove him early to school. He was subdued. His hands were clenched. I dropped him off and wished him luck.

His phrases came back to me: he had said, "I've almost mastered it." What did he mean?

When I got home, Toby's wife Debbie phoned. It was she who had introduced Danny to her friend, Daphne. But she now regretted it. "Danny was perfectly OK until his love affair with Daphne. Daphne was playing with a child's mind."

Debbie said that she didn't want Danny to come round when she was not there. I felt like weeping at the thought that there was *someone* I could trust.

Danny lasted the day at school, but came home a bit depressed. He swam about ten lengths, then played his guitar.

I took him tea and said, "Oh by the way Debbie phoned."

He was very pleased: "Oh, really!"

"Ja—she's worried about the brain damage, and about you coming round when she's out. I invited them to lunch on Sunday."

"That's really nice. Thanks very much Mom."

He came in for first study period at 5.30, did his hour; and then we had supper. Then at 8 pm he came to me very nicely to ask to be let off the second hour.

"I don't want you to think I'm just trying to get out of it like I used to. It's just been a long day. I could do about ten more minutes, but ..."

"No, it's all right love—you've done well."

"You think so?"

"Ja, sure."

On Tuesday morning he went off to the bus-stop for school. I made some coffee and sat in the living room reading the paper. The bell rang. Who could this be?

It was Danny. He burst into tears. I led him to the living room and sat with my arm round him on the couch, and he let himself be comforted for a long time.

"The thing is—I don't know how to handle all the levels: the practical details, the school-work, and the interpretations I *have* to do. They all do talk in these double voices and I have to understand both the ordinary things they are saying and the other things they are saying about me."

"Well my love, it does seem like a mild form of temporary insanity."

"Yes, I agree. But I can't not do it. I've acquired a special talent for opening up packets of words and predicting what people will say."

"Don't worry about it. Dad and I will protect you for the moment."

"I'm quite willing to be protected."

"Will a squash lesson be OK?"

"Ja, I think so—I can't very well predict everything the teacher says while I am hitting the balls."

We went to the Doll's House for lunch. We got on to the voices again:

Danny said, with great certainty and warmth: "Well *you* know what I am talking about."

"No, I really don't my sweetheart. I think you are having verbal hallucinations."

"The pot might have *helped* me, but now I can do it without pot. These waiters hear everything that everybody says. That's how they get their kicks."

"They may hear some of it physically, but they can't possibly interpret it all."

"Yes they can. When Max and I were sitting in the car right at the back they heard what we were saying."

"I feel very uncomfortable at the thought that you are interpreting everything I say at a double level."

"Oh I try not to do it with you."

At the squash lesson all the depression and madness simply disappeared. He threw himself into it, and for the first time for weeks, he laughed!

It is 2009. I am editing this book. Danny told me about a teacher at a later school.

"You didn't hear any voices at that time?"

"No I didn't." Then he added, "The voices were very terrible. And adults have had them too you know. Virginia Woolf, for instance."

"And yet you didn't want to take that medication that made them go."

"Oh, I do remember profound relief at one time."

HOME AND CAMPING

So the decision was no more school for this term. I would get the material for Damelin's Correspondence Course. No going to school—but also: no dagga.

He had a quiet day at home. At the end of it I said, "You look a bit depressed."

He sighed, "Ja well—I'm just preparing myself for six weeks solitary confinement. But I've done some positive things today—fixed my hi-fi, got back to clarinet."

That evening he asked for a pill—the same Surmontil anti-depressant which was given for withdrawal symptoms. I brought it and hot milk for us both and we talked in the dark.

Danny said, "I'm so longing for my next squash lesson. I need to get on top of things. I need to get my confidence back. I was always king in the classroom. I was always the one the teachers could relate to. When I walked in the door I knew I was the one who would know all the answers. And when it came to Standard 8 I was quite shocked. Everyone else seemed to have caught up with me. There were so many people in the class who could give opinions that were perfectly valid."

He was invited by Mark G to go away for the weekend in the mountains with "totally straight people" including Dion, whom Nicky liked very much. Dion wanted him to go. I thought no, not because of possible drugs—I trust Mark and Dion—but because he's still so fragile. However, Danny himself is keen and insists that it will be comfortable and right for him.

On Sunday evening he returned from this trip looking very fit. He was proud of his excessive muscular exertion and he sounded completely normal.

On the Monday morning I woke him up cheerfully. He said, "In this dream I had a difficult science lesson at Damelin, then I had this homework to do and I wanted to get it over with."

In the dream his brain was last year's brain.

He did some of the correspondence work.

He seemed confident again. But it didn't last. Later that week while he was getting ready for squash he found he had left his takkies (gym shoes) at somebody's house. He was suddenly acutely depressed. And then came the outburst:

"Why does everyone know what is going on in my mind? It's as if my mind is up on a movie-screen and everyone can read it. Even Mark G knows! Eight people on that camping trip and they all *knew* all the time what was going on in my mind. Everyone all over Jo'burg knows about me. Why don't I know?"

Probably just because they are older and have experienced more."

"Even six-year-olds know!"

I laughed and managed to make him laugh—a break in the storm.

"Why's it so *complicated*? Why does everything link up? I have to think about it 24 hours a day and you still want me to go to school!"

"Well, not at the moment we don't. Shall I read to you for a while to help you calm down?"

"Every book, every magazine I open, it all links up."

We went on a drive to look at Phoenix House. This was the only drug rehabilitation place at the time, as far as I knew. It looked peaceful and pleasant. Danny thought it might be quite a nice place to spend a few weeks in. No school demands. Kind grown-ups.

Sanca stands for South African National Council for Alcohol and Drug Abuse. They counselled addicts as outpatients and they ran Phoenix House. I phoned them up. They said not to worry about the voices—they were very usual—a few pills would fix him up. I made an appointment for Danny. We were to see Miss H, the superintendent of the Jo'burg clinic.

We went in together to see Miss H. Danny told her that pot had helped him with his jazz and creativity, but that he no longer needed it. Miss H was alarmed that he could get effects without it. She felt that meant he was heading for a breakdown.

He had some time with her alone, and then she saw me alone. She said, "He is in a very bad way—unable to structure his thoughts. He would not be able to do schoolwork. He would also not be able to take the structure of Phoenix House. He is not following through his thoughts."

Her voice and manner implied that his brain damage is irreversible. I was in shock. I didn't know how to find the car. Danny was cheerful and found it easily, and told me to drive carefully. He persuaded me to let him have an hour with Shaun Fourie, saying that I always know when he has been smoking pot. I dropped him off there, and he was fine when he came home.

"Johnny Fourie was there," he told me. "Shaun told him that I was giving up drugs. Johnny admitted that drugs didn't do him any good. He said that his memory used to be fantastic and that because of drugs it isn't any more. He wants Shaun to stop altogether."

He added, in a sad voice, "They should have just told me if I was too bumptious, not used double-talk. Everyone in Jo'burg used it—not just the Fouries."

He has lost that total confidence in his own rightness.

"It will never end," he said.

"Oh it will, it will—that's one thing that is certain."

The Damelin Correspondence course was discouraging. The text was closely typed and very black, with no spaces or questions along the way. Danny started on the Biology one. He read through it quickly and then said he couldn't answer the questions at the back. I said he hadn't read it properly, but then he insisted that I do it. So I did—and I couldn't answer the questions either! These notes would discourage an eager, sane student forced to spend a term in bed with a broken leg.

I discovered Master Maths. This was a small tutorial place which had a very systematic programme going from one clear step to another. A lot of people who "couldn't do maths" had been helped there. They tested the students, took them back to the level where their maths was secure, gave them a lot of practice at that level, and then went on from there. In the mornings there were very few people there: it was quiet and unthreatening.

Danny went there a few times a week and didn't mind going and didn't hear voices. One morning I myself was catatonic—too exhausted to get going. I phoned the Serviceable Sisters—a group which would take anyone anywhere: placid middle-aged women. From then on they often took Danny to Maths. He didn't mind.

The idea of British O-Levels took over from battling with Damelin Standard 8. He could do two or three subjects through the British Council. It seemed a better answer; but he found it extremely difficult to start studying, or to keep going for any length of time.

Squash was the only activity that he enjoyed every time. One day after squash he phoned his old teacher, Lucky. He came to me and said, "You don't even feel like cigarettes after something aerobic. D'you mind if I go out for about an hour tonight?"

"Where to?"

"To Lucky—I want to work something out with him."

"Does he smoke pot?"

"Not at all! He doesn't even smoke cigarettes!"

So he did that. And another time he spent a night at Mark G's house—a family house, not a commune of pot smokers.

Of his "mind thing" he said: "I'll just let this other thing drop—I'll let my mind get on with it, but I won't focus on it."

I bought *The Lord of the Rings* for him. A reading time was built into his quiet programme. I asked him, "How is the Tolkien?"

"Oh it's marvellous—it's a real escape world. The first real escape book I've read."

So that's how life was for a while. But we had made an appointment for him to be assessed at Tara, and we thought we'd better stick to it.

TARA

In Johannesburg everyone knows someone who has spent some time in Tara. It's a pleasant place with low buildings and large grounds. You don't go there for life but simply to get through a bad time. If you are certified as insane you go to a forbidding, locked-up institution out in the country, called Sterkfontein.

Oliver and Danny and I drove there without talking. We were called into a room with Dr T, the head of the adolescent section; and two ladies who said nothing at all. Dr T asked us what the problem was.

Oliver started: his slight uneasiness at Danny's December holiday non-eating. The running-away. The note about the police. Oliver gets bogged down in details, so I interrupted and went on with the story, not really knowing what to emphasize. Danny interrupted me at one point and said the drugs were entirely his own fault and he didn't want others to be blamed.

Dr T asked, "Who makes the decisions?"

Oliver answered, "We both do."

I said, "Oh I think mostly I do, but Oliver supports me."

Dr T asked Danny: "What is your family like?"

"Well it's a tightly-cohesive family. Yes, definitely. Mum is sometimes out of it because she's busy with housewifely things and Dad and Nicky and I are more interested in art. But of course I have been outside the family for some time because of smoking dope."

"Do you have any interests besides music?"

Danny smiled shyly, "Well ... um ... psychology."

"You are interested in the human mind?"

"Well, yes."

Then Danny went off with the two silent ladies and Oliver and I walked around and chatted and had tea. Then we went home. I was to come a week later to hear what they had found out about Danny.

On the Saturday night Danny saw *Altered States* at Brett's house, another safe, non-pot place. I had heard about this movie from Nicky and knew that it celebrated craziness, so was not happy about it, but Danny seemed OK when he came home.

On the Monday he was ill with a lung infection and on anti-biotics. He was cosily in bed, with a duvet as well as his blankets—"warm-at-last"—and his Tolkien. There were no issues.

It was Friday morning. Danny was over his infection. He dressed for breakfast, had a Tolkien read and was now really practising his clarinet in the Oliver's studio in a structured way. I went for a run. I was jittery about going to Tara for the results, and the run did me good.

Driving there I was relaxed, expecting kindness and information.

I went in to Dr T. What happened next felt like an attack, as if I was being accused:

Dr T: This boy needs immediate hospitalization. He is very disturbed—quite switched-off from reality. Incoherent. He has a high IQ—120, university level— probably would be higher if he wasn't disturbed.

His drawings show abnormal thinking—lack of boundaries—incomplete definition. No communication whatsoever in the family. Father powerful and unapproachable. Mother vague. World alien and hostile. There is confusion between reality and fantasy—flight into chaotic unreal thinking. His resolution of problems in the stories was inappropriate. The inkblots show him completely cut off and living in his own world. He is wrapped up in his intellectual thinking, which does not seem to be in touch with reality.

Your son shows the typical protocol of a psychotic person. It will get worse if it is not treated. We will admit him at any time.

I sat there being given a life sentence. I had hoped so much of Dr T: I had expected to be put at ease and given helpful advice.

I drove back feeling shattered. I phoned my dominant friend, Jo S. She had never seen Danny being frightened of his thoughts. She thought he was probably amusing himself in the tests: "Adolescents do that all the time."

I stood in my room in a daze, with my head between these two noisy people with their emphatic opposite opinions. I was crazed with doubt.

Danny wanted to know everything Dr T had said. I simply said that he wanted him to come into Tara for a few weeks.

Danny thought that would be fun: "Lots of painting and drawing and music. Do you know that Joe Pass learned to play the guitar in his three years in a mental home?"

(Joe Pass was a leading London jazz guitar player. I had once gone into Oliver's studio and thought I was listening to Joe Pass. In fact it was Daniel himself, aged about ten, recorded by Oliver.)

I dropped Danny off at Debbie and then fetched him again.

"Debbie thinks it's a good idea to go in."

"And you? Just because it will be fun?"

"Well, yes. But also because *they* think it would be good for me—because I can't be with people and so on. All this started after December you know. Until then I was happy jamming and everything."

Danny was as disorganized at supper as I have ever heard him. There is nothing like being told you are mad for making you disorganized!

A therapy friend warned me against labels.

A book I was reading suggested that the child's psychic structure "dissolves" during adolescence. "Don't let an episode become something permanent by allowing the child to 'use' it."

One of the most difficult things about Danny's breakdown was doubt about what to do. He was still only on pot-withdrawal medication, whereas Dr T wanted to put him on to anti-psychotic medication. Danny often got small pupils in the evenings and a faraway look. He couldn't watch television because it sent him evil messages. Debbie said he was not asking for pot any more and we had no reason to think he was getting it elsewhere.

We decided to hand him over to the experts—since Danny accepted the idea. I took him in on a Sunday. He was put in a room with five beds, but no one else there. When I left, Danny was lying on his bed listening to a tape—looking quite contented.

Oliver visited him in the evening. He came back and said, "Horrible place, horrible room—it's like a barracks!" It was raining. We felt miserable about Danny being in there.

The next day when I visited him I found all his friends there: Toby and Debbie—and Max—and a couple of others. They were sitting there looking absolutely stunned. They had had fun experimenting—and now their young friend had gone crazy.

Tara phoned me the next day—very sternly: only his parents could visit him. They were worried about his friends bringing drugs in. They were not letting him out of his room because there were drugs on the property.

Terry, his Saheti teacher, wanted to visit him. They said no. She went anyway—with her young son Lucien, and luckily whoever was on duty thought it OK.

Terry phoned me. "He's all right—just a bit bored and depressed. I'd love to see those stories he wrote for the tests." She thought his stories might reflect the Danny who wrote stories for her back in his Saheti days—often "way out". She also knew a lot about the psychedelic age and its images. She was not, of course, allowed to see the stories!

On the Wednesday Danny phoned and asked me to take him to his Maths lesson! Tara of course refused this too.

Dr T shouted at me on the phone: "You don't seem to *realize* how disturbed this boy has been! I can't *understand* why you want to whisk him out to a Maths lesson. He needs to *relax*."

"But he himself *feels* that a Maths lesson would be right."

"Do you think he's in any position to judge?"

"I think one has to work with him when he's feeling right and good."

"We want him in Tara for a little longer so that we don't label him the wrong way."

Danny's friend Max phoned me—the one we had distrusted the most. He said he had felt he should keep away. He admitted that Danny was depressed, had lost confidence, and said some very strange things. He said he was very very sorry about what has happened.

Oliver and I went out to dinner—steak and wine. We agreed not to talk about Danny. Oliver had another problem: his sister was married to a man who was obsessed by a cult called "Science of Mind": the mind can do anything, including make you lots of money!

"I hate that materialism," said Oliver.

"But then you also hate the drug culture, which is the opposite."

"Man is an animal: he should have clear goals, live in small groups, and do what his parents did. That's my last word!"

In bed every night I wrote my diary. That night I wrote: "I have spoken to three doctors at Tara and they all sound anxious and alarmist. Surely that's not right?"

On the next Tuesday evening, Danny's tenth day there, I went to visit him with his cousin Hector. On the way there Hector said that during that period last year—when he ran away from school and told lies to his father—he could definitely have been regarded as "psychotic".

When we got there Daniel was extremely restless and wanted to come out immediately. I explained that Dr T had said that if he came out Tara would wash their hands of him.

I left them alone and went to the duty-room. I explained to the sister that it was not that I thought there was *nothing* wrong with Danny, but just that the social atmosphere had to be taken into consideration and Daniel was now in a non-environment.

Sister Z said, "He is kept in his room because of the danger of getting drugs in the grounds of Tara. They want to check whether his condition is caused by drugs or not."

I went back to Danny who said, "I am locked in. They keep me portraying the same line of thought 24 hours a day. I need to talk about *different* things. Brian and Vivien—two young psychologists who came on the second day—I could talk to them. They were organic. But they didn't come again, and I have had this brick wall man talking to me for an hour every day ... and I *hate* these drugs. They put a barbed-wire fence around my mind."

Danny said he would sign contracts about not smoking pot; he readily agreed that Hector could be a watch-dog.

We laughed a lot. Danny said that he felt himself again and that he was definitely coming out. With strength and vehemence he said, "I'll come myself and talk to them."

I thought ja, OK—let them see if they can handle Danny in this mood! We went to the duty-room and there found Dr T!

Danny demanded: "Why are you keeping me in here?"

Dr T answered: "Because you have been very sick."

"Well all I need is *rest*."

"Which you can get here."

"But this is not a *natural* atmosphere for me."

"The life you were leading was much less natural."

"Yes, well I'm going to sign a contract."

Dr T said to me, "These pot-smokers don't keep their word."

"Smoking pot was not Daniel's whole world!"

"No, I realize that. But we feel it is quite wrong that he has been associating with all these adults. He should be in an ordinary school associating with his own age group."

"Yes indeed," I said. "But we have to deal with him as he is now."

"And we feel that smoking seven joints of pot a day indicated something abnormal. A lot of adolescents experiment, but they don't go to extremes."

"Well, he's an extreme sort of personality. But he hasn't been doing that recently you know. He exaggerates to prove that he's not a sissy and to put one over the grown-ups."

"You can take him out. I'm not stopping you."

"Yes, but you put me in an impossible position by saying you wouldn't take him back if he really needed it."

"No, I would *never* say that!"

Danny (fully alert): "So it's all right then! You would take me back so I can go?"

Dr T (to me): "You have to take the responsibility. He's your child. I don't feel it's right. I can't give you my consent."

"But perhaps your goodwill?"

"Yes, all right. Talk to Dr L tomorrow about the pill dosage."

AFTER TARA: DANNY'S THEORIES

The next day I dropped Danny off at Maths and went to see Dr L—the doctor who had talked daily to Danny. I saw immediately why Danny had called him "a brick wall": he was frighteningly stiff and unsmiling. He said that Tara had decided that they would only take Danny in again if we agreed not to interfere.

I drove to fetch Danny thinking, "Nevermore". And nevermore it was. Dr L gave me a prescription for anti-psychotic drugs—"the major tranquillisers" they were called: Stelazine and Largactil. I fetched them from my chemist, but put them in my cupboard for the moment. That night I gave him one of my own sleeping-pills—Mogadon, the one currently used. Even this I was uncertain about, since he had been on these other pills. When to give and not give pills, and which pills to give, became a major agonizing thing for me.

Danny the next day was very relaxed. Toby came round. We didn't often see him because he was studying for a Music Degree at Wits. He had a delicate face and sensitive expressions. His father was very rich and had paid for the Orange Grove house for Toby and Debbie. Toby told me later that he never smoked much pot himself because of his studies.

The three of us were having coffee at the kitchen table. Danny said gloomily, "At Tara even the furthest walls were talking about me."

Toby and I burst out laughing and couldn't stop. I think we were hysterical with relief at having him there with us. In the end Danny joined in.

I thought to myself: Maybe when Danny looks back he may remember the warmth of this time, as well as the panic and depression. There is so much sheer good human feeling—in him and in us.

But Danny was determined now to "solve the problem" of what people were doing to his mind. He wrote his ideas down on little pieces of paper. They were nonsense: "word salad": unrelated words with correct grammar but no sense.

He came to me and Oliver: "Did you people read what I wrote?"

"Ja," I said.

"What did you get out of it?"

"Well," I said, carefully. "It seemed like a mixture of metaphysics and parapsychology."

But that night at supper Oliver and Danny and I had a good conversation about capitalism and communism. Danny wanted to abstract abstractions, but he was not talking in word salad.

"What takes *everything* into consideration?" asked Danny.

Oliver answered, "Pragmatism perhaps."

Everyone thinks he should "talk to someone"—a therapist. Except his Jewish grandmother, Sally: She said, "I had a friend who took her husband out of Tara and off pills and she talked to him quietly and sensibly every evening and he came right."

The next day Danny and a friend spent the afternoon drumming in the garage, with Mark and Hector listening. He came in looking relaxed and happy. He and Oliver were going to a rubbishy movie that night: "I'm really going to enjoy it in a human way."

Oliver said, "Oh we'll have a good laugh."

"I *need* that. I've had to work so *hard* interpreting things."

"Do you have to do that *all* the time?" I asked.

"Oh yes—it's like an instinct—you can't turn it off. I just want to know what's going on."

"Well you can't solve it all at once," I said.

Danny wrote on the toilet wall: TRUE EGOTISM: STAYING WHERE YOU ARE, WITH THE KNOWLEDGE THAT YOU CAN GO FURTHER. (We used to write messages on the toilet walls in Koki pens. But this year no one had done that.)

Debbie phoned: "Danny told me about the Tara tests: he said they showed him a picture of two people kissing and he started off saying: 'Well these two look like two average people in love,'—but then he got bored and decided to freak them out so went on a flight of fancy about the war in China!"

I read up about the "major tranquillisers"—the anti-psychotic drugs—but they had side effects, and also Danny had refused even to consider them after he had been given them at Tara. Better somewhat mad than a zombie. Most of the time now his delusions were not making him anxious but making him feel special.

I spoke to my own doctor, Dr van Niftrik, who thought that Danny's psychosis was almost certainly a dagga after-effect and would gradually fade. He prescribed sleeping-pills (the same Mogadon), which I gave to Danny when he seemed to need them.

The next week one morning at 4 am Danny and I were both awake and wandering around. Danny said, "I'm going to make early breakfast. Can I make you some?" "Ja, sure." "Scramble or cheese toast?" "Scramble."

Then he asked me questions about Oliver's family and ended with: "I don't want to be any nationality—I just want to jump around and try them all."

He sounded and looked totally sane. At 5.15 am he walked off to Toby and Debbie's house, wearing his dressing-gown. I fetched him there, brought him home to change and took him to Maths and home to lunch and then to squash in the afternoon. Oliver came home, knowing nothing about Danny's very early start. I was too tired to explain it to him, or to notice what he was planning: he had decided to take Danny to another movie so that he would be too tired to need a sleeping-pill. So that's what they did.

But I think the day had been just too long for Danny, and the next day he was very paranoiac: raging up and down the passage, shouting about evil forces and wanting to know what was going on.

One calm morning Daniel and I were talking quietly in the living room:

"I wish the hell someone would just tell me what is going on."

"The only reason I don't tell you is that you wouldn't believe it."

"Well I wish someone *would* tell me."

"OK."

So I told him about the unconscious mind and projections.

Danny, still very calm, said, "Well, I've *told* myself that this force is just in my head. But there's just *too* much coincidence."

Then Oliver came in and told him all about the hippies and the drug culture—linking Eastern philosophy with the taking of drugs.

I told him that all his notions about thoughts coming from the outside were in fact "thought hallucinations"—but that it was more difficult to check them against reality than visual hallucinations.

He took all this quite calmly.

He then told us about "understanding African languages". He was using this to show us that what happened in his mind was real. He turns on the radio and listens to African speech and then all of a sudden he hears two kugel voices talking about him. He illustrated this.

Oliver said that the reason they seemed to be talking about him was because the memories of them talking are in his head. Danny considered this but was unconvinced.

Unfortunately they then went on to the kitchen and the discussion got more heated. Oliver came to me. "I think you'd better give him a pill to calm him down."

"When Ivor comes for him he will change direction and then he will be OK. We should only discuss it with him for short calm periods."

Oliver said heatedly, "I don't want to discuss it with him at all!"

His uncle Ivor, Hector's dad, was doing some work on a house he had just bought and Danny was able to help him. When I went to fetch him I waited at the top of the drive and he waited at the bottom—a mistake—and when we finally met he gave me his beautiful smile: his real one, not his mystic one.

I said, "That was something good. I've been thinking all afternoon about the Forces of Good."

"How d'you mean?"

"Well all the religions recognize a Force of Evil, but they also recognize a Force of Good. And I wondered where that was in your philosophy."

"Well ... I ..."

"For instance the message I have been picking up from you over this time of helping out is that it is OK."

He was puzzled: "Me helping you?"

"No—I mean me helping you—I sort of get the vibe that you think that's OK—and that you are, well, grateful."

"Yes I am."

We didn't talk for the rest of the journey. At our house he said, comfortably, "Shall I shut the gate?" "Ja, would you?"

He was quiet and friendly at supper. Apologized for clearing before I had finished. He seemed very tired—reaction perhaps to our complete denial of his theories.

It's such a very adolescent thing: imagining that people are talking about you. Just not usually so loudly and clearly. In a way he has learnt to live with it. But he also says he is very TIRED of it.

The next day he asked me, "So then I would have to start from scratch?"

He said to me that *everyone* can do it—from 2-year-olds to 90-year-olds.

"Do you do it to them?"

"No, that's the funny thing. At one time I thought things did it as well—buildings—everything."

And another day he said, "If I had never had pot I wouldn't *know* all this. I would just be walking around like an ordinary person."

"It's all in your imagination."

"If it's all my imagination then I must have a fantastic one!"

LUCY WONDERS WHY

I went to visit my Aunt Freda. She was hospitalised for episodes of insanity for a few months every two or three years. She had now been diagnosed as "manic-depressive" and was on lithium. I had never understood this diagnosis, because I had never seen her depressed. She was an intelligent aunt whom I loved talking to. On this occasion, because of Danny, she explained to me about her disorder. Both the mania and the subsequent depression were her "mad times". During her manic phases she felt she could do anything; then came disaster and failure—and these were her depressed phases when she suffered from paranoia.

I thought how when Danny was in a manic phase, pot "did him no harm". In the subsequent depressed phase, pot immediately brought on the paranoia. As a child he had often been either wildly enthusiastic or almost ill with lethargy.

In a manic phase he doesn't *need* to try: in a depressed phase he doesn't *want* to try

I told various experts about my manic-depressive aunt, but they didn't think the relationship was close enough genetically: Freda was Daniel's grandmother's sister—his great-aunt.

Freda had not become insane during adolescence. She was a great success as a teenager—a gifted ballet dancer who was also very beautiful. She went up, up, up at the East Rand eisteddfods. She was also a star academically. But in her thirties she found she could not have children of her own, and this disappointment triggered off her first attack of insanity.

Debbie, Toby's wife, from the Orange Grove "House of Pot", came to visit me when Danny was out. "I've had Daphne on my mind. There's something I want to tell you about that time."

Daphne was Debbie's 26-year-old friend who had fallen for Daniel during the Christmas holidays. Danny's earlier girlfriend, Sandy, only about three years older than he was, had disappeared in about September. She was about to write Matric, and possibly was sent to relatives in Durban to get her away from sinful Jo'burg. Danny had waited and waited and asked and asked, but there was no news of her. By the end of November, after his exams, Danny felt quite thrilled that here was this new woman in his life. But at one party, when the couple were being shown off to everyone, Sandy walked in! Danny was stunned: this was his real girlfriend! But what was he to do? The two looked at each other in a bemused way, and then Sandy left.

When Daphne discovered that Danny was only fourteen, she felt both worried and humiliated. Perhaps Danny sensed this, because one evening at her flat, he simply couldn't perform.

I was hearing this for the first time—from Debbie. She said that the next day their crowd were all sitting around in a circle. Suddenly Daphne started to mock Danny for his inability to perform.

"She just went on and on and on. Danny sat there looking at the ground."

"It could have been pot of course—that's known to affect performance."

"Yes—and that was another thing with Daphne. She never smoked pot, and once she discovered that Danny was smoking it she tried to get him to stop."

I asked Debbie where Daphne was now, but she didn't know. Daphne had stopped seeing her after the disaster of Danny running away from home and school and evidently not in his right mind.

I thought: One day perhaps he will bring home a girlfriend who is younger than he is, and whom he can instruct about real life without bluff and pretence. Then we will know that he has caught up with himself.

I thought about Danny and his four manic "highs", and then toppling off all of them. The first was triumphing over drugs. He had smoked pot while writing his exams and had passed. His older friends had given up pot during exam time. This made him feel, in that one way, superior to them.

Danny and I drove to Midrand to collect band equipment he had left in Jan K's barn.

"Ja, we were a bit mad last year to smoke so much dope. But the others gave up at exam time. I was the *only* one to smoke all through the exams and still pass!"

So there he was, the baby of the group, outshining them!

The second high/low was status-symbol Daphne and her rejection of him.

The third was being called "the greatest young guitar-player in South Africa"—yet having nowhere to play. No steady ladder to climb. Friends often saying they would come round for a jam, and then not showing up; and Jan K's rock band never getting off the ground. Danny thought he could crack it by forming his own band, but he believed that would only be possible if he left school. School was holding him back.

And the fourth was returning to Damelin, and finding he didn't know what was going on either academically or socially. But by then he was already psychotic—so this can't be called a cause. But it was another high/low situation, since he had been so very confident in Standard 7.

BACK TO POT

In later years Danny was very clear about the reasons for his pot-smoking: "The first time it was for excitement and adventure. The second time it was for depression."

This is what Toby told me years later: "I never saw Danny as an addict. He never seemed to go for it compulsively. If I was there when he arrived and I could steer him into the piano room, then he would sit down and play quietly. At other times he smoked first and then sat down at the piano as if to attack it. He would play in an aggressive and out-of-control way and I feared for the piano."

Immediately after Tara, Danny was not smoking. Debbie invited him over when no one else was there. We didn't let him go to that house at the weekends when all the friends sat around and smoked.

I took Danny and his now trustworthy older cousin Hector to my parents' farm. They stayed there for the weekend and never left their room unless they were famished. These two as boys of eight and ten had roamed the hills and talked about sex and life and saving wild animals.

Hector told me afterwards that Danny had not smoked pot, nor asked for it. He had also not talked about "evil forces". Danny told me that he had finished *The Lord of the Rings* and read *Kramer versus Kramer*.

But Danny was tired of being controlled by his new jailers (his old equals) at the Orange Grove house. One day when he came back from

Maths he walked towards the car jauntily—grinning: "That was a *most* enjoyable Maths lesson—well, I mean, quite enjoyable."

I thought that day would go on being fine. Debbie was alone and Danny said he would be back at 5. But while he was there she phoned in great distress: "Lucy, I think you ought to come over here and hear what Daniel has to say. Max came—they had a terrible row about pot and now Danny is just pulling out every argument under the sun about why he should be given another chance." (Because, of course, he "ought" to be able to handle it.)

It sounded as if he was on one of his collision courses—driven, maniacal.

I said to Debbie, "Get Max to go, and point Danny in another direction if possible."

"We'll do some gardening. I was so angry with him that I asked him why he didn't just go to the street corner and buy some!"

I suppose that Max, his most daring fellow-adventurer, turning against him by refusing him pot, was the last straw.

That night he raged at me for opening his door while he was trying to work something out on the guitar. I interrupted him a second time to give him his pill and he was again revolting and horrible to me. Later I said, "I was upset. I've never seen you like that."

"Ja—well it was my fault. I should have asked you to leave the pill outside or something."

"Oh well, that's OK."

"I'm actually not very nice. I should start a company like JR (of "Dallas"). If you just let me smoke one joint a week I could be nice again."

Dried leaves or resin of Cannabis form a hallucinogen which may be smoked, made into a drink, or eaten. Use of the drug results in loss of inhibitions and impairment of judgement and memory. Long-term effects have yet to be fully studied, but it soon creates great psychological dependence. Also known as dagga, hashish, kif, pot and marijuana. (Hutchinson's Encyclopedia 1986)

There were only two rehabilitation places that we heard about at that time. One was a government institution in the Magaliesberg Mountains which sounded punitive and soul-destroying. Phoenix House, in contrast, sounded benign—and we had heard of people going there and being helped. Danny thought the idea was OK: he would be with people who were not smoking pot at all, instead of with his friends who smoked themselves but wouldn't give him any. And Oliver and I needed a rest.

Oliver and Danny and I went to see Dr R, the chief boss of Sanca, at the town office. He, like Dr T of Tara, had a good reputation. But Daniel that day was in a bad mood—sunken, sullen and depressed. Dr R disliked him instantly, and used a hostile manner with him, which increased Daniel's negativity. Dr R said he would let us know about Phoenix House. Then he got in touch with his friend Dr T at Tara. Dr T told him that Daniel was schizophrenic and therefore unsuitable for Phoenix House.

So Dr R refused us, saying that Danny wouldn't manage the structure of Phoenix House. I was puzzled, since Danny wasn't dangerous, and Phoenix House must have seen hallucinating people coming off drugs. Danny's lack of structure was in his head—he would have complied with a simple external structure and simply played his guitar in some corner. Daniel of course might not have stayed—he might simply have walked out after a week or two. But those two weeks would have given his main carer, me, time off to recover.

Perhaps I should have tried to arrange all this through our own doctor—Dr van Niftrik—who knew the family and knew Daniel. Dr van N told me to tell Danny to look at adult pot-users who had smoked for a long time, and judge them as people. But Danny was not that rational, and we knew no adult junkies.

Danny *did* know how to get pot from street-corners and service stations. His mind was not organized enough to earn money or to deal in drugs, but he could swop a few cigarettes for a joint.

Oliver found him smoking pot in the garage. Father confronted son, but son just grinned inanely and said he was working on his own system.

"Don't you *want* to get well," I moaned. And to myself I said: What can one do with him?

Oliver said to him, "Look at you! You are just a zombie. You are no good to yourself or anyone else."

That night Danny came to me:

"Ma, can I have a sleeping-pill?"

I was firmly angry: "Do you want a home and love and protection and music and a sleeping-pill when you need it? Or do you want pot? You have to decide."

Danny replied blearily: "I don't want pot. I don't know why I ever started it."

"Give me the rest of the pot."

He reached into the drawer next to his bed and drew out an envelope. In it was what looked like a twisted piece of brown paper. I took it, gave him a sleeping-pill, chucked away the envelope without looking at it and went back to bed.

Meanwhile, in America, my sister Hilary was having trouble with her son Neil's pot smoking. Neil didn't go mad, but he was troublesome.

Danny was difficult to wake the next day and I had to cancel his appointment with the physiotherapist.

On the way to Maths:

"Mrs Wenham assumed you have an infection and I didn't tell her the truth."

"Why not?"

"What is the truth?"

"That I smoked pot."

"Good."

Mrs Wenham was a physiotherapist whom he went to before Maths. He often walked from her to Maths. She was helping him with massage and posture and relaxation.

On the way back from Maths, Danny asked me, "I wonder what Neil thinks about pot now?"

"So do I. I asked Hilary but haven't heard from her yet. Do you know about Nicola's reaction to Neil?"

"Ja. He wrote to her when she was studying in Oxford."

"I think he expected her to approve."

"Oh I don't think any addict would expect that."

Oliver mostly just assumed that any negative or fragile behaviour was due to pot. Danny stayed away from pot for a while and Oliver noticed that his guitar playing was better. He complimented him and Danny said, "Yes, I've just realized all I've been through this year—the running away, into drugs ... and I've realized what you and Ma have been through ... and that I don't need daily narcotics."

He and Oliver went off and bought some jazz books.

Lesley, a friend of Nicola's, offered to help Danny. She took him with her to help out at a Saturday morning drama class for Indian children. The first time he was very self-conscious and anxious.

Since he was not allowed to go and visit his pot friends or go out with them, he now had to find other things to do at the weekend. Lesley invited him to spend the night at her place. We said that was OK. When it was time to go he looked a bit disintegrated and funny ... I gave him a Surmontil (anti-depression and anti-anxiety) and off he went.

Oliver (puzzled): "Why do you say he is frightened? He just seemed excited."

"I don't know. I just know that there was an underlying panic, instability—he was holding himself together. I don't think he's quite stabilized yet."

"Well no, I don't suppose he would be."

On the Sunday morning we both went to Lesley to fetch him. Lesley made tea for us. Daniel looked pretty heavy and depressed. I asked him, "How was last night?"

Daniel replied negatively: "OK."

In the car he cheered up:

"Will it be all right if I play at the Wits Jazz Club tonight?"

"How late would that be?"

"Oh not later than about 10.30, 11."

"That's fine. Who are you playing with?"

"I thought I would do a solo—but I'm not quite ready to handle that."

Later that day I phoned Lesley. I asked her whether the social situation had been threatening for Danny the night before. She said a group of dope-smokers had turned up—they had been "adolescent" about it. Daniel had argued about it—asking for pot—but Lesley felt it was more for the sake of the argument than because he really wanted to smoke. They didn't let him, and Lesley herself didn't smoke.

Lesley and Danny talked about his situation this morning. Lesley gets the impression that he *knows* he has been ill and wants to get better.

He *knows* that the Saturday morning drama class is good for him. He was very uptight with the supervisor girl last week, but this week much better.

Danny told Lesley that his whole problem started with the acid (LSD) on New Year's Eve, and then went on with the pot. This is actually something of a breakthrough.

Oliver took him to the Wits Jazz Club. He didn't play himself, and was not quite comfortable socially, but survived.

However, the next morning he was in an extremely angry, black mood—trapped; low self-esteem. Therefore society was keeping something from him. I knew that the weekend had just been too much for his coping mechanisms. He worked up to tears and talk of running away. I put my arm around him.

I dropped him off at physio, after which he was to walk to Maths. But I got into a panic and I went early to the Maths place and sat in the car trying to wait: I just wanted him to come so much that I could think of nothing else. I imagined him running away with no money, and none of his friends taking him in: all he could do would be to find some pot and get stoned. Eventually I was mindlessly compelled upstairs to the Mastermaths place. Danny was discussing his work with Linda, quite matter of fact. In the car he said:

"Listen. I am prepared to do O-levels, but I don't know about A's. I am prepared to work for six good O-levels, but I doubt very much whether I'll go on to A's.

"That's fine."

IN CAHOOTS WITH MR S

I found a therapist with a good reputation for being friendly with teenagers, so I made an appointment to see him. He worked in Parkhurst—quite far from us, but I had an old friend nearby with whom I could have coffee while Danny was at his sessions.

I was very optimistic about therapy in general and Mr S in particular. In the diary I wrote, "Mr S can help you: maximize your potential; integrate your personality; have far more *real* good feelings; cope with society; cope with reality."

I told Mr S about Danny and then said I assumed he wouldn't plunge into Daniel's delusions straight away. He said that's precisely what he *would* do and that you don't usually get the opportunity to attack someone's delusions straight away. He says that Danny's "evil force" is a "delusion"—not a hallucination. A delusion is when you carry on believing something without any proof. He says that provided a person is capable of logical thought the best way of changing a belief is to dispute it. He burst out laughing when I said Tara hadn't allowed Daniel to see any of his friends.

Danny came out of his first session beaming:

"Excellent! He just knew straight away what I was getting at. Do you think I could go to Exclusive to get some books, or the library? I need some books on psychology."

"Do you mean right now? No maths?"

"Well I just feel so inspired now."

"OK. It's fairly close to here."

"He's sort of brilliant. When I came in he said, 'So what's the news?' and I said, 'Oh nothing special'—and he seemed quite annoyed that I had come for no specific reason. After ten minutes he said, 'You could write a book!' I said '10 volumes!' Does he know how *old* I am?"

At Exclusive Books he bought a book called *Alien Intelligence* on the paranormal and came home and started reading it.

Later that day we went to Mrs Wenham, the physiotherapist. In the car going there he talked to me about his new book—Darwin, Eugene Marais, the brain. Mrs Wenham worked with Danny for one-and-a-half hours. Danny was co-operative, natural and open, not stiff and held together as he so often is.

Mrs Wenham said to me, "There is a lot of good in this boy."

Danny often hallucinated in a benign way in the evenings. His pupils were tiny, he was far away from us and didn't communicate; and he had a smile which could only have indicated heavenly bliss. I didn't like this state particularly, but it was easier to deal with than his paranoiac rages. I called it "hallucinatory happiness".

What he was doing this evening as a result of his session with Mr S may have been reading a mystic book, but his happiness was in this world and not hallucinatory.

After a few sessions with Mr S he had changed his "terrifying box" (society's conspiracy against him) to "the Game". The dangerous, terrifying thing that he discovered and which could destroy him and everything else is, say, Level 4. But now he is moving on to another level where he plays "The Game" and deals with social embarrassment in some sort of oblique and metaphorical way.

After he sees Mr S he feels good and has positive ideas. Even if these ideas have no follow-through, at least I feel happy to see him positive. All the recent criticism—both real from us and his friends—and imagined in his head—has not helped.

One evening after supper he started on "the Game" while doing the washing up. He said he had reached the point where he knew absolutely everything there was to know. (He has kept the sequence going from "double voices" to this "game").

"As I was telling my psychologist this morning ... people being reduced to atoms ... and *yet* there are emotions. It's such fun. We are really getting somewhere. We don't talk about me at all. We just talk about society—I talk and he agrees now and then."

Things were going so well that I went to the farm for the weekend to see my aged and neglected parents. At home, Danny's old friend from Woodmead, Adrian (who went to Eden and never smoked dope), stayed for the weekend.

As I drove in he shouted, "Hi Ma!"

"Hi my love. Dad says you had an excellent week-end—that you were actually in the presence of stoned people and not stoned yourself!"

"Ja, that was pretty good, wasn't it!"

He had been off all pills and undepressed.

"Happy Mother's Day" said Hector—well it really did seem like one!

One day he laughed a lot at squash, and then said: "Do I have to go to Mr S? I feel much happier now. I felt very confused, but after three sessions of talking it out I'm all right. I wouldn't have anything to say to him today."

He went a few more times, but found it more and more frustrating. Mr S seemed to have become a total Rogerian—sitting there and saying nothing. (Carl Rogers had formed a whole theory after a woman "cured herself" by talking for an hour while Rogers said nothing at all.)

Finally Danny refused to go any more. I took his last appointment myself, but found it equally frustrating:

Lucy: So how do you see him now? What do you think is wrong with him?
Mr S: Well what do *you* think Lucy?
Lucy: I don't know. That's why I am asking you.
Mr S: He'll probably always be a bit weird.

Which turned out not to be true at all!

Erikson: Adolescents are completely egocentric. In the brain of an adolescent is the whole world. They are often testing the rock-bottom of some truth.

Lucy: Adolescents have sometimes had visions which make sense to the adults of their tribe, like Joan of Arc in France and Nomquase in the Transkei.

MAY/JUNE 1982

By May of this year, 1982, Danny was only officially doing three O-Levels: English Language, English Literature and Maths. The English I had simply assumed he would cope with, since it had always been an easy subject for him. He had a lesson once a week with Mrs R—an elderly, disabled woman who lived in a high-up flat somewhere. Danny didn't mind the lessons—this was one-on-one with a friendly, non-threatening person. But Mrs R, who had probably not taken in the extent of his disorder, said he would never manage O-Level English by the end of the year unless he did more homework.

Danny used to sit down at his desk to do this homework, but when I saw the short, tight, forced paragraphs that he was doing—in contrast to his flowing essays of the year before—I knew that it was "too much" for him. I think now that it was the language centre of his brain that was disorganized, and that too much interference blocked his ability to answer Mrs R's irrelevant (to him) questions. Maths must have happened somewhere else in his brain.

One afternoon after lunch Danny was supposed to be finishing some English homework for his lesson, but he asked for an atlas and for the telephone. I tried to rest, but felt worried. I heard him slam the kitchen door and went after him.

"Danny, I can't help feeling anxious. I can't really rest when I feel you may be going off somewhere to get pot or running away."

"Can I talk to you about these O-Levels?"

Well he thought them a complete waste of time. When he went out of the kitchen door he had been off to make arrangements for going to Cape Town. He would stay with Nicola and get a job.

We compromised on a programme which included only Maths as an O-Level, since that is the only subject he couldn't easily come back to if he wanted to pursue his education and also because he can do it easily. He will give up pot, do squash and physio daily, and not run away.

"Do you think a 15-year-old who could think out theories like I do *needs* O-Levels?"

This was "grandiose", yet spoken in a normal voice. It referred to his psychotic fantasies, yet his question did not come from that mad place.

I felt that at least this was *his* new plan, which would perhaps carry him through the pot-recovery months. Being so controlled by us has made him feel powerless.

In the car going to squash he said, "Can I change my room around?"

"It's your room."

"I feel so much better already. I'm going to be like Nicky now—I'll probably get depressed like Nicky."

"Then you'll have to learn to deal with it."

"I'll just change my room round again!"

Gary, a friend of Nicola's, came around. He said that when you come off dope you get a surge of energy and start tidying your room.

Danny has put his mattress on the floor and used the under-board as a room-divider. Then he put drapes all over. "It's a designer's room—or a musician's."

Jo S feels Danny has manipulated me. But since he has also manipulated himself out of a depression, it doesn't much matter.

In his spirit of boundless optimism he invented a method of writing down everything: The 12 notes of the scale, written over and over, corresponding to the 24(!) letters of the alphabet and to the 24 hours of the day and the 7 days of the week: "Amazing isn't it? Now I can translate Shakespeare into music."

On the way to squash one day I started making up a story with him:

"Imagine that you have got a son. Your wife has died and you are solely responsible for the boy ... How old is he?"

"35."

"If he was 35 you wouldn't be responsible for him!"

"Oh I would—because he would be a vegetable."

"OK now seriously—he's about ten. What's his name?"

"Maximillian."

"OK. Max for short."

"No! I *hate* that name."

I hated that name because Max had given him LSD. Danny probably hated that name because Max refused to give him pot.

"Let's have Maxwell," suggested Danny.

"OK—now—Maxwell is 15."

I told him all about how Maxwell spiralled up and spiralled down. Danny refused to go into squash until the story was finished.

But the story at that stage had no ending.

The May truce did not last: winter set in. Jo'burg in June and July is freezing, except at midday when a stunning sun warms us up.

Daniel's times of feeling better were when he felt hope. But these episodes of hope—feeling Mr S believed in him, or giving up O-Levels—had no lasting quality to them. And now the Wits Jazz Club, which he had been to a few times with his dad, suddenly fizzled out. Danny had been working himself up to playing there himself, but before that happened the half-year exams loomed for the students, and the jazz club didn't exist any more.

Everyone else had something real to get on with. Often, getting together for a jam couldn't be worked out—because other people had jobs or studies to do.

Danny stopped writing things down and became more silent. He said, "So you think I'm unresourceful?"

"Not in all situations, no. You are resourceful in music. But your thinking seems to have got stuck. When you came out of Tara you wrote down your thoughts and they weren't stuck at all. You were airing them. And you don't talk much."

"I don't state things for fear of being contradicted. There is a ten to one chance you may be wrong."

I stood at the stove stirring the scrambled eggs. "You and I thought that nothing could go wrong. Both of us. We both flew too near the sun."

I thought: He feels very alienated, strange and different—the more he feels like this the more difficult it is for him to enter society again. (However, I can now see, in 2009, that this was an important phase.)

His voice had become tight and high. His movements no longer looked in control. Mrs Wenham, the physiotherapist, said to me in private: "This boy has no reserves. Everything is done with utmost effort. Very slowly. A desperate effort for him. It is as if he is suffering from nervous exhaustion. Not so much physical as mental."

Danny's arm began shaking. He had to hold it still with his other hand.

He was mostly too tired for squash.

Sometimes Oliver and I took Danny out somewhere. But we saw other young people giving him funny looks.

I myself have become frail and despairing. I know that this will not do—and I write myself stern notes.

I watch a film on a deaf child named Jonah. I think: Jonah's mother went on and on looking for solutions. Only mothers do that. Only mothers will put all their thought and time and energy into one child.

Oliver and I went to see a play called "Buried Child". I felt close to madness myself and had to hold myself together and dissociate from it. Oliver felt none of that—and in discussing the situation on the way back I started to feel strong again. I knew that Daniel needed my togetherness and that I had at least to pretend to be cheerful and confident.

In the past Oliver had had a migraine about once every two years. Now he started to have frequent migraines. We had to stay away from him as any noise, even of sympathy, aggravated the situation. He took anti-migraine pills which sedated him somewhat but he still wanted no visits. He lay on his bed in the dark.

My father dies. My mother is senile and alcoholic and refuses to move from the farm.

My daughter returns from Cape Town University. She says I look anorexic. I weigh myself: from my middle-aged weight of around 150 pounds, I am now my schoolgirl weight of 125 pounds.

Chapter Nine

BREAKDOWN PART II

NOBODY LIKES ME

Back in 1982 I read that in adolescence strong drives develop; they grow taller and more powerful—and this may drive them to break away from authority. They feel themselves to be stronger than the forces which once held them.

The talk therapists don't see the adolescent in this mood. I had one session with a therapist who thought that Daniel needed to "get into touch with the primitive". I thought, driving home from this session, that Daniel needed rather to control and shape his impulses, and to know that he could control them.

One evening Oliver said he was "gated" because he had come home late the night before. I don't think Danny even knew the word! Immediately off he went in his wild strong way—and didn't come home all night.

Another thing I read was that adolescents don't push their parents beyond their endurance. But we were beyond our endurance!—and Danny, being not only an adolescent but a disturbed one, probably simply didn't know it. He lived in his own head.

Oliver said, "I don't even like him any more. I just think: Who is this guy?"

I agreed. "Ja, me too. One just feels that we have this practical problem of how to deal with this person."

Danny himself was feeling very isolated. He said as usual that he didn't trust society—but added that he didn't trust anyone. Today I said I would give him a lift—and wasn't I "society"?

"Well you're my *mother* and I have to trust someone a bit."

One day Lucky, his old jazz teacher, phoned. I answered. Danny heard me saying that he was not really fit.

"What do you mean by saying I'm not really fit?" he said, indignantly.

"Well, why aren't you doing a full day's work?"

"Because I've been mentally ill."

"Why?"

"Because society has imposed things on me for the last six months."

One day Danny played his guitar at a club with Oliver there. The next week Oliver said, in his hearing: "He must be on dope if he thinks he played well on Sunday night."

Oliver found it difficult to understand that everything Danny did wrong was not necessarily due to current pot smoking—although the whole condition might have been triggered off by pot smoking originally.

Lucy to herself: Nowadays I worry more about the nervous voice, the sighs and the tiredness than about the psychosis. I long for him to fling himself into the pool or into some joyful therapy. He says that when he has finished coming to his "conclusions" he will start again—on "reality".

Danny had been passionately looking forward to Nicky coming home. He had asked me many times when she was arriving, and never remembered the answer. He had been convinced that Nicky would understand his theories. They had always played fantasy word games and he thought they would always be on the same wavelength.

I remember the first time since December that my two children sat at the kitchen table together. I was washing up and glancing across at them. Danny in a serious voice said one of his weird, meaningless things, and Nicky got a look of absolute horror on her face. She had not taken in that he "really was mad".

After that he took very little notice of her. She was another one he "couldn't trust".

Danny was now "on holiday"—which made things more difficult because he didn't know what to do with himself.

Oliver, also "on holiday", came into my room. "Daniel is on the roof, leaning against the parapet, smoking a cigarette and listening to some rock. Sounds crazy to me. Do you think it's a protest or what?"

"That sounds harmlessly crazy to me—nicely crazy."

Danny spent two whole nights out and came back at 7 am. I thought he had stayed with Toby and Debbie in Orange Grove, but it seems he simply spent the nights "out" somewhere.

Not having his regular programme is making him more manic; he looks full of power and he is grinning in his superior way.

It seems impossible for him to be moderate. He either submits to Mark being in charge of him and bringing him home at 11 pm, or he breaks out completely and stays out all night.

My sister Hilary saw him for the first time since his breakdown. He was in his "other state"—weak and shaky.

"He desperately needs some successes," she said. "Even small things."

I talked to Debbie. She and Toby are fed up with Danny. They found him at an adult club at 4 am, dancing by the speaker all alone!

But not smoking pot, or fighting with anyone—so I just laughed to myself.

"Everyone's against me," he complained to me.

"Yes of course!" I said cheerfully. "If you are a law unto yourself you cannot expect other people to like you."

"Yes, I do see that."

The next day he left a note for us before he went out:

WENT OUT. VARIOUS PLACES. WILL CONTACT. WILL SEE. DANNY

Danny was now in fact a lot more normal. He was thinking of ways in which he could perhaps satisfy us and himself. He put a proposition to me—that he should spend his time finding professional musicians and putting a group together. He sounded completely articulate—so we discussed it and I said I would ask Oliver. Who was against it—not at present a workable idea.

It was very cold. Danny got up late, cleared up the kitchen, practised for an hour or more. At lunch only he and I were there:

Danny: Hey, chocolate! Amazing!
Lucy: Ja—well, I felt depressed.
Danny: I trust not because of me?
Lucy: Oh that is always there.

Danny: I don't see why.

Lucy: I'm certainly not worried about your physical or mental health at the moment. You seem to have given up pot—which is a huge thing.

Danny: Oh it wasn't difficult—I just moved out of those circles.

Lucy: Well now it's the education problem. I don't want you to miss opportunities. I think you might very well want to study psychology alongside of music at Wits.

Danny: I would have to write essays, take lecture notes, and read books. I could do that now.

Lucy: Well they don't know that.

Danny: I'll forge a certificate.

He started to go for long walks at midnight—all alone. If I was awake I would see him unstoned and cheerful when he returned. One night a friendly policeman brought him home. "He needs help," said the policeman.

His cousin Hector noticed that he was better—at least by his and my standards: "He's making much more sense." "Ja," I said, "I think so too."

Danny thinks that Jo'burg is tapping some benevolent vibe at the moment. Perhaps this is because there are no pressures on him and no one has been annoyed with him.

However, this did not last. Toby told Nicola that Danny was driving them bonkers. They shut him out last week and he climbed over the wall. He begged for pot and went through Toby's drawers looking for it. He is in love with Esmé whom he met there, but she has her own boyfriend and doesn't want him. The more he is rejected the more obsessional he gets.

No women have been interested in Danny this year. After four years of all girls, and particularly older girls, finding him enchanting, his breakdown has changed all that. They flee from him.

"Next week we are going to Molozi," I told Danny.

"Really?" said Danny amazed and delighted. "Just the four of us?"

"Yes."

Molozi was the family pine farm in the Zoutpansberg Mountains north-east of Louis Trichardt in the northern Transvaal. It was the place (much warmer than Jo'burg) where we had spent every July holiday in the past, when the children were young—where we had gone for forest walks and Oliver had painted and cooked and we had sat around the fire at night and read a book aloud. It seemed a miracle to Daniel that this place and that life still existed, away from the terrors of school and the problems with "society".

Nicola was not only cut off from Danny, she was also extremely disturbed by him—was having spastic colon and other digestive disorders. She heard that Toby and Max took acid (LSD) at the weekend, which didn't help her peace of mind.

From my point of view Danny was a lot better. One morning he hadn't slept at all the night before but I found him sitting in the kitchen and thinking and noting down a few thoughts—abstract and philosophical, but not "psychotic".

The first night up at the farm, Oliver, Danny and I talked at length, Danny with his slow, stuttering abstractions. Nicola walked out. I knew that Danny was doing better than when he had delusions or hallucinations or spoke in "word salad". But his very abstract utterances simply irritated Nicola.

"Too great a diffusion of interests is wrong. I am a musician—I live in a certain house, go to a certain school. My six squares—I can touch on others occasionally, but most people jet-set over all the squares."

The next day however, something went right for all of us: Nicola and Oliver found out that Danny could not only drive, but could drive well. They were impressed with his driving and this was a great morale boost for him. Each of them went out driving with him.

My driving lessons in the late afternoon north of Jo'burg had not been a deliberate secret. It had simply not come out. Oliver had been at work and then often had migraines in the evening. Nicola had been in Cape Town.

I had found that Danny listened well to driving help from me. And if he had been driving in the afternoon, he didn't have his faraway look at supper.

Nicky started having solutions for Danny: "Danny should stay with me in Cape Town—there's a good school opposite and a beautifully equipped new Technical High School across the Gardens."

"Ja." I said. "A lot of people on hearing that Danny is non-academic say we should send him to a Technical High—but he is even less technical than academic.

Oliver said, "He's a non-academic intellectual—and there's only one thing people like that can do—carry on with academic work.

Danny talked a lot to himself about Esmé—the young woman he had fallen for at Toby's house.

Sometimes he wanted to talk to us about her: "Let's talk about Esmé."

"Does she smoke dope?" I asked.

"That's none of your business."

"There's only one person at that Orange Grove house who doesn't seem like a dope-smoker and that's Shelley."

"Ja, Shelley's great."

"She's still got an edge to her personality, which dope-smokers lose."

"Yes—that's quite right!" agreed Nicola. "They lose their sparkle."

Danny mumbled, "I've got my sparkle."

"Well it's coming back," said Nicky generously. "Your eyes are getting clearer."

Danny even gave up smoking cigarettes up there, because there were no shops to buy them at. He endured this with no fuss at all. He had brought his little ideas book with him and frequently wrote in it.

He and Nicky sang "Noggin-a-nog"—a game from their past: each one would say it at a different pitch—going lower and lower or higher or higher—and then laughing.

Oliver was so pleased with Danny that one afternoon, when I was resting, he gave him permission to go by himself by car to Louis Trichardt—about half-an-hour's drive away. I was anxious and disapproving. Only I seemed to sense his fragility—plus I was worried about the cops. Danny came back from Louis Trichardt, car and boy undamaged, but he vomited violently and had an evening of sighs. Was it too much? Too much power and control?

One evening Danny said, "In America there are these groups of acid-taking people who are doctors and philosophers."

I exploded: "Oh Danny, that's been blown-up long ago. That was Timothy Leary in the 60s and the results are sitting in asylums all over America."

"Why won't you let me finish my sentence? Do you think I would run off and join an acid commune? I only smoked acid once in my whole life and look what it did to me!"

Danny, in this saner state, needed a lot of praise, often asking: "Did I drive well today?" or "How was my reading?" We were reading aloud every evening as usual, but I don't remember what book.

On the way back from Molozi we talked about Danny's future—what was possible and not possible for him in the jazz world. He spoke of his ambition to form a group, the type of musicians he would need and what type of music he would play. Anyone would have taken him for a sane 20-year-old. But it is an article of faith for him that he must "be advanced". This is absolutely and unquestionably "good". And this limits his chances of making a beginning.

Back home he wanted Nicky to go with him to a club called "The Deviate".

"Oh no! I couldn't bear it. I don't like the people—they are pretentious. I don't like the music. I would rather stay home and read a book—or go to a play."

"Oh. OK."

Nicky, once she had got over her first horror of Danny, was good for us. Extrovert and immediate and noisy. A feeling of life going on. But the day came for her to go back to Cape Town. She was going by train and we took her to the station.

"Well Ma," she said to me privately, "You must look after yourself. This family depends on you. I depend on you. I wouldn't be who I am if it wasn't for you."

Oliver, still on holiday, tried to get Danny to practise guitar chords every day, but anything that organized was beyond him. Then Mark, his "Streetkids" band friend, entered a band for "The Battle of the Bands"—the same competition that they had done so well in two years before. Danny was going to be part of it, Mark hoped. Mark was now in the Police College Band in Pretoria, doing his army service that way, but he had some leave. He called it the Damelin band, and this seems to have been accepted by the organizers.

One lunchtime Danny was anxiously trying to contact Mark for a practice—very frustrated. Suddenly I heard the car—he was driving it out of the gate—I ran after him and jumped into the passenger seat. I sat there breathing and he drove carefully to Mark's house. "This is very good for learning self-control," he said. But he accepted that this was not going to be allowed again. I kept my car-key safely in my possession. He often asked to drive in the suburbs—I said no—he accepted it.

I didn't tell anyone about this episode. I knew that teaching a disturbed 15-year-old boy to drive a car had been irresponsible. But I needed answers.

PROFESSIONAL MUSICIAN

In August we held our breaths. Danny was no longer rushing off like a bomb. Band friend Mark G, with helpful determination, held his "Battle" rehearsals. Danny had not played formally with a band this year. The occasional jamming he had done with his friends was loose— it didn't really matter if Danny was not listening to the others, because they were not going to play in public. Mark said he was now forcing Danny to focus better during rehearsals, and they were definitely going to play in the Battle.

Danny told me that the headmaster of King David rang up Mark and said he'd heard he wasn't going to play because he was in Tara.

"Why did he think that?"

"Oh it's all over the town. Everyone is talking about me. I'm becoming well known and that's great."

Debbie from the Orange Grove drug house (friendly helper, not girlfriend) invited Danny to go away with her to the Drakensberg for a few days. Alone with her. Away from us. No social or work pressures. No drugs.

Lucy(to herself): Well the boy left with great enthusiasm, armed with camera, books and good intentions—to walk—and of course with tapes and guitar—to a wintry 5-day holiday in the Drakensberg with Debbie.

I was well able to relax completely when someone else took over. I didn't think about him at all. Debbie would have phoned if anything had gone wrong.

Danny came back in a good state, walked in and gave me a kiss. He said he had spent most of his time in his room but went for the odd walk and even the odd run.

"Did you and Debbie manage to stay friends?"

"We only had one argument."

"What was it about?"

"Musicians—and I brought her a little flower to apologize."

"If you were both arguing surely you should both have apologized?"

"Oh it was just that we had a small conflict and it came out too big."

"Well they say it's not bad to express anger. I think I don't express it easily—and then I explode."

"I usually express too much when I play—but I *can* let out just enough to play well. I let out little samples of feelings and follow that through until the next one comes."

"It's like witches and princesses—the witches are our angry feelings and the princesses are our good ones."

"That's probably what it was like long ago. Society has just become too complicated now. Like in *The Lord of the Rings* there was the white force and the evil force and it was more glamorous. I mean now we have Dallas, and JR is sometimes bad and sometimes OK."

A week went by with no hallucinations and no delusions. We were nervously hopeful.

His cousin Hector said, "He puts himself over as very cool and rather tired, and I wonder whatever happened to the child with the raging temper and the wild enthusiasms."

He was odder now in his looks and mannerisms since he first got ill, which I thought was perhaps the effect of being too much away from society.

Oliver was encouraging him to think of himself as a working musician: "Well if you come to me with a recording contract then I will send you to America."

This seemed to me an impossible demand. I heard Danny on the phone to Hector saying that next year he would either go back to school or go to America.

The day came for the Battle of the Bands: "Ma, can I ask you a special favour—a long visit to Shaun. It will help me a lot."

"How will it help you?"

"With tonight."

"Will it help you feel a part of society?"

"Oh I'll be accepted by society tonight all right!"

So he had his visit to Shaun Fourie—dangerous because he might be offered pot there, but he seemed not to be smoking pot at all in this period.

And then there is a blank in my diary. I say nothing about the Battle and I remember nothing about the Battle. I think now that I simply delivered Danny to Mark and didn't go myself.

Last week—2006—I phoned Mark in Cape Town and asked him what had happened. Mark said: "It was chaotic. We got up there on stage, and it seemed to be going OK. But Danny, as lead guitarist, was supposed to play an eight-bar solo in the middle—and he went on to play sixteen bars, and I thought well OK that is sometimes done, but then he went on playing and playing—32 bars—64 bars. I just didn't know how to stop him."

"So what happened?"

"I can't remember."

In September, Danny was more responsible—and definitely not smoking pot. He was always home before 11 pm.

We sent him to a weekend Communications Course. This was the first time all year that he had been with a group of young strangers and survived. It was "communication through drama" with Mark Rittenberg.

"I may not last out the whole day," said Danny. "12 hours is a very long time."

He did survive the whole day. He survived the whole weekend.

"What are the other people like?" I asked him on the way back on the first day.

"Nice."

"What sort of age?"

"Oh, all older than me—probably all about 24. I like that."

"I thought there was another 15-year-old?"

"Oh yes—a girl from Damelin."

To Oliver who fetched him the second night he raved about the course and how wonderful the people were, and how Mark R was "fantastic". But to me he said, "Do I have to go tomorrow?"

On the Sunday when I fetched him at the end of the course he smiled and waved at everyone as we left. He couldn't stop talking about how amazing it had all been.

"That was a very romantic day!"

Danny was also taking more initiative, but just how much he was now going to take astonished me then and still astonishes me now.

Oliver had a week's break and everything was so calm that I decided to go to Cape Town to see Nicola as Gwendoline in *The Importance of Being Earnest* at the Little Theatre in Cape Town. Nicola had a flat with a friend in Gardens suburb—next to the original Van Riebeeck vegetable gardens for feeding sailors, which were now botanical gardens for healing Lucy. I stayed with Nicola in her flat, and walked around and breathed. I had once sung in the chorus of an opera at the Little Theatre, so there was nostalgia, as well as joy in Nicky's performance, and spring, and freedom from the boy.

When I returned, Danny had exchanged his two guitars—one electric and one acoustic—for a bass guitar! My first reaction was dismay. But he said, "You don't have to worry about me. I am going to lock myself in the garage and practise for 8 hours a day for 5 weeks."

In fact it only needed one week of intense practising to master the bass guitar. At the end of the week, on a Sunday evening, he phoned his old jazz teacher, Lucky, and told him he could now play bass guitar and if anyone needed a bass he was available.

The very next evening someone rang him up and offered him a band job if he passed an audition. He was scared shitless.

Lucy: What's the worst that can happen?

Danny: He'll give me an audition and then kick me out.

Lucy: Well you'll still be alive the next day.

After the phone call he gazed for a long time in the bathroom mirror and then lay silent and white-faced on his bed.

The next day he auditioned and was accepted.

"So now I've got a sussed-out pretty good life. They're older guys. It's called "Bandit"—they play progressive rock. It's really good—if people ask me I'll be able to say, "I'm a musician,"—and the money is good too.

I phoned Ernie, the leader, and he confirmed that the band did not smoke dope—and so it must have been, because Danny did not fall off the world during this time. Danny also confirmed later that this band, amazingly, did not touch pot. They were middle-aged and had families and did ordinary jobs during the day. We dropped Danny every weekday evening at Ernie's flat in Hillbrow, from where they went to a hotel in Alberton where they had a bandroom and held their rehearsals. Ernie brought him home.

This went on for a couple of months and they played a couple of gigs, for which they did not get paid. Then some other gigs were cancelled and their Xmas venue closed down. Danny started to get frustrated and eventually left.

JEFF AND FAMILY THERAPY

One of his delusions was that he could read my mind. Mostly this was benign, and he smiled happily to himself. But now that his self-esteem and sense of reality were growing he was able to question himself:

I was sitting quietly in the living-room. No one else was home. Danny came in and asked me, "Ma, what question am I going to ask you next?"

"Do you love me mother dear?"

"No," said Danny glumly, "What are you feeling now?" That was the question.

"I didn't know."

"Do you *promise*?"

"Yes. A few months ago you would have said I was lying. But now you have to choose between whether to hang on to your theory or to trust me. It's called cognitive dissonance. It's uncomfortable."

"Yes, it is."

Later that day he came to me and asked, "So you don't think I have special powers?"

"No."

The next day he said, "Ma—I want to go for an EEG."

"Why particularly?"

"I want to see whether my mind has improved."

"Oh I'm sure it has. It shows in your behaviour."

It was now October. Way back in August someone had arranged for us to have a family assessment at the Wits University Psychology Department. It was for research and for students, and now in October we hardly remembered doing it. Living with day-to-day problems which needed constant solving was an efficient way of deleting memory. We remembered sitting in a small lecture room with a few other people, and video cameras, but nothing about what any of us had said.

Now the results came. Their report said:

Daniel is too powerful … the family would benefit from Family Therapy.

Danny said, "I wish I could see that video!" Well, so did I! I also thought, "Different days, different ways," since Danny was now so co-operative.

Nevertheless Oliver and I were always curious and keen to learn anything that would be helpful so we decided to go for family therapy. Danny of course felt got at. I remember walking through the Wits grounds, where I had experienced so much youthful happiness, with Oliver and me walking ahead and Danny slouching behind.

And then we met Jeff Cumes, who was almost shocking in his charisma and his springtime, intelligent warmth. Jeff was a beautiful man. In all my dealings with experts during this terrible year—many of which I have not burdened the reader with—I had not met any really nice people. I fell for Jeff, and Jeff fell for Oliver (who was himself a charismatic person).

I remember thinking that we were doing this at the wrong time. Danny had not smoked pot since before August, he was going to his rehearsals every evening without complaining, and he was sticking to our requests.

But from Jeff's point of view we were a really weird family—allowing him to drop out of school and to smoke cigarettes. A lot of the early sessions were simply trying to explain that we had not done that lightly and casually and permissively.

Jeff thought that Danny had tried to be too weird too soon, whereas we three —Oliver and myself and Nicola—had postponed "artiness" until we were stable. But Jeff knew nothing about the psychedelic scene. He may have read about it, but he and his wife had small children in an ordinary primary school, and he had never been offered pot.

Daniel himself in retrospect says his breakdown was due to his peer group (or "groups" rather, since there were many different groups he participated in, all of whom were pot smokers). He doesn't think we were in any way to blame. He said that even at the time, when he was just fourteen and starting at Damelin, he was critical of Damelin for allowing cigarette-smoking in the canteen. Smoking was something you tried to get away with behind the backs of the grown-ups. But Damelin was trying to give the students respect for being young adults—and this had mostly worked in earlier times.

But Jeff felt that Daniel had tried to be too different and out of the ordinary long before he was ready for it—and I agreed that his growing up had been too speeded up. Until the age of 12 he had been fine. Nicola had even said, "I hope you're not going to turn into a typical South African boy who goes to the army."

But a lot of things had happened to him in this year of 1982 and the months that preceded it. He had been a desirable youth and a famous musician, and then had become a magician with special powers. Now he was none of those things, and I thought he needed time to consolidate.

Lucy's diary: I liked Jeff very much—friendly, relaxed, attractive— and a good person. But I think any sudden imposition of "structure" would be wrong (supposing we could!). Any complete reversal of our attitude to him would surely be very disturbing at this stage. Danny goes to his rehearsals at night and does not behave badly in any way, so nothing sudden is called for.

I again felt hopelessly guilty yesterday—all my vaunted mothering abilities gone for naught. But I think it's more complicated than that—a whole family and society interaction. So it doesn't necessarily mean that my handling of him—my love, support and encouragement—was a wrong element in the picture.

We went out to supper and talked about the Cumes session. Danny was very restless. He seemed somewhat callous and indifferent. But I wonder whether it wasn't a "hurt child" syndrome—for however much we see the session as a useful exploration, he sees it as criticism—that he cannot live up to our expectations—that he has to be "weird" simply because he can't succeed in the "straight" world. But at the moment I am really only concerned with his social awkwardness—with people in general, whether druggies or not.

Jeff in the end turned out to be a good thing. After about our third session with him, Danny's middle-aged band started not working out. Danny had absolutely nothing to do. Jeff's idea that we should be "normal" parents, and that Danny should definitely go back to school, started to take shape. I was relieved to have a group to help me—Oliver and Jeff as well as myself. It made me feel not so anxious about my decisions, and it was also good for Oliver and for Daniel himself. Oliver was helped to be a firmer, more authoritative father. And he was encouraged to take Daniel out for beers.

BACK TO SCHOOL?

Oliver, with his new-found confidence and firmness, said to Danny, "Well my boy— either you go out to work and earn your living, or you go back to school. And that's my last word."

Oliver seemed to have forgotten that Danny had ever been psychotic—and Jeff simply saw Danny's madness as part of the confusion of having been given too much freedom too soon.

But I knew that Danny's mind was not anywhere near where it had been in his Standard 7 year. Complex academic tasks would be too much for him. Whether I called it "a disorganized mind" or "blocked off psychotic material that he still tries to make sense of", I knew that he wasn't able to use his whole, freely-flowing brain at this stage. I longed for some friendly rehabilitation place which would give him tasks and training at the level he was at, and plenty of "communication through drama".

He and Oliver sometimes went off for beers in the evenings, but Oliver mostly hated it. Danny would get up from the table and waft and weave in his hebephrenic, drunken-hairdresser way to another table to ask for a light for his cigarette. "Hebephrenia" is an adolescent form of schizophrenia characterised by silly gestures and inappropriate smiles. If I took Danny shopping, everyone turned and looked at him. (Hebe was the goddess of youth.)

At one therapy session Jeff asked how the Oliver outings were going. Oliver replied that he was very embarrassed by Danny. "We went to the Carlton Hotel. In the foyer we were sitting on a couch. But Danny wasn't sitting at all, he was lying there with his head way back and his legs stretched out."

"Why didn't you tell him to sit up?"

"I just can't do that. It doesn't feel right to me."

I knew what he meant. Liberals were allowed to scold their children for hurting other people. They were not allowed to object to individual mannerisms.

In my diary I wrote: "Man without content is a bag of bones."

I hear him prowling around the kitchen. He eats mounds of food in the middle of the night. I ask him what he thinks about in these lonely late-night sessions.

Danny: Mouldy elves. Spotty elves with ingrown toenails.
Lucy: Let's talk about plans.
Danny: What about Cape Town?
Lucy: But what would you do there while everyone else was going about their business?
Danny: How about the Drakensberg?
Lucy: Yes—fine—with people who were climbing mountains and so on. What would be good would be to be with people who are younger than you.
Danny: Younger people are very relaxing.
Lucy: You could go to Happy Acres?
Danny: Well I might try phoning up the gang and seeing what's going on there.

This is a change. Before he just assumed "they" would be against him. I think he's run dry. All his schemes for getting out of school and into music have led him nowhere. He's got nothing to fight against and nothing to fight for. He no longer feels that rushing off to night-clubs is such a marvellous idea. He doesn't seem depressed. He doesn't seem lost. He's just a bundle of adolescent energies with no place to go. He doesn't say these days that he is "adult". It seems that his hallucinating world has also lost some of its charms. If he does refer to it it's just in a mechanical way.

I apologized to him today for the putting-down. I feel I have become worse than Oliver. I told him I believed in discipline but not in putting-down and continual criticism. He seemed to appreciate this.

Danny: I *must* go to Cape Town!

Lucy: Everyone in Cape Town will be working for exams—just like everyone here.

Danny (feelingly): Do you think I don't *know* that! Can't we talk about Cape Town?

Lucy: I'm not supposed to talk about your wild plans. Your future has to be decided first.

Danny: Let's talk about Cape Town.

Lucy: First we have to find a school.

Danny: I'm not going to school.

Lucy: Why don't you want to?

Danny (hesitates): I'm scared that the kids will tease me—(softly) because of my mouth. I wouldn't feel secure.

Lucy: You will get used to it though. Do you like Standard 8 children?

Danny: I don't know. I haven't seen many of them lately.

Lucy: Anyway you cannot become mature by just staying at home with your family. And you really don't want to take on adult responsibilities Danny—it's not much fun.

Danny was now cradled in a sort of game, where he sat there in Jeff's sessions listening to quiet, considered, professional Jeff telling us how "Tough Love" worked. We, Danny's parents, had to decide what we thought was in his interests, and then if he wouldn't co-operate we were to impose consequences.

I went to the school authorities and found out that Danny did have to be at school legally until the end of the year he turned 16—which was the next year.

Danny had now completely left the middle-aged band, and was doing nothing at all.

Danny: Let's talk about Cape Town
Lucy: There's no question of Cape Town unless you comply with certain things.
Danny: What things?
Lucy: Preparing for school.
Danny (very convincingly): I am not going to school!

I broke down and wept. I put my arm round him and said, "Don't you think you still need parents?"

"I suppose so."

I went to the government high school down the road from us—Highlands North School. My heart sank. Just noticing little interactions made me see immediately that Daniel wouldn't fit there. Everything is cut and dried. No art. No drama. No music. The headmaster said he should go to the Arts School.

Oliver says that Jeff has given him great strength. Whenever he wavers he thinks of having to confront Jeff next week.

Daniel was getting no lifts or money or cigarettes from us, despite much pleading. One day he said, "D'you want me to starve or something?" When I ignored him he walked around the house singing. After my bath I found him sitting on my bed with a dictionary!

"Ma—what does 'nonchalantly' mean?"

"What you would call 'cool' or 'laid-back'."

"He sauntered nonchalantly to the door," said Danny, doing just that.

His reaction to this new situation has been to be extremely boisterous. Up at 7 am, flinging himself into the kitchen:

"Hiya Ma, what sort of a night did you have?"

He paces up and down, backwards and forwards to Oliver's dresser where he usually finds a few coins. Then says to me, "Can I borrow a couple of rand?"

"No. At least you're good for a laugh."

"You're not going to?"

"No," I said, laughing.

He wrote a love-letter to Esmé, attached a beautiful spray of yellow spring flowers to it, and went off walking with it. Esmé lives in Benoni which is miles away. He tried to get there once, but didn't have the proper address—and at some level he must have known that Esmé wasn't in the least interested in him.

He phoned Nicola, suggesting that he hitch down to Cape Town and come and stay with her. He came to me gloomily: "Nicky doesn't want me moving in."

The fight is on now! He has no cigarettes left. He asked us both for money. He asked Oliver what he had to do to get it. Oliver said, "Start your rehabilitation programme." No emotions. Everyone cool. It's a bit like the pot story—it does at least wake him up out of his dream world. Oliver and I could have fought him like this before—but then it was always my lone fight, with Oliver not even noticing.

He's bolshy this morning. I have to learn the extreme self-control of *not* saying things to him just because I think of saying them.

I called him out from the garage to clear his room. He "shot" at me with his guitar, with an ugly expression.

I stood there, very relaxed and said, "It's OK—you're allowed to feel hostile. I can take it. You can come and talk if you like."

"Ja, OK."

He cleaned his room and came.

We sat outside. I began, "The first thing I want to say is that I am not fragile. I get weepy and I get hysterical and I condemn you completely, but that is all temporary. Basically I am very strong—and whatever you are—hostile, disgusting, whatever—I will not disintegrate."

"Ja. That's good."

"I realize you must be feeling very frustrated—with Nicky too, now that she has said she doesn't want you—but what I have realized is that we must stand firm. In the past I have bended every which-way with your plans, and Dad has largely stayed out of it and been a buddy, but now we realize that you must have a stable background in which to experiment. You can be bland and friendly one day and aggressive the next and that is all OK because Jeff and Dad and I are forming a strong structure to contain you.

"Ja, right."

CAPITULATION

1 November, 1982. 1 pm. In a very, very roundabout way he has now capitulated. He slept at Debs last night and came back just now and curled up at the end of my bed. He asked me, "So what have you been doing?"

"Oh this and that—I've made a few schools enquiries. There's the drama department at the Arts School. It would be a second string for you, rather than the commercial music route. And there's the Waldorf School—where Hector was in primary school. They emphasize creativity."

"Can I go to Cape Town now and then go to school next year?"

At supper I said to him, "Danny I told you to get dressed." (He was wrapped in a towel.)

"And if I refuse?"

"What sort of a childish thing is that?"

"I feel as if I was three years old."

Oliver shouted at him: "Danny! Go and get dressed!" (He went.)

2 November:

Danny: Can I steal a rand?

Lucy: No.

Danny: I'm not going back to school and that's that. You can't *make* me.

Lucy: We want you to be more than a hack musician—we want you to be a fulfilled person, disciplined enough to study composition, if that's what you want to do in five years time.

Danny: All right. So if I tell you I'll go back to school can I have a rand for cigarettes?

Lucy: If you write it down.

He wrote down: "I WILL GO BACK TO SCHOOL BEGINNING OF 1983. Signed: Danny." I gave him a rand.

Whatever Jeff says, Danny is still terrified of any social situation or anything new. I think that someone, through sheer force of personality, has to get him going—carry him along on an enthusiastic plan.

He came into the kitchen.

Lucy: Momentum is what you need, my boy. Once the stone falls over the cliff it keeps going. But how to get it there?
Danny: Push and shove.
Lucy: Right! And that's what I'm going to do to you.

Later I stormed into his room.
Lucy: Look, Danny—let me organize a programme, and you won't even know what it entails. You are too much of a thinker—you paralyse yourself. I'll organize a programme for November, you'll get your money back and your trip to Cape Town—but instead of questioning each step you just go along with the whole programme.
Danny: OK. Organize away!
Lucy: It will be like that game we used to play when you were about seven, where you pull out one thing at a time and what it says, you do. Some things awful, some things nice. But all geared to get you back to school.
Danny: OK.

Suppertime. Danny and I had started eating:
"So tell me something about this programme."
"Not a word! You'll only argue with every point."
We ate in silence for a while. Oliver came in and sat down.
"So aren't you going to tell Da?"
"Danny has decided:
1) To go back to school
2) To follow any programme I design for him in November without questioning each part of it.
In return for which (subject to your approval) he:
1) Goes to Cape Town for two weeks in December.
2) Gets all his privileges back."

Oliver stretched his hand across the table and shook Danny's: he was quite overcome; near to tears; couldn't eat. He said, "Danny my boy, you will never regret this decision."

"I suppose not."

Oliver beamed and laughed and yoo-hoo'd. "This calls for a celebration ... But tell me, how did you suddenly—I mean what made you ... There must have been ..."

"It was Mother Dear actually."

We went to the Oxford Hotel for a drink, all silent on the way there, Danny and I manic on the way back.

SCHOOLS AND CAPE TOWN

Five schools rejected him. The two I remember are the Waldorf School and the Arts School.

I didn't understand the Waldorf system of education, but I knew that they respected the individual, had small classes and emphasised the arts. They accepted Danny for an interview although they already knew his age. After he had had his interview they told me he was too old for the Waldorf system to work. It was too late.

The drama department of the Arts School was recent, and they were on the lookout for promising pupils. I spoke to a pleasant, expressive Jewish woman and collected the material for his audition. Danny had to learn a speech from a play.

The audition was on a Thursday afternoon. Oliver said he would hear Danny's speech on Wednesday evening. However, when Wednesday evening came, Danny had done nothing about the speech. He either couldn't or wouldn't learn it—perhaps was afraid that he wouldn't be able to learn it.

Oliver came after him in a rage. Danny fled into his room and locked the door. Oliver broke down the door and started fighting Danny, and Danny started fighting back. Jeff had told Oliver that this would not be a bad thing to do. I stopped the fight and Oliver disappeared.

Danny stood there white-faced and washed-out, as if his ego had totally vanished and he had become a dead thing. It frightened me. I thought, "Now he really is truly mad." I led him to the car and drove him to the nearby Savoy Hotel. He liked being alone in a hotel bedroom and I thought this might feel right. A hotel bedroom was immediately comprehensible to him: there were not too many data coming at him at the same time. I ordered tea and we sat in the bedroom quietly drinking it. Then he said he was OK and I told him I would fetch him the next morning.

That fight had nothing good about it. It neither "cleared the air" nor did it advance his recovery. It never happened again and no one talked about it. The only thing Danny said when he saw his door off its hinges was, "Now we are quits", because he himself had broken the kitchen door off its hinges when we locked him out of the kitchen earlier that year for having pot in the house.

He was still learning his speech on the way to the Arts School the next day—but that of course was often how he had done things long before his breakdown.

There were two pleasant Jewish women there to give him his audition. I waited outside. Afterwards one of them said she would phone me.

That evening the phone call came. The woman said they had found him strange but very talented and they had decided to take him on.

I knew there was still another hurdle to face: the headmaster of the whole ABMD school (Art, Ballet, Music and Drama). The trouble was that Oliver worked in the Music department—and Oliver had talked to his fellow staff members all year about Danny's breakdown. The headmaster had simply heard the word "drugs"—and refused absolutely to take Daniel.

So that was that.

Apart from the fight, November had gone past quietly, with Danny quite calm about visits to schools. He had also gone to a six-week course—a session once a week on a Wednesday night—called "Smoke-Enders". Danny didn't particularly want to go on smoking and went to this course without panic or resistance. There were adults of all ages there and Danny handled the situation. His smoking of cigarettes after that was uneven—sometimes none at all, sometimes a few a day, sometimes more—depending on his stress levels. He knew he wouldn't be able to smoke during the day at school.

We didn't do any thinking about Cape Town. Nicky would be in charge of him. He had been promised this visit—his Holy Grail—so it had to happen.

He went for the first two weeks of December, when Nicky's exams were over. Her flatmate was still there, so Nicky arranged for Danny to stay at her friend Jeremy's place down the road, because he had a spare room where Danny could play his guitar. Jeremy was "great" and he didn't smoke pot. Nor did Nicky or her flatmate.

But Cape Town in December is a mecca for Jo'burg students, who pour down there into empty bottles which rapidly fill up. They expect to be put up and entertained—and they bring the drugs. Danny went on a few happy outings alone with Nicky, but he felt very out of place with her friends and these older visiting students. It was an out-of-control situation in which Jeremy could not prevent his friends bringing drugs nor offering them to Danny—which Danny of course accepted—and felt instant relief. But the dagga plus the awkward situation threw him out of his current calmer state, and he was soon walking around Cape Town through the night and shouting and talking nonsense. Once again he was brought home by a friendly policeman. Jeremy told Nicky he couldn't cope; Danny slept on Nicky's couch for a few days and then came home to Jo'burg.

Back home his structure was in place and he settled down immediately.

DIAGNOSIS

Nicky decided to stay in Cape Town for Christmas. Xmas-on-the-farm with the extended family no longer existed: Granddad had died that year; I had found a house for Grandma near us in Norwood; the farm was sold; my sisters were not visiting. My mother lived within cycling distance for me—I would bounce down a path through a sloping park, spend some time with her, and then push the bike back up.

Christmas Day was just the four of us: grandmother, one daughter, one son-in-law, one grandchild, quietly having a lunch cooked by Oliver. No concert.

My mother handed a cheque for R50 to Daniel. She didn't know how he had spent the previous R50 Xmas present (on a cap of acid), but she knew he was now not allowed to keep money. (When he got his privileges back, that did not include the freedom to keep his own money.) Danny handed the cheque to me to keep for him.

Between Xmas and New Year Danny and I had an appointment with Dr F—"the best psychiatric diagnostician in South Africa".

The appointment consisted of three parts: first I went in alone and told about what had happened to Danny; then Danny went in and had a session alone; then I went in again alone to hear his verdict.

Dr F said, calmly and firmly, "I'm afraid your son has schizophrenia."

I was shattered. My first instinct is always to believe what I am told. Nevertheless I said, "But it could be drugs, it could be adolescence!"

"I don't believe that. I will explain to you how he thinks." He cleared his large desk of objects. "I give your son a problem here (pointing to one end of his desk). Now normal people might zig and zag along my desk, but they come back to the problem and end up here (pointing to the other end of his desk) with some sort of solution. Your son simply falls off the side, and never comes back to the problem. There is no cure for schizophrenia."

"But what if he comes right?"

"Then my diagnosis would have been proved wrong."

"So how can I help him?"

"He will have to be permanently on medication."

"Isn't there a support group I could join?"

"Not that I know of."

I came out of that room unable to solve problems myself. I had no idea how to find the car. Danny found it easily. While we were driving home he said, "Ma—you know the R50 Grandma gave me for Christmas?"

"Ja."

"Well what if I took the money up to Hillbrow—I'll go by bus and keep the bus tickets—and then I'll go to the record shop, choose what I want, and come home with the receipt and the change."

I smiled to myself, "That sounds fine."

I knew he could do it—and he did. I lay on my bed and laughed. Dr F might be an expert in diagnosis; but I was an expert on Danny.

This terrible year of 1982 had ended, but not entirely without hope.

Chapter Ten

ST MARTIN'S SCHOOL
(AGED SIXTEEN, 1983)

White Johannesburg was divided into two parts: north and south. To the north lived the rich show-offs, in the middle was the city with its offices and flats, and in the south was a less fancy area with English-speaking artisans and immigrant Greeks. My dad said that property there was less expensive because the wind blew the mine dump sand in that direction.

In these southern suburbs had been a well-known school for black Christian boys, connected with Father Huddleston and the Community of the Resurrection: St Peter's School. I had known black journalists and musicians who had been to that school. But when Bantu Education was imposed, the school closed down. The staff were too disgusted and too principled to operate in that way. I thought this was wrong, because the excellent teachers would still be there for discussions, and they could teach creatively, around the corners of the silly new system: their influence would outshine "Bantu Education".

I don't know how long the school stayed empty. But then it started up again as an Anglican school for boys and girls: "whites only" for the moment. It was now called St Martin's. Pupils came to this school from all over Johannesburg.

While Danny was in Cape Town in December I went to visit the school. The sun shone; the buildings were modest; and Christmas singing poured out of the chapel. Then it was break, and I found myself back forty years amongst the classmates of my youth. They were genial, open and natural. There was no flirting or flaunting. The school had an ethos of simple and kind Christianity, and the pupils were part of it.

The headmaster, Mr Wigmore, accepted Daniel for the school sight unseen. "He will be a challenge to us. I will decide after I meet him whether he should go into Standard 8 or Standard 9."

I don't think he asked me whether I was a Christian! I had been one in my youth, and since then I had valued its values while not believing its beliefs. And Danny had accepted its rituals and its stories at his previous schools. At St Martin's the teachers and pupils went out of their way to express goodwill and kindness rather than cynicism and hedonism.

In January I took Danny to the school. He liked it immediately.

After Mr Wigmore had interviewed Danny he decided that he should go into Standard 9. In a one-on-one conversation Danny could come across as articulate and sophisticated. Jeff Cumes, our family therapist, disagreed with Wigmore: he thought Danny should go into Standard 8. They argued it out on the phone, but Wigmore won in the end.

I thought Danny could write sentences at about Standard 5 level. His mind was still far too blocked for anything more complicated. But I didn't express an opinion. For me the important thing was for Danny to fit in with other people of his own age, and gradually to regrow his mind.

Danny had two states which were not useful: he could rush around in a manic state, curse everyone, break things, hallucinate: be uncontrollable. Or he could opt out and be unable to get out of bed. I could no more control this second state than the first.

I went to see Dr F—the psychiatrist who had diagnosed Danny as schizophrenic, but who had no views on practical management. I was prepared to try medication. I asked him whether Danny could possibly be "manic/depressive". He thought not. At any rate the phenothiazines were appropriate for that disorder as well.

By now I knew about the famous phenothiazines: they had emptied the psychiatric hospitals worldwide. No more were psychotic people thrown into padded cells or tied down on to beds. On this medication they stayed quietly at home. But they were not cured. They were not able to work or to love or to interact with the world.

However, for the immediate problem of getting Danny to regulate his sleep/wake times and to get him over his terror of school, the phenothiazines were worth a try: Stelazine and Melleril were the two we used for Danny. We started them at the beginning of January. Danny immediately recognized that they were the same pills he had been given at Tara—not by the look of them, but by the feeling of being damped down. But he accepted that they would calm him for school so he didn't object too strenuously at this time.

Danny at this stage, even before the pills, had no views of his own: his former strong lifestyle had disintegrated and there was nothing to replace it. So he asked us what to think and what to do. He still sometimes referred to his "system" (the fantasy world he had created from his delusions), but not in any detail. It was safer to say nothing.

We went for school clothes. He tossed his hair back in front of the mirror. All the assistants giggled. I called him to me and said quietly that the mannerisms of tossing his hair and posing in front of the mirror were not appropriate. He was silent.

In the car he said I had been hostile. I said that I was just anxious and that I couldn't be perfect. "When we get home, go and do that gesture deliberately in front of the mirror. Then you'll see how ridiculous it is and laugh at yourself."

"I don't promise."

Peddie, our twice-a-week helper, hadn't seen him since before Christmas. She found him transformed. No more "Gimme, gimme!" And no more spitting, shaking or weaving.

Lucy (to herself): He looks pretty well all right now. Not strange. Rather handsome in fact. It's as if the pills and our direction for him and the discipline have released some new maturity all of a sudden.

Mr Wigmore, the headmaster, said, "I think he himself is sick of the underworld."

I said to myself: But it all depends on whether he feels accepted.

It was a week before school was due to start. Oliver took Daniel to the Wigwam—a mountain resort—for a few days. On their return Oliver said to me, "He is improving all the time; but not ready for school. No one thought him odd in any way; just quiet. And he did talk once or twice, in the billiard room. And we played ping-pong: he was hopeless at the beginning—all over the place, but he gradually became more focused. On the drive back he asked me to tell him a story. I told him about Eugene Marais' baboon and otter."

A therapist friend told me that a non-anxious person taking the phenothiazines feels completely bombed out. So the thing to do is to find a balance between anxiety and being bombed out.

Minor tragedy: good haircut man gone; lady cut it; looks awful. Danny said, "Weird isn't it?"

He has never looked good with very short hair.

"Am I going into Standard 8 or 9?"

"Jeff thinks 8. Wigmore thinks 9, provided you don't do subjects like Maths, where missing Standard 8 would matter. What do you think?

"Oh I actually think Standard 9 would be quite a good idea."

Oliver took him to meet Mr Van der Walt, who would be his housemaster.

Afterwards, Oliver said to me, "Well he may not admit it, but I think he struck up a rapport with this guy. Van der Walt said, 'I don't mind telling you Daniel, but I would like you for my choir. I'm short of basses.' And then later he said, 'I think this is the right school for you Daniel.'"

Van der Walt said that all the staff will know about Daniel's medication but none of the children. The pills will be given to the matron. Daniel insisted that he had nothing against sport. There's this assumption that arty people don't like sport.

At home the next day Danny smoked only four cigarettes and felt good about this. He swam and put on his St Martin's tracksuit. Looks great!

He came to me and asked, "Ma—if I can't face St Martin's can I do Correspondence?"

"No. Because then you would never get over your fear. What's the worst thing that could happen?"

"Mmm—I suppose not finding my way to the right classroom and being called lazy and being kicked out."

"They'll assign you someone to show you where to go. If you lose that person just go to the office."

"No problem! I know where the office is and the church. But what if I can't handle St Martin's socially? Can I do Correspondence then?"

"No. Jeff feels that would be quite wrong. He wants you to try to handle things and then if things go wrong to tell him about it. I'll tell you what I'll do: I'll turn you into a frog. Frogs haven't got the imagination to be anxious."

Van der Walt phoned me. He said that two things concerned him about Danny:

1) Not being able to repeat simple instructions.
2) Gobbledygook about religion.

BACK TO SCHOOL

The day before Danny was due to go to school Oliver woke with a massive migraine. He took his beta-blockers but it got worse. The doctor came and gave him a Stelazine injection and for the rest of the day he lay on his bed in a drugged state.

It was sweltering weather and Danny had slept on the roof the night before. He and I had breakfast outside. I was determined to stay completely and absolutely relaxed.

"So I go back to school tomorrow?"

"That's right. How d'you feel?"

"Terrible!"

"Why particularly?"

"It's so long since I went to school."

I said, light-heartedly, "Here's a lucky charm for you." (It was a little guitar-man.)

"Thanks."

"I just catch the anxiety and tension and impatience the moment I feel it starting and chuck it out."

"How do you chuck it out?"

"Stop dwelling on it. Go and do something different."

Danny and I went to Dr F. Danny went in first. Then I went in.

Dr F (surprised), "He seems much better."

"He is very anxious."

"It's not a question of anxiety. His condition is more a question of disorganization and fragmentation. Will he be able to sit through lessons? He may just walk out after half-an-hour. His attention-span is not good. He should sit in front—and teachers should ask him at least one question per lesson."

Back home he swam 20 lengths, then tried on his uniform. He looked very good.

"All the little girls will fall for you." He grinned.

Later he said, "It's not the teachers or finding my way around. It's that the work is so different. I've been doing such different work." (He meant the "work" that he did in his head when he was trying to make sense of his psychotic fantasies.)

The day before this last day Oliver and I had seen Jeff.

"What's the worst that could happen?" Jeff asked us.

"Well that he'll go psychotic," I replied.

"How does that manifest itself?"

"Well he is cut off from reality. He hears things that are not really being said."

Jeff asked Oliver, "What worries you most?"

"That he will get into such a panic that he will just feel he has to escape."

Back to the last day: friends came, and he visited friends for short times. I popped into Oliver from time to time. He remained knocked out. I remained cheerful and relaxed. I gave Danny his medication, which was three Stelazines a day and a Melleril at bedtime. At 9 pm I got both my patients into bed, and by 9.30 pm they were both asleep.

I went to bed. I wrote my diary.

He went to school the next day. He did not hallucinate. He did not run away.

One small battle was won: Danny was accepted by the other pupils. They didn't know that he had ever been "odd" and he found enough of his friendly self from the past to get on with them. Interestingly his friends tended to be in Standard 8—the 15-year-olds. And on the small school bus that collected pupils from the north the average age was even younger. The children looked at tall Danny with interest the first time he boarded this bus.

In the second week the school secretary phoned me and said she could see Danny from her window. He was sitting on the lawn laughing and chatting with some girls. They were of course this pleasant, giving, Anglo-Saxon Christian group, who simply didn't know how to be "nasty". So it was a good place to get his social confidence back.

I used to fetch him after school. One day he said, "Can I have some money?"

"What for?" I asked, suspiciously.

"They keep asking for donations in chapel and I feel bad because I haven't got anything."

Nicky came home. "Danny gets younger every day! And when we went out on Saturday he didn't say anything at all that wasn't perfectly OK, whereas in Cape Town I couldn't communicate with him at any level."

But schoolwork was an immense effort for him and on his worst days he didn't go to school at all. Sometimes I would take him late.

His Biology teacher told me, "His class couldn't be nicer; they are a very special group. The girls realize that he has suffered in some way and they want to help. They clapped when he returned. He is definitely improving. I couldn't understand his speech or read his handwriting at first. Now I do. After he has been away he asks boldly in front of everyone about what he has missed."

His English teacher said, "He's terrific! When I walk into the classroom and he's not there my heart sinks."

"Do you understand what he says?"

"Not always. I go back to the staffroom and look up the words he uses! Sometimes I realize that he had made sense."

"Well it's an amazing school. No other school would have accepted him so well."

Danny needed enormous quantities of rest for small quantities of concentration. Sometimes he could manage, often not. He said to me, "Last year I was in a little tiny hole in the wall, from which I refused to come out, until I was forced out to school."

Daniel knew from his first day at St Martin's that he would not pass Standard 9. He had a good awareness of what was too difficult for him. We, Jeff and Oliver and I, said it didn't matter: it was enough for him to be going to school and doing what he could.

The ability to cope with an essay question is light years away from the ability to do exercises, one point at a time. He and one other student were doing Music as a subject. The teacher started them from the beginning on theory: Danny could do it easily, and he also felt it was relevant to his future music career.

History, once one of his favourite subjects, was impossible for him to grasp: the muchness of it overwhelmed him.

The teacher said, "He's a nice boy. The only problem is that he doesn't answer the question."

A new aspect of Danny being at school was that he didn't at all mind being helped. I remember one morning sitting on the floor of the living room and bringing his mind back into focus over and over again. He had a history test later that day and he and I were both motivated for him to pass it. All the way to the southern suburbs I coached and questioned him in a good-humoured way. He just passed the exam— and we both rejoiced.

Art was going well. In the mid-term report the teacher said, "Daniel has made a great effort and is working well."

Mr Wigmore, the headmaster, said that Daniel had flashes of brilliance. In the report he wrote: "A fair number of nettles still to be grasped, but the challenge to him and to us is certainly worthwhile."

What about English, the subject in which he had once soared? Well English was also the subject where most of the garbled material appeared.

Lucy (to herself): Well, he got 70% for his essay on love (the second highest in the class). We'll have to overlook the fact that Nicky discussed it with him for two hours! And Mr B seems to have overlooked his eccentric expressions.

From Danny's essay: "It varies from a life orientated sporting determination to an applied discipline. Its general acceptance through the years tended to converge towards soppiness and energetic malfunction."

Later in the year he wrote this essay on "Freedom":

When people say the word "freedom" they probably mean something like "escape" or "feeling free". I do not think "freedom" is too much of a hard word to define, seeing that it is probably the most valued priority and need of millions of people in the world today.

The one thing about freedom is that everybody's always looking for it. Most people in the world work for a living, and enjoy time away from their work e.g. an afternoon with the kids, a morning of golf etc. This is their personal freedom and enjoyment. It gives them time to think, or just to laze about, killing time or indulging in their favourite pastime. But on the other hand there are the spoiled brats of society who are always looking for, or demanding the absolute freedom, which is a bit like hanging a carrot in front of a donkey's nose. Once you find the ultimate freedom, there is always some other aspect of it that you would rather have.

So it turns out in the end that you should make do with what you have, and not be choosy. The way to obtain freedom is to do other things at the same time. It's like if you don't think about it, it will come to you twice as easy.

GOOD TIMES

Middle moods were best—when he was neither catatonic nor manic. I took Nicola's friend Lesley to fetch him from school. Danny had undone his shirt and tie.

He sauntered over to the car. "Hey! You look relaxed!" I said.

"Ja I am—totally relaxed. Hey Les. I've got such a sexy Biology teacher. Such beautiful legs!"

"Describe her," said Lesley.

"About five foot ten, sort of like Vanessa Redgrave—and such style! Such charisma. She makes you *want* to learn."

"Who's the next best?"

"Mr Boyle. He's so vivacious! Big eyes. He's our English teacher."

Mr Boyle said to me, "He's relaxing more now. He even got the whole class off a test! He's getting a bit cheeky, but not in a bad way."

I bought Danny a punchball. He punched it for so long that his knuckles were bleeding.

"You'll have to wear gloves."

"But then I wouldn't be trained in manliness."

For the mid-term break (a week), Oliver brought home the Arts School double bass. Danny was enchanted. Once again he couldn't stop. By the end of the week his fingers were badly blistered.

At supper he said, "I really want to do ice-hockey ..."

"There you go again," said his father irritably. "Always some new thing."

"Oh tell him he's a wet blanket."

"Dad, you're just a soppy blanket."

It was 8 o'clock. He lay in bed.

"I can't get to sleep."

"You don't have to. It's early. I'll help you with some music theory."

I had bought him a "note-speller", in which he could make words from the music notes. He was thrilled because it was so easy.

"I'm just writing them as I go." Then he added, "You know, Ma, I don't really know what to think."

"Oh that's easy—don't! Just take it easy. You've had such a change. It's bound to feel strange. You couldn't have thought, last year ..."

"Yech!"

"Why 'yech'"?

"That's what I would have thought last year about my life now."

Neither of us thought back to the year before last year, when he was sleeping with a 26-year-old model.

He often asked for incentives to get down to work. Oliver thought this would impair taking initiative, but I thought it was a step on the way.

He's full of beans. He tells me he's worried about not being hungry. I tell him not to be melodramatic about it:

"One's brain is very suggestible. If you say, 'I don't know why I'm never hungry,' in that anxious way, it thinks it's a terrible thing. Now you also haven't much appetite for cigarettes and you aren't even noticing it."

"Now you are making me feel guilty. I smoke at school."

"Well it's good that you can feel guilt again. Last year you couldn't."

"Last year I was mad. That's why."

I found the little gadget which you click to go up a number. Danny was fascinated by this tally-counter. It is a friendly little thing. He gets a punch when he does some small thing to help him with the future. He has punched up the nine points he has already.

Danny agonizes: "I feel nauseous."

"Say it again in an ordinary voice."

"I feel nauseous," he says, with an enormous grin.

"Well done! I'll get the tally-counter. Wow! Double figures!"

"Is it just for me?"

"Yes."

"That's nice."

My Canadian sister Jenny and her daughters were staying at my mother's new house in Norwood. Bess, once such an irritant to four-year-old Danny, was now thirteen. She was calm and pretty, and in Toronto she was learning the flute. Danny was learning the clarinet with Oliver, for his Matric music.

One day he went for a run—better than a Stelazine for getting him into the middle mood; and when he came back Bess was here playing her flute with Oliver. Danny joined in and was a star on his clarinet. Absolute concentration. He sight-read new material which he hasn't been able to do up to now. I think he was at exactly the right level of arousal, and enchanted by Bess.

Wednesday: He fell asleep in the afternoon then felt depressed. Found him high in the Australian Chestnut tree.

"I'm very depressed and I'm not coming down."

"I bet you five cigarettes that when you have swum, done a Biology session and played music with Bess you will not feel depressed."

He did all that and felt better, but at supper he sat there being very gloomy. I told him it was unchristian and he laughed. After supper he decided to grow a moustache. At this level of depression he can easily get out of it.

That night I gave him a whole Mellerin (the sleep-inducing phenothiazine) because of the afternoon sleep. I didn't want him raging around the house all night and then unable to go to school. But that didn't work. The next morning he was in a lumpen state. He could not focus or smile. In the end I abandoned getting him to school and even doing Biology at home and instead got him to sort toys, which he did willingly.

Talking about his situation:

"I put on my ear-phones and listen to my sort of music for an hour and then as I take them off everything hits me."

"What exactly?"

"Having to get up in the morning, school, classical music."

"What is so dreadful about getting up in the morning?"

"Well I get tired, and I'm not the type, and ..."

"Well those may be reasons why, but what I'm asking is exactly how you feel."

"I look out of the window and I'm confused by what I see."

"And then at school?"

"There I keep myself together by relating to the class and the teachers and everything that goes on."

"So then what happens in the mornings is worse than school itself?"

"Yes."

One day he was up before me. He dressed in jeans with a hole in one knee and a kerchief tied around the hole, and a jersey and braces. I looked at him with astonishment.

"It's Civvies Day!"

"Surely "civvies" doesn't mean clothes with holes in?"

"Civvies means ANYTHING!"

He got into the car looking scared and excited, pink and bright-eyed.

"You look great! At least it's woken you up."

"Just see me walking into chapel!"

He got out of the car, adjusted his kerchief, walked jauntily to the bus-stop. The bus rolled up, bearing a neat load of respectably casually dressed children.

Lucy (to herself): If school can only provide enough outlet for his sense of drama and fun and rebellion, he will survive it.

SENSITIVITIES AND MOTIVATION

I read Mark Vonnegut's *The Eden Express*—about his slow recovery from a schizophrenic breakdown. I saw many parallels with Danny.

Vonnegut: "I was so distractible that even very simple tasks were impossible to complete. I was so sensitive that the slightest hint of negativity was utterly crushing."

Sometimes Danny found Oliver crushing. Oliver had never had a breakdown, but his youth had been a crushing one: his father had mocked and despised him. A successful career and a successful marriage had changed him into a happy person, but the scars were still there. When Danny behaved inadequately, Oliver would sometimes forget to be patient and would let out some cutting sarcasm.

One day Danny was doing Art Theory with Oliver, and then afterwards he came to me in the studio where I was practising *The Messiah*. I was going to sing in a "Messiah from Scratch" performance.

Danny: Does Dad ever scare you?

Lucy: No of course not! He's my buddy. Have you ever been scared by someone your own age?

Danny: I don't mean physically. We had that fight and I beat him. I'm stronger than he is. But when he draws himself up ... He's a fucking good teacher—puts things across in a powerful way. He's so intelligent. An intelligent person must *know* when he is being evil.

Lucy: I know what you mean. I do talk to him about it; that crushing tone. But it seems he can't sense himself doing it.

Danny: He seems to be attacking the fibres of my brain.

Lucy: But Danny, when I get angry and hysterical, surely that's also ...

Danny: No. That's quite different. I *know* you so much better. I don't really *know* Dad. Well I know that sounds funny ...

Lucy: That's why Jeff said it was a good idea for you two to go off without me.

Danny: The word for Dad when he's like that is "mysterious".

Later he and I were watching a pianist on telly playing Liszt.

Lucy: Is he scary?

Danny: No. He's more jolly. You can *see* him concentrating. Pianists are never mysterious.

Lucy: They express their feelings directly?

Danny: Yes, that's it!

Yesterday Danny came into the kitchen after his clarinet lesson with Oliver. I was cooking. Oliver came in. He said, in a tone somewhat cool and aggressive, "If you're browning that meat, the heat should be higher—and it only needs a few seconds."

He left.

Lucy (to make a point): Oh dear I'll *never* be able to cook.
Danny (immediately tuned in): Yes you will. Dad only knows a *little* about cooking. That's what makes him so off.
Lucy: He knows a lot. Teachers can't *always* be in a perfect mood.
Danny: They should always be HUMAN.

At school Danny wrote a history test. Here is one of his answers:

My personal belief about the Industrial Revolution is that the time factor involved was almost nothing, compared to a change, similar in structure and similar in social manipulation. My opinion, taking into consideration the need for a social involvement as opposed to being thrown in at the deep end, would probably be a wary one. A need for change, I think, comes only when it's needed. The Industrial Revolution was, I think, a crime toying with the social and political acceptance of almost half the world. How can an ethical existence, formulated over thousands of years, suddenly come to an end? I think not only of the physical losses (men, women and children lost their lives down mines) but of the whole mental personal status. It is very wrong; which closes my personal opinion. The Industrial Revolution was the end of free-work, natural teamsmanship and a lot of life.

This is more out of control than the "Freedom" essay, yet he does get across some feeling for the displaced people—mirroring his own displaced feelings perhaps.

People said it was time to leave him alone. Let him get on with things in his own way. Of course I often tried that, but at this stage he still did nothing unless there was a programme and rewards. Whether it was a punch on the tally-counter, or an appreciative comment, or a chocolate—every tiny immediate reward worked.

It was May and everything was going well. I reduced the phenothiazines and had some anti-depressants to give him only if necessary.

One day he was lying down and looking depressed. "I'm allowed to give you this pill if you are feeling depressed." "Mmm … I don't know."

"I'll give it to you and then later perhaps we can talk about what is causing it."

"I'm not feeling strange in any way—but if you want to give me the pill ..."

"How about the book?" I asked, for he was allowed rewards to encourage him to read. "You don't have any money in the bank, and then if you are into it when I come back from my run you can have some chocolate."

He started reading straight away.

I came back from my run.

"How did the read go?"

"Very well! I almost finished the book."

Then he had his second bath of the day—on his own initiative!

Lucy (to herself): He functions well under good supervision and constant checking, i.e. he is not expected to exercise inner controls. It is only if he is expected to and then fails that he feels bad about himself and goes wrong.

That night Danny was to have friends round—reliable ones, so Oliver and I went to the movie "Ghandi". When we got back he had left a note: "Gone with Mark. Back at 11 pm."

"What do we do now!" I asked Oliver.

"Well what are you going to do?"

"What are you?"

"I'm not going to get all upset about it."

We went to sleep. Danny came back and seemed OK the next day. He came to my room: "Ma, did you mind my going out last night?"

"Well, we did have an arrangement."

"Ja, but nothing worked out. They couldn't come. And I did come back at a reasonable time."

Wow! I went to his room: "I've come to give you a kiss for developing a conscience. (Gave one). Is that allowed?"

"Ma, you only ask if that's allowed *before* you give a kiss!"

"Well, I can't ungive it now."

Adrian, his one non-pot-smoking friend, spent a Saturday night with us. In the morning I went to their room. He and Adrian were chattering away, Daniel pink-cheeked. (This is mentioned because Danny was so often grey-faced.)

"Don't forget Grandma's birthday party."

"Yay! (To Adrian): This lunch at the Country Club is a real jol."

"So you'll dress up smart and shave and everything?"

"Ja, of course!" (He hugged himself and bounced on the bed.)

At the Country Club he looked extremely elegant in white pants and an off-white jacket. My aunt Freda said, "My goodness Daniel I didn't even recognize you!"

He behaved impeccably. He asked Grandma politely if she minded if he had a smoke. He had a Tequila before, and wine at the meal. Became red in the face and did a certain amount of grimacing and smiling, but in response to us, not privately.

That afternoon he said he felt sick. I sent him to bed. I refused to give him cigarettes. They were for working and I decided he'd probably feel better later.

"I think it's just a down-swing after feeling hyped-up today."

Danny gave me a "power-stare", which was what I called a strong aggressive look.

Later he came to me and said, "Since I'm not really sick and I'm going to school tomorrow can I have my cigs?"

"Not until you've done some Afrikaans with Dad."

"But I just feel slightly down."

"There's no better cure for depression than work. Dad will work kindly with you like he did the other day. He's promised to do that now."

Now he is doing Afrikaans with Oliver—and his self-esteem is saved because Oliver doesn't know about the cigs reward in this instance.

Afrikaans at school was not too bad. He was in a small class for weaker pupils. They often sat outside on the lawn and the teacher read them stories which they then discussed.

That evening at supper I said, "When we were looking for a school for you, Dad and I did decide that we believed in Christian principles."

Danny was amazed: "You did?"

"Not believed in God as such ..."

"Oh you mean *ethical* principles."

Oliver and Lucy together: "Hey! You used that word correctly!"

An ethical system was what we wanted to be his inner guide in the end, but for the moment he mostly needed cigs and chocs and clicks and hugs.

DEFEATED BY DAGGA

In the new culture that Danny was experimenting with he did not play his guitar at all. Oliver asked him why. Danny said that he could not think about two instruments at the same time and that classical music was more pure.

He also didn't go out at the weekends. He said that he only wanted to work.

It was a nice idea. But the strength of the young male pot culture was all around him. His friends hovered like evil shadows wanting to sway him from his new course. And Danny was not only a recovering schizophrenic: he was also a young adolescent male with strong impulses and wanting to fit in with his peer group.

One day I took him driving. While I was driving him out of town he simply seemed placid, so I wasn't worrying. But when he took over the driving he couldn't stay in his lane but meandered over the centre of the road. I took over the driving. He was still mild. I had never seen him behaving in this way, but I thought it might be the immediate effect of dagga smoking.

When he was at school the next day I searched the house and his garage. I found pot in his garage: his refuge providing he didn't smoke pot. Who had given it to him? Why was he smoking again?

After school I called him in for a meeting. He made coffee for us and I pulled out the phone.

Lucy: We were talking yesterday about goals. Wouldn't you say that one of the goals of this house—yours and mine—would be to help Dad get over his migraines?
Danny: Yes, definitely.
Lucy: So what is it going to do to his migraines if he comes home and I tell him I found pot in the garage?
Danny: So don't tell him. Just lie. I don't smoke pot in the garage any more. It must be from before.
Lucy: So if Peddie clears out the garage tomorrow and then next week...
Danny: Oh you mean you haven't found pot in the garage? You shouldn't have done that to me ... my pulse is racing.

Lucy: Calm down. I did find pot in the garage.
Danny: Well someone else must have left it there.

Later I took him his cigarette. He was lying on his bed in the dark.
Lucy: Danny I don't want you to shout at me and I'm just going to say this quite calmly: I don't believe you.
Danny: Ma, what if I said, "Maybe that pot belonged to me and maybe it belonged to someone else but I really don't know anything about it and that's the absolute truth."
Lucy: That's just a way of getting around telling the truth.
Danny (desperately): Ma I need reassurance. I'll say that it was my pot if that will please you. Is that all right?
Lucy: No, not if you are just saying it to please me.

The next day when I took him to the bus-stop I was still unfriendly. Sister Smith, the school nurse, phoned me up from the school: "Daniel is in a great state. I have never seen him like this. Very restless. I don't think he will settle to work."

I fetched him from school. He stared at me in a hallucinatory way. He wants my forgiveness.
Danny: Why don't you trust me? You must learn to trust people.
Lucy: Only if they prove trustworthy.

I had thrown that pot away and after about a week things calmed down again.

Danny: If I work hard today can I go and hear Shaun tonight? I promise I won't smoke dope. The last time I smoked dope I couldn't even hear properly. Smoking dope fucks up my concentration. I have to concentrate twice as hard if I smoke dope.
Lucy: Well you seem to be getting some insight.
Danny: Oh I've always had insight.
Lucy: No. Last year you didn't.
Danny (grinning): Well perhaps that was because I was smoking dope.

He seemed to be acknowledging the immediate effect of smoking dagga but had no insight into the broader effects. He was like a beer drinker who doesn't actually drink beer while he is driving. He simply thought that pot was something to deny and hide from the grown-ups, but was not seriously damaging. Toby, who owned the drug house in Orange Grove but who was seven years older than Danny and had tried to keep him from pot, now said to me that he still thought that pot was better than alcohol: it was the mantra of the age.

I spoke to Toby recently (2006). He is now 46, has a new wife and a new house and a good job in computers. He himself had never "done drugs" to excess. I told him I would protect his privacy in my book by changing his name. "But I don't regret anything at all about the drug culture," said Toby, who had sold LSD for years.

People today who say that pot by itself is harmful, i.e. not only because it leads to "harder" drugs, but because they have lived with its longer term effects, are often rejected by the liberal establishment as stuffy and out of touch.

Back to the story. I was defeated. My resentment showed, and Danny's resentment mirrored mine. All that hard work and support. But pot exacerbated the very problems he already had: sluggishness; inability to concentrate; moodiness. It was at any rate difficult for him to stay focused: pot made it impossible. Jeff said it must simply be an absolute taboo in our structuring of his life. This might have worked if we had known about the urine tests. These show any pot-taking in the past two weeks. We could have built it into our structure for him and this might have worked, because the tests can be done at a quiet time. He could have seen friendly Dr van N every two weeks to get the results.

Since I didn't have that solution I went on searching for pot in the house more systematically than before.

Danny (lying in bed): Why are you looking through my jackets?
Lucy (matter-of-factly): For pot. I have to check.
Danny: Well I don't like it.
Lucy: If you want more privacy you'll have to give up pot.
Danny: Well don't check while I'm here. I don't like it.

The next time I found pot in his room I took it away and locked him in the house and went to visit my mother, shouting back at him, "Danny I don't mind if you break the house down but we won't let you damage your mind."

While I was away he broke open my locked cupboard and took cigarettes. I found him lying on his bed smoking. "Well you said I could break the house down."

I called the friendly sergeant from Norwood Police station and he talked to him, saying afterwards, "That boy should see a psychiatrist. He doesn't look as if he has a grip on things."

I had dreams of dead children. In one I gave birth to quins, all deformed. They all died. In another it was older children falling over cliffs.

One day I fetched him from Adrian—the non-pot-smoker. He was somewhat nervy and excited.

Danny: I've got a new way of handling my pills (i.e. the effect of his medication.)
Lucy: Without pot?
Danny: Pot doesn't make any difference to that.
Lucy: Of course it does. All those extra chemicals.
Danny: That's why I'm careful with pot. Anyway I may be giving up pot. I told Adrian I was giving up pot.
Lucy: Super!
Danny: You mustn't connect pot and hallucinations. They are completely different things.

In the car a few days later:
Lucy: You seem very bitter about me.
Danny: I don't feel anything any more. You've destroyed everything for me. You never try to understand my point of view. You think it's all right to talk to my friends about me and look through my pockets.
Lucy: Only because you smoke pot. I don't like doing it.

And then later I heard him talking on the phone to his cousin Hector in a strong voice:

Danny: Hey! I've been put on a suspended sentence!

Hector: …

Danny: For two weeks or so. They were going to the police and....

Hector: …

Danny: Well I was busted. I've been busted four times already this year.

Hector: …

Danny: I'm not going to get busted again.

Hector: …

Danny: No, well I'm definitely not going to get busted again.

When the holidays came Danny said that he would like to spend them at Tara. He seemed to have forgotten his bad experience there. Now he thought of it as a happy rest-camp, where he would not be made to concentrate. But above all where his friends would not tempt him with pot, nor keep it from him when they were smoking. I wish there had been a friendly pot-free rest camp for him.

To Nicky on the phone he said: "I don't like the tension at home. I think I'll give up dope."

WINTER TERM

In the April/May holidays Danny was more bored than bad. On the eve of the winter term he told Oliver that he was looking forward to going back to school. Unfortunately St Martin's, like the other private schools in South Africa, was a three-term school, with the middle term covering the freezing highveld winter. At a similar school in my youth I got chilblains, rheumatism and frequent infections. At fourteen I spent a whole winter term away with sinusitis.

We were coming to the end of our family therapy sessions with Jeff. At one of the last ones Danny said, "If I become an educated person will it not chip from my character? Will there not be less innovation?"

At home he played very loud music. If he went straight from this music to a clarinet lesson he was less focused. I asked him about this loud music. "Don't you think music affects mood? Sometimes when you are supposed to be calming down you play this loud, stimulating, nervy music."

"Schizophrenics don't play music in conformist ways. They are likely to do the opposite."

"Schizophrenics can't even look after themselves."

There were no psychotic symptoms this holiday, so I tried leaving out the medication.

"Do you realize I haven't given you any pills for two whole days?"

"Yes, and I do appreciate that."

Jeff suggested that Danny have a therapist to himself, whom I wouldn't talk to. Danny couldn't see the point at first, but in the end he agreed.

"OK Ma, you can phone up and make an appointment for me."

"You'll have to do that. I'm not allowed to talk to her even on the phone."

"You'll never keep that up!"

But he did phone her himself. Sandy G. He talked to her in a very natural way—friendly and confident—no one would say disturbed. He cycled to a once-a-week appointment and said he liked her set-up.

At school he played hockey for the first time, got the hang of it very quickly and loved it.

But unfortunately physical illness messed up this term. Smoking cigarettes and dagga, missing the previous winter's germs because he hadn't been at school, and also the evening pill, Melleril, which gave him a stuffy nose—all this had perhaps lowered his resistance. He had a bright red throat with little white spots dotting it, so I had to accept that this time he really was sick. Then each time he went back to school the infection came back, so he had very little schooling that winter.

One special happening on some of his few winter school days was that Mrs Goudemond was taking him for Art. She had been his Art teacher at Saheti, and when I had met her the previous year, when Danny was at his worst, she had said, "Of all that class Daniel was the one I would least have expected to go wrong."

Now she said, "Daniel contributed more than the others today. I asked them whether they had frozen brains! We were discussing Greek temples and he asked interesting questions."

Halfway through this term I seem to have been quite pleased with him, in spite of the illness.

Lucy's diary: I showed him his current account today, with R3 credit, and his capital account with R10. I think he feels altogether better about himself now and things should go well. I feel exalted! Like my father and his trees, I plant 300—and one grows.

(Oliver used to say, despairingly, of each of my new plans, "What good do you expect that will do?")

But the term and the illness and the absences from school dragged on. In less happy mood I said to myself: All regularity has vanished from his life, except eating, smoking cigarettes and sleeping.

School when he did go he found discouraging. He had an English test in which he did not understand the comprehension part at all.

But he was not on his medication any more and this had not led back to psychosis. As the August holiday approached he got into an exuberant holiday mood, shouting and singing.

Instead of being paranoid about outside forces he was often quite nasty to me. As his illness wore off the problem of his outings came back.

Danny: If you are not going to give me lifts then I am not following your rules.
Oliver and Lucy: Everyone has to follow rules.
Lucy: Shaun is not as responsible as some of your other friends.
Danny (menacing, pointing): If you compare my friends then I've got it in for you.
Lucy (getting up): I do not tolerate threats. If you do that I quit.
Danny (needing a lift): Come on Ma! I'm sorry!
Lucy: Well this time you get a warning, but don't do that again.

Oliver was impressed and said to me later, "You were *marvellous*!"

Neither of us was good at taking this sort of firm line. We could shout at him in an angry mood, but not take these clear, parental moral lines with him.

On another day I was driving him somewhere and he was being obnoxious, so I stopped the car.

Danny shouted at me aggressively, "I want to tell you this: if you stop the car again I will hit you. I'm not going to stand for it."

I turned the car round and started going home. He apologized and I took him to his friend.

To encourage myself in the face of all this I wrote a list of how he had improved:

> *He is not on pot.*
> *He is not running away.*
> *He is formulating attacks on me instead of being paranoiac.*
> *His body and personality show greater strength.*
> *His arm doesn't shake.*
> *He doesn't spit inside the house.*

I took him to Dr Tuomi, a hearing therapist.

Dr T: He may be hiding a comprehension difficulty under all that bluster. A cover-up. He has a bad case of adolescence. I had two years like that myself.

Lucy: So what did you find?

Dr T: His physical hearing is perfect. But as soon as I give him a more complex sentence he can't get it.

Lucy: Can he be helped?

Dr T: Oh yes—but first he has to want to learn. At the moment when you overload his memory his brain refuses to work. But also he has chosen to represent himself in a bad light. However, in social chat he can function well.

I wept and wept that night for him and for me, and for all the mothers of children who can never become independent. The weird behaviour has gone, but the non-coping child is still with us.

I looked, again in vain, for some place where he could safely and pleasantly spend his August holidays. He thought "America"! This was because America was now competing with Cape Town as a mecca in his mind.

The money I had inherited from my father had now finally been processed, so we no longer had money worries. Once I would have thought it wrong to have money, but now I rejoiced.

Lucy: How about Canada?

Danny: Canada! Do you mean it? Stay with Aunt Jenny?

Lucy: It's just a possibility. I'll give you her number and then you can phone her yourself at a suitable time—not the middle of her night!

Danny: OK!

Chapter Eleven

CANADA AND EXPULSION

VISITING CANADA

On Friday 29 July Daniel phoned Jenny at midnight our time, when she who worked all day would be home. At 2.30 am he woke me for a cigarette. (For the last 18 months I had allowed him to wake me at night, wanting him not to feel all alone in his fragile neediness. But nowadays when he seemed more bad than mad, I often felt quite cross.)

He said, excitedly, "She says that's tremendous!"

This trip is gripping him, not allowing him to slip back into switched-off answers. He is all focus and clarity. But I have lost his passport! And I am in danger of being so fixated by this that I lose sight of other factors.

I confirmed with my sister Jenny that it was OK: a two-week holiday with her and her family. I booked his ticket.

I had hidden his passport to prevent him running away with it. Now I spent four days looking for it. Danny was in a euphoric state, smiling like one in love. ("If this be madness," I thought, "play on".)

He phoned Nicky in Cape Town and said: "Hey you know what? Mum's lost my passport. I can't understand it!" He is jubilant that I am fallible.

Jenny phoned with misgivings. She has talked to two friends whose sons' groups "smoke pot like we drink wine". (She and her husband had wine every evening.)

I phoned Nicky. She had found Danny not bad at all on her recent trip home. She said now, "He will just have to have the courage to face up to it, or there will be nowhere he can go. He must just say: Hi! I'm Daniel! I know the dope scene, but I can't take it: it freaks my head out."

Oliver says that Jenny really has nothing to worry about, because she can just send him home. I phoned Jenny again and this time she said, "Well if your family are all in agreement, then he's welcome." In fact we three, Oliver and Nicky and I, were the only ones supporting the trip—and of course Danny himself. Other adults thought we were being rash.

On the Thursday, less than a week since his phone call to Jenny, I was snugly in bed after my bath, reading a book. Danny came in—so childlike and open. "Am I *really* going?"

"Yes you are."

"When?"

"On Sunday."

He sat on my bed, hugging himself.

The next evening:

Danny: Ma, where did you put all that dope you collected?

Lucy: Different places—my filing-cabinet, my summer clothes suitcase
... Shall we throw it all away, symbolically?

Danny: Yes.

Lucy: All right. We can do it tomorrow.

Danny: I want to do it now!

Lucy: Where would you throw it?

Danny: In the swimming-pool.

I put on my dressing gown and found the pot, hoping all the time that the hidden passport would be with it. We put on the outside light and went to the swimming pool. I gave the pot to Danny and he threw it in:

> *Danny: Ashes to ashes*
> *Lucy: Dust to dust*
> *If the policeman doesn't get it*
> *the swimming-pool must.*

The next morning I knew there must be a De Bono answer to the lost passport—something completely different from just having hidden it away. I sat on the floor fingering our three passports. I idly turned the pages of Daniel's "aged 10" passport with his "aged 10" photo. Suddenly I saw the date, 1987, and turned further and found his 15-year-old photo from last year. The old passport and the new passport were the same thing.

My concept: Passports have the photo on the front page.

My false memory: He got a *new* passport and I hid it away.

I took him to the bank with his ticket and his passport to get his travellers' cheques. When we came back I wrote a poem:

Daniel in Nedbank, Fairmount, July 1983

> *Ignored small queues,*
> *but was not ignored.*
> *Paced with lop-sided ease*
> *over light wiped tiles,*
> *Fixed for ever in his pacing,*
> *until his turn should come.*
>
> *Grilles separated*
> *the front-facing faces*
> *focused comfortably*
> *on slips and cheques and rands,*
> *While his furiously fixated mind*
> *avoided their numbing accusations,*
> *and longed for Canada.*

On the Sunday of his departure Danny was rational and coped with his own packing. Even packed a spare pair of glasses. Only on the way to the airport could I sense his nervousness. At the airport he couldn't collect himself. He walked off very determinedly without knowing where to. But in the end he handled the luggage situation on his own.

But I was by now all too aware of his anxiety and regretting not having made some plan for the air-hostess to help him. I imagined all sorts of disasters: pot being found in his luggage; not hearing the final call; hallucinating everything the other passengers said to him; forgetting, or not wanting to take, the sleeping pill I have given him; and arriving in Canada a total wreck.

I thought he would be fine once in Canada. Jenny and her husband and children are calmer, more conformist people than we are, and I think Danny will do well with them.

Monday. Well Jenny phoned and he has arrived! But he had difficulty with the immigration authorities through non-communication, and is very, very tired. "The sleeping pill didn't work," he told Jenny. He is watching telly. Too tired even to talk to me.

If I had absolutely insisted on his run yesterday, he probably would have slept. But everything I insist on these days is seen and dominance and control.

> Lucy's diary: The strange business of being Daniel. Cut off from the world a lot of the time and in those times autistic, so not able to develop. I think he would thrive in some sort of fairly strict remedial community where he was forced to be active in many ways: community work, dancing, athletics; and then given a lot of individual help with his thinking and comprehension.

Thursday. Three days gone past and no phone call. I dare to hope that this might go on. I have relaxed and got on with the rest of my life.

Jenny of course did not introduce him to the pot-smoking children of her friends, so that situation never arose. Instead she arranged a wind-surfing course for him on Lake Ontario, and this was a great success. Jenny herself worked full-time so she simply gave Danny instructions on how to get there—bus, train, tube, ferry. A transit system with tokens. I later found it muddling, but Danny apparently mastered it easily.

At the end of the two weeks Jenny phoned:

"Everything has been fine. We've had confrontations over cigarettes, that's all."

"Has he behaved reasonably well apart from that?"

"Oh yes, he's been fine—for a 16-year-old boy! Lots of civilizing still to come."

Jenny later wrote me a report on the holiday. She said that the wind-surfing and shopping were a great success. He spent all his shopping money at the beginning. The major clash was smoking: "He didn't seem to be able to consider our needs and that made it difficult to be nice to him." (Jenny and her husband were recent ex-smokers and extremely sensitive about smoking.) There was no "inappropriate behaviour"—nothing one would call "disturbed". He didn't take initiative once the planned things were over, and he didn't talk much. He related well to the cat. Always took it on his lap when watching telly. She took Danny to a jazz concert—famous old jazz players, and Danny took photos.

Danny planned to take "lots" of sleeping pills on the journey back, but Jenny saw him decanting them into his pocket and prevented that.

Lucy's diary: Yesterday I drove alone to the airport. The time was grey shapes and sporadic twinkles. I watched the robots relaxing from red to green. I arrived at the airport at 6 pm, at the same time as the plane. Slight unease was nibbling at me now. I went and had a kit-kat and some coffee. At 6.15 I went down to the arrival hall. I like the atmosphere of the waiting people. There are always a few black people, smartly-dressed and confident.

No one reads. People chat quietly. If they need information or are sufficiently bored and sociable they talk to strangers.

Two blonde children chase each other around. Nobody minds. The girl, about four, says, "Oops, sorry!" when she suddenly finds herself face-to-face with me. She chases her seven-year-old brother, who indulges her by not out-pacing her. They are there with their grandfather. Who are they meeting? The girl is lively and yet not a show-off. How *are* they made that way?

Staff start emerging. I contemplate asking them whether the plane was delayed by the craziness of my tall, delinquent son. They are all neat and purposeful, and my crazy question is quickly suppressed.

The first passengers come out. I relish the relief and joy of the meetings. One woman is not met. Her eyes scan the audience. She moves out of our ambience.

The audience gets thinner. The passengers come out more slowly. I think, "The coping people are all out." I know now that Daniel will be last—retained by customs officials, unable to fill in forms correctly, switched-off, numb.

The grandfather and the two blonde children are still there. The girl sits on the post at the emergence-point. The boy stands beside her. They are both solemn now—peering in. A woman comes out, elderly yet still strong. She lifts the girl up and hugs her, pats the boy on the head. The grandfather moves forward. The grandmother says, anxiously, "Have they really been all right?" My heart sinks. What has happened to their parents?

It is now 7.15 pm. I cannot stand up any longer. I cannot be interested any longer. I walk back to the seats and put my feet up. My gaze never leaves the exit point, but it's unfocused now. From this new vantage-point I find I can see the shoes and strides of the passengers underneath the panel before they emerge. Him? Not him? Him? Not him?

I am expecting a wavy, light-shirted, effeminate blonde boy. I do not at first recognize the black-jacketed, dark-haired, reg-op guy who walks out. I walk towards him, uncertain. Recognition focuses. We hug, smile, walk off together, centre-stage. He is all right! We walk off comfortably into the night, all hostilities forgotten.

In the car he talked and talked and talked, transformed for the moment from the sullen, nervous spitting adolescent of two weeks ago into the charming male companion he may one day permanently become.

"My God he's sane!" I thought. "His mind is working quite clearly, his voice is deep, he sounds strong."

At home he bared his breast proudly, revealing *Playboy* and *Penthouse*. He said, grinning, "They made me open my jacket. I thought I'd had it! I had them in my case from Canada to New York, but then I decided they'd be better under my shirt."

SEPTEMBER: EXPELLED

September is spring here in South Africa. I now, in 2006, have welcomed the warmth and gazed at the flowering tree that overhangs my cottage (which was once Oliver's studio). It's a syringa tree, holding out to the sky its masses of pale purple clusters of flowers, while clutching its way up the trunk is a creeper which takes its bright yellow bells up to shout amongst the purple florets. I love this unusual mixture of bold and delicate.

But in September 1983 I would not have noticed.

On the last day of August in that year I wept and raged: How will it end? Will he ever come right? Is there perhaps just too far to go? The distance between the present opter-out and a possible future coper is scarcely imaginable.

Canada had worked, but only one week separated Canada from school. Danny's sleep pattern was easily thrown out and jet-lag didn't help. But on the day before school started he seemed fine, and went for a long cycle ride and had his hair cut without fuss.

The problem was that he had done nothing academic for weeks—months perhaps; not even read a book. Often his brain didn't work properly. And now he was going back to a school who were no longer paying him any special attention. The teachers were gearing up for exams: chatty lessons belonged to the earlier part of the year.

Danny came back from school that first day looking exhausted and fed up. However, he managed to cycle to Sandy for his therapy session. When he came back at 4.30 pm he lay on his tummy on his bed, smiling slightly, and went to sleep. He slept around the clock and the next morning said he thought he was ill. He got up for breakfast and then went back to bed and to sleep. I poured cold water on him. He chased me and hit me on the chin. At 11 am he was asleep on the couch in the living room.

Two days later Oliver and I were drinking coffee in the kitchen: "Well," I said, "he's on the bus."

"I feel sorry for the bus, that's all," said Oliver.

We had had a frenetic night. I had locked my door after several "last cigarettes". Then at 4 am he woke me to make him breakfast. He said that his watch said 6.30 am.

In the chaos of not sleeping and not coping at school he had no resistance when a boarder at St Martin's invited him into the boarding house to smoke pot. Poor sleep patterns, oceans of missed schoolwork; dysfunctional thinking—and now this.

I was shouting at him a lot. I seem to have lost the plot at that stage. He would say anything to get out of doing anything and I felt hopeless. I did not hear about the St Martin's' pot-smoking until later, nor that when he did go to school he spent most of the time in the sick room.

However, I worked on myself and got back to sane, loving mothering and things went better. He went to buy chocolate and brought back the right change. A pebble of accountability. "You know Danny," I said, "It is worth any amount of other suffering to get this honesty thing straight between us."

I asked him what I should do to get him up in the morning and he said the water throwing idea was a good one and he would accept it.

A few days later he came home from school very cheerful—said he had had a very good day. They had started athletics and he had passed all his required standards: long jumps, high jumps and different distances of running. But he was hyped up. At 10 pm he was very restless so I gave him a Normison sleeping pill. By 11 pm he had scratched the top of his body all over with a razor blade in some sort of pattern.

I said, angrily, "What are you doing!"

He smiled: "Toughening myself up for the army!"

"Just don't do it that's all."

By then he was starting to feel sleepy and said a calm goodnight and went off to sleep. But he had been sniffing for days—the type of sniffing that I knew was from dagga. So now I knew.

On Sunday 11 September he visited a friend and came back very stoned and was incapable of doing anything to prepare for school. He announced that there were failures in communication at home and he would like to go to Toby's house for a week. Toby was at Wits doing a music degree, so Danny felt he could work there with Toby. And Toby did later say that Danny had done some history in the evening when he himself was busy with an essay.

Danny got himself to school in the mornings—but Toby was not supervising, so Danny went without his books and without shaving.

On the Wednesday the headmaster, Mr Wigmore, phoned me and said: "I'll have to ask you to take him away. He spends all his time in the sick room, and then today he phoned for a taxi in the office without his shoes, and with his shirt out. And he has not shaved this week. We can't handle him any more I'm afraid."

I went to the school to fetch him. He was sleeping in the sick room.

Lucy: Danny!

Danny (astonished): What are you doing here?

Lucy: I've come to fetch you. You're expelled.

Danny: Why?

Lucy: You haven't shaved, you miss most of your classes. Just everything,
  my love.
Danny: I did two hours of history last night. You can ask Toby. I'm a
  perfectly good student. I could go to Damelin.
Lucy: They won't have you.
Danny: Of course they will. I was the best student in Standard 7.

In the car going home we continued talking in a calm and rational
way, as if life was completely normal.
Danny: What will happen if I don't get into Damelin?
Lucy: You'll have to get a job that's all.
Danny: Will you still send me to America?
Lucy: Not unless you've proved yourself here.
Danny: I'll cycle to Sandy tomorrow. Will that please you?
Lucy: Yes.

The next day he kept his appointment with Sandy. On the Friday
of that week he worked with the Yellow Pages and the phone all day,
and eventually came up with an appointment for Monday with a TV
agency.

I took him for his audition and a very nice lady ushered us both
in. Danny had been nervous before, but not too overwhelmingly. He
read too quickly. Then he gave an excellent impromptu short speech
on his hobby: "I have a hobby which is more than just a hobby. It's my
music..."

The pleasant lady said his audition was "average" but that he had a
good telly face so they would take him on. They straightaway gave him
a part as a British soldier in some TV series.

For the next seven weeks Danny had work for the SABC about two
days a week. I remember Oliver taking him to a shoot in the country
and I took him to the Victory Cinema where he was a prominent
member of the audience. I also remember taking him to spend two
whole days at the SABC building in Auckland Park. What a relief!
That was for an Afrikaans series. One of the plays was called *Time and
the Wood*, but apart from these scattered memories the whole thing is a
bit of a blur. I don't remember ever seeing him on television, but these
productions do take a long time to get screened.

In the meantime I myself had found a weekly release: I went walking with three friends every Sunday morning at Emmarentia Dam. It's a place where you are far from houses, with streams and dams and parkland. We talked and talked, but I think never about Daniel! Two of these friends were a couple and after the walk we went to Mr Crusty and got freshly baked rolls which we took to their house and had with home-made jam and newly-brewed coffee. Back home Danny was probably still asleep, but Oliver was there if needed.

OCTOBER: KNIVES AND BOTTLES

On the Friday night of the week when Danny was expelled, Oliver and I went to a play, *The Long Journey of Poppie Nongena*. It was about the terrible times that "Poppie", based on a real person, had experienced under apartheid. For 40 years she had been moved around, or had struggled to resist being moved around.

Coming home in the car both Oliver and I wept—for Danny and for Poppie.

Even though there were now so many Afrikaners who were questioning apartheid, the fact that people were still being shifted around, that the diehards were still in power, made my usual optimism shift. Oliver and I were now on the same side. Both of us were pessimistic about Danny and pessimistic about apartheid. But I still recorded any hopeful signs:

> Stellenbosch has talked about *Poppie* for months. Jean was at a Cape Town performance where Koornhof (a Nat minister) wept throughout the second half. But the removals are ruthless and continuous and no one can stop them. Yet in Pretoria a largely Afrikaans audience stood up and sang *Nkosi Sikelel'i* at the end of *Poppie*.

On the Wednesday after this I went alone to hear Koornhof himself speaking at the Houghton Primary School. I sensed his confusion. When I got home there was a message from Debbie of the Drug House: Danny had left their house and gone off with a friend who had a "button". This was a new problem: a button was a Mandrax sleeping-pill—but crushed and smoked with dagga (in a broken-off bottle) it had a shocking effect, like being shot. Toby only once smoked a "white pipe", as they were called, finding the effect too powerful. He was that delicate sensitive boy, with a quick, expressive face, studying classical music. I asked him this year (2006) why he had sold LSD and he replied, "But someone would have sold it."

"Buttons" were difficult to get—and expensive. In our house on another occasion I picked up the second phone in a different room from Danny and heard a sweet young girl's voice saying eagerly to him, "Hey Danny! Guess what! I've got a button! Come over!" It was a new excitement for Danny in his failed state.

On the night after hearing Koornhof and hearing for the first time about Danny smoking a white pipe, I slept for about four hours. Before and after this sleep I alternated between the two themes: the disaster and degradation of forced removals and the disaster and degradation of Danny.

Danny was high from Canada and school expulsion and his acting jobs. In earlier times all this wild young masculine daring would have got him to do heroic deeds in battle. Now he simply did a heroic deed on himself.

This was one night when I was doing the washing-up in the kitchen and he was doing a wild dance outside while shouting a trance-like song. In the rain. It seemed harmless enough. He came inside, dripping with rain, and went to his room. I went to bed.

The next morning I saw that he had written on the message-pad:

Danny: I'm a little GIRL (gurgle!)
Go Fucken STAB
YOUR HEAD NEXT TIME!

I went into his room. He was lying there white-faced and awake. He confessed that he had hurt himself while dancing, but that it was nothing to worry about. In fact he had plunged a knife three inches into his thigh, while doing his wild dance in the rain.

The doctor said he was lucky that no muscles or arteries were damaged. The leg was bound up and the wound healed quickly.

One day we were in the car going shopping. He was in the back with a cold drink. He chucked the empty bottle down and it rattled around. We were about to turn into a parking lot at the Pick and Pay shopping centre. I said, "Can you do something with that bottle? Like get rid of it for instance."

He opened the door onto the middle of the road and threw it out. The glass scattered all over the main road. I was furious.

"You're just paranoiac," said Danny.

"It was an extremely anti-social act. I represent society and I have a right to get angry."

Back home he raged around for a while, then came to my room: "I admit it was a wrong thing to do, and I'm sorry, but I don't want to talk about it. I'll take a taxi to Sandy. (He had some taxi coupons for emergencies. His wound hadn't healed enough for cycling.)

I wondered why he was packing his rucksack. I heard him phoning the taxi. An hour later I decided that he had probably gone off somewhere and so I decided to take his appointment with Sandy. As I drove out I found him with his rucksack and his guitar standing on the pavement. He had been waiting there all that time for the taxi which was going to take him to Cape Town. We went to Sandy together. I was startled by her consulting room: it was a conversation-pit—a carpeted cube sunk into the floor. We sat at one level and put our feet on another. Tea and biscuits were brought. Sandy treated my wild and sulky son as a real human. And in two minutes that was what he was.

But Nicky and Oliver no longer thought him human. Nicky said, "He just seems to have a sub-human personality. Up to now I've felt desperately sorry for him, but now I don't know. I just feel like giving up. This thing of not having values really disturbs me. That he should come from our family and not have values. All my compassion went to Daniel, but not any more."

Oliver had stomach acid and migraines, and found himself raging at his pupils. One afternoon he was teaching a young girl the flute when Danny came pounding on the door with some raging complaint or demand. (The yellow and purple flowers were now plopping on the roof.) That night Oliver said to me: "I can't go on. It's him or me. Either he goes or I go. He is a drug addict. We must not bluff ourselves that he can come off."

And Characters, the acting agency, they too had had enough of him:

Characters agent: "We've had bad reports of him. They say he was selfish and they didn't know what was the matter with him. He doesn't care about other people and he's a spoiled brat. They don't want him back."

I phoned my friends and contacts for support and suggestions. They all gave me sympathy, but none had any solutions. Two of my Christian friends belonged to weekly prayer groups which were including Daniel in their prayers.

NOVEMBER: A MOTORBIKE?

I too was giving up. I felt defeated and hopeless. At the same time I knew I could not give up, so I talked myself into being committed and cheerful.

One day I was walking through a hypermarket and saw a hug-sized teddy-bear. Without thinking about it I took it with my other shopping to the check-out counter, paid the bill and brought the teddy home. For myself.

Another thing I did was to get Oliver to look through all his bits and parts of hi-fi systems and see if he could make me a record player for my bedroom. He did. I had not bought records for myself since I was a teenager. In the days when we didn't have extra money, if I did have some I would buy a book. If Oliver had some he would buy a record. So I listened to his records which were his taste in music and performance. I now went to the Hillbrow Record Shop and bought myself a few records which were entirely satisfying for me. There were new pianists like Murray Peraiha, Barenboim and Ashkenazy, whom I hadn't heard before, and orchestras recorded so well that you could hear the inner voices. I bought Mendelssohn and Schumann and Beethoven: one-piano and two-piano concertos.

Then I closed my curtains, switched off the lights, turned upside-down on my relaxator, put my teddy under my chin and between my breasts, and lost myself in the music. "Danny-sadness" was still somewhere in the background, but muted.

Danny also had a release: playing the piano in Oliver's studio. Mostly he wasn't allowed in there. Oliver was not a tidy man: cords trailed around and books and papers were scattered everywhere. Danny on a bad day could wreak havoc. But late at night when he couldn't sleep he would wake me and I would let him in there to play the piano. He would do this without disturbing anything.

Earlier that year, in the winter, Danny and I had gone to the Doll's House on a day when he was sullen and sarcastic—bitter about something or other. As we arrived there was a hoot—and there was Robbie Robb! Robbie was Danny's hero from when he was ten years old. Robbie had been 15-year-old Nicola's boyfriend. He was able to put together rock bands that worked: ones that got written about in newspapers: "Tribe after Tribe" was one of them. He was a hippy in style and had in the past taken drugs. He was the one who had a bright red Afro hairstyle shaved off for the army—and then got out of the army by using old hallucinations to bluff the authorities that he was mad. But Robbie was now focused and ambitious and could get things done.

Lucy's account of this meeting: Danny went straight over and started talking, then they both came over to me and Robbie and I talked. Then Danny went over to them again. Then followed something beautiful to behold:

Robbie and Danny were in a sort of dance of communication. I could only see them, not hear them. It was a very dramatic exchange: two bodies making points with great emphasis, and yet they were at that subtle point between being strangers and knowing each other too well.

I imagine they talked mostly about music, but also about pot, which Robbie has now given up. Robbie said later: "Those people like Kerouac did a lot of damage. They themselves could smoke dope and come to no harm. As I was telling Danny, my friend Peter can smoke dope and remember and focus afterwards. I can't do that at all."

As we drove home Danny was pink and absorbed: "Robbie is fantastic!" he said. When we got back he walked to Adrian instead of nagging for a lift. Robbie had pointed to the sky and the world. I imagine he was telling Danny: "It's all there, brother!"

Since neither Robbie, his hero, nor Nicola, his heroine, could smoke dope and focus the next day, Danny could somehow have got over his own humiliation at not being able to do so. But once he was with friends in a ritual situation, he would not have thought that way.

I phoned Robbie and told him that Danny had left school and was free.

Robbie said, "I can't have anyone in my group who is on drugs. He must dress neatly and shave properly."

Robbie phoned Danny. Danny was excited. He said to me: "I'm so glad Robbie phoned. I lay awake last night wondering what I was going to do for the rest of the year."

Danny went to Robbie's house in Westdene and played with Robbie's band. But it was no good. Robbie told us that he wouldn't be able to use Danny because of poor concentration. He is the best guitar player Robbie knows, but he switches off.

However, Robbie was prepared to have him over about once a week to help out with instruments and have a play and a chat. On three occasions he even let him stay the night. This was a great relief to us. At this stage Danny either didn't know, or hadn't accepted, that Robbie was not actually going to use him in his band.

Danny now developed another new passionate idea: a motorbike! In normal times we would just have said no, but we and he were living in a time of emergency. He needed another focus. On the days that he didn't go to Robbie he was still out of control and often violent. How could we let a violent adolescent boy have a motorbike?

We heard about a bike school, but never found it. We told him that every day without pot (and of course white pipes!) and with co-operative behaviour he would get points towards his bike. He tried hard.

We knew that the slightest slip after he got the bike could cost him or someone else a life, so the deal was that the bike would be immediately removed if there were setbacks.

His behaviour was not perfect. He continued to wake me at night and I let him do this. I realized that he couldn't work out what else to do on those occasions. One night he woke me for the motorbike picture—the one we had decided on. It was a "scrambler", not a big, powerful bike.

To myself I said: I think he has smoked some pot. But he has not been manic, so I continue to put ticks on the bike chart. I intend not to accuse him of things, but to find every possible way to increase his sense of self-worth.

But I suppose he smoked a little more, because he started being hostile towards me again. One morning I asked him not to come into the little room next to mine in the middle of the night, "opening cupboards and looking at yourself in the mirror". He stormed out of the house and came back apparently stoned. I said we would just have to start the bike programme again.

He got vicious. He stood in front of this wall-to-ceiling, corner-to-corner mirror in the little spare room next to mine. "How much does this mirror cost? A lot hey?"

He grabbed his squash racket, pushed me out of the door and locked it, and then in a few minutes he had smashed the mirror to pieces with the handle of the squash racket. I watched him doing this from outside the window. I was terrified that he would go on to cut himself to pieces. The police came. He wouldn't come out. I talked to him through the window. He said he would calm down if we gave him the bike tomorrow. Eventually he came out. He said he would really give up pot if he got a bike *now*. I saw the sense in this. Oliver at first said "no". Then he came into Danny's room and agreed.

It worked. He drove his bike safely and well and was proud and cheerful.

FINDING HABILITAT

At the end of November I was standing in a check-out queue. There was a pile of *You* magazines next to me. I saw on the cover: *Griffin O'Neal goes to Rehab in Hawaii.*

I picked it up and turned to the article. There was Hawaii, and there was the sea, and there was Griffin O'Neal smiling. I read a bit of the article, bought the magazine and brought it home. I read the rest of the article in a trance. It was my imagined place for Danny. But was it real? Was it affordable?

I phoned my brother-in-law in Toronto. He did research for documentaries and had access to almost any information. The next day he phoned back: "Habilitat has the best record in the States for rehabilitating drug addicts and difficult teenagers." He gave me the phone number. It was exactly 12 hours away, on the other side of the world. I phoned at 11 pm (Hawaiian time: 11 am) and was told to phone again at noon—our midnight.

I spoke to Guy, who had the friendliest voice in the world. He told me all about Habilitat and said they would take Danny. The cost is reasonable, because the residents do the work themselves—both the work to keep the place going, and work to get money from the outside world. And they train people for jobs for when they leave. We did have to pay fees, but the dollar in those days only cost one rand.

I was stunned at first—it sounded too good! Would Danny go? Would Danny stay? I told Danny about it. He said, "Well, I've got nothing to do at the moment, so I might as well lie in the sun in Hawaii."

He talked to his friend Toby about it and Toby told him about the Polynesians and then the British coming. It's now an American state.

For Oliver it was end of term at both the schools he taught at. He was determined to spend his holidays being a good father to Danny. He first got him to accept the reality that Robbie didn't want him in his band. Danny said he had been getting bored anyway because he had been doing repetitive stuff, not his own songs. (Long ago, before his breakdown, he had given Robbie a present of one of his own songs, and Robbie had recorded it and put it in one of his albums.)

Oliver tried to explain to Danny about Habilitat, although we didn't know much ourselves at this stage. He asked Danny if he would like him to take him to Los Angeles. There was a flight going via Brazil, and they could spend a few days in Rio. Danny was jubilant. Oliver put enthusiasm into preparing for the trip and keeping Danny busy.

But then Danny visited his friends, and came back disillusioned and thinking he would miss his friends unbearably.

He said to Oliver, "Jan K says it's a con—that it's just a reformatory."

"It's a place for people who have problems."

Lucy (to herself): Oliver had a good chat to him about Hawaii. Danny conceded that we do have authority to tell him to go. But he asked for the right to tell his friends that he was going there to study, so that they wouldn't look down on him or laugh at him.

Griffin O'Neal, the boy on the *You* cover, is the son of the film star, Ryan O'Neal, and the brother of Tatum O'Neal, whom I saw when she was the child in *Paper Moon*. Griffin and Daniel: two troubled boys with gifted sisters.

FORCED TO BEHAVE

Everything was organized. They were leaving on December 30. It was now December 14. Two weeks and two days to go. How to get through them?

We never went up to Molozi in December, both because it was too hot and because we had Christmas traditions down here. But now it seemed like a good idea. My sisters weren't here, so there was no competition for the Molozi house.

Oliver said that I could stay in Johannesburg! A blessed rest. He would take Danny with a few friends who seemed fairly reasonable. They all smoked some pot, but were not addicts or difficult people.

But before they left there was a small crisis. We still had to motivate Danny to do things that were good for him and especially things which would make his sleep patterns right. Oliver's holiday plan for him was that he had to swim 20 lengths before he got his pocket money. Oliver didn't trust him to do this unless he was watching. One day Oliver wasn't there. Danny asked me for money.

"You'll have to do your lengths first. I'll watch."

"I refuse to be watched by you."

He then went and swam and I heard him shouting out the numbers of lengths.

He came to me and said, viciously, "Now give me my money or I'll kill you."

"Calm down and apologize first."

"I'm sorry, I'm sorry, I'm sorry. What more do you want?"

Oliver came home at that point and gave him his money. Danny rode off furiously for petrol and cigarettes, minus helmet and shoes. A policeman saw him and accompanied him home. He let him off, but forced Danny to look at him. Oliver witnessed this.

Oliver was triumphantly self-righteous: "Ja, he let you off but I've got his name and he says he'll willingly come and flatten you."

"Cool it, both of you," I said.

"Well it just shows doesn't it? We think he *cannot* behave properly, but when someone *forces* him too ... then he can.

I was very tired. I said, "I'm confused. I don't really know what you're saying. He's always been able to do things when someone is forcing him to."

But we didn't believe in force.

Oliver and Danny recovered and went off happily to do their Xmas shopping.

Danny, wearing shoes and helmet, went to fetch Esmé, his make-believe girlfriend, from Benoni. He had tried to visit her earlier in the year but had got lost. This time he brought her back on his bike, very gleeful. She is pretty and young and does not look like an addict, in spite of being part of the Drug House set. They lay together by the pool like two innocent teenagers of long ago.

Danny now talked about pot and psychosis as if they were past history.

Lucy: I wondered why, the other day, you felt that having a bad reaction to pot made you somehow inferior.

Danny: Well it was what the others said, especially the older ones—that I couldn't handle it. They really degraded you for that. It was destructive.

Oliver and Danny went to a movie, "Superman III". Oliver said that only his speech after the movie was loose. "He finishes sentences with any words which sound like the end of a sentence."

At supper Danny said, "Debbie used to be caring, but the drugs have changed her. For me dope was a tremendous challenge—because your parents are so against it and it's illegal and because you risk messing up your mind."

Later, alone with me, he was talking about his psychosis:

Danny: You would never believe the speeding-up that happens. It's like a screen with lines in front of your eyes. Can you believe that I used to think I could read your mind?

Lucy: Some of your experiences seemed quite good. You would smile.

Danny: No, it was all bad. It was so bad that I used to think I was dead. Even though I was brought up an atheist I used to lie in bed in the morning and think I was on my way to Heaven.

Lucy: But Heaven's supposed to be nice!

Danny: Or Hell. I didn't know how I would get good again. I felt very powerful. But I knew nothing about morals and ethics. Sometimes I still get scared that I'm not going to be able to consider all the things someone says. You know what? I'd like to go by bike to Molozi—two days before the others. Then I can have two days by myself to think about Hawaii.

Oliver agreed to him going up by bike, but not to him getting to the farm house first. There were too many things to see to there. So Danny would set off first, then Oliver would pass him north of Pretoria, then Danny would have a night to himself at the Holiday Inn in Pietersburg and then ride to Molozi the next day.

The day before, Oliver said, fed-up, "He hasn't done any of his packing."

"Well go to him now and say that you are just about to pack the car and could he do his packing. He can get things right if they are immediate and there is warmth. I don't think it's our job now to reform him, just to give him support and warmth.

So that's what Oliver did. And Danny said to Nicky, "If Dad always spoke to me as nicely as that I would never need to raise my voice."

Oliver talked to him about what to do if he had bike trouble or was stopped by police. There were no cell phones yet at that time.

On the Sunday morning, December 19, Danny was ready to go at about 9.30 am, but didn't go. He went to the garage and put on music. I went to him.

Lucy: The rain's going to come soon.

Danny: I think I'll go later.

Lucy: Well it's your decision, but you'll get very wet.

He collected up his spit, moving it forward into his pursed lips, and spat on the ground. But he then collected his things, including bacon and egg sandwiches which Oliver had made for him. Oliver left soon afterwards and passed him on the road.

At 7 pm I heard that he had arrived safely at the Holiday Inn in Pietersburg, after a wet ride.

LAST DAYS

Nicola was going up to the farm the next day, with her new boyfriend, Bob. She usually worshipped Oliver, but was now seeing him through Bob's eyes: "Dad is very dogmatic. He keeps interrupting Bob. And it's taken me years to get over copying Dad's sloppiness and rudeness. But you, Ma, are the most sussed-out intelligent woman I know. I think it must be hard for Danny and Dad to live with you."

And then I was home alone, breathing in the silence, and writing poems.

I visited my mother. We talked about my uncle Hal. Grandma said, "Hal says he doesn't want to come to lunch at the same time as Oliver."

"Whyever not?"

"Oliver is too arrogant, too bombastic, too loud and too opinionated."

"Oh! Well yes he can be. It's just as well that I'm quite strong, but it can be hard on Danny. Anyway Oliver is being marvellous with Danny at the moment. How did you like Nicky's Bob?"

"Yes he's all right, but he's just very ordinary, and Nicola's not."

"What about Oliver? Is he ordinary?"

"Yes"

"And me?"

Grandma hesitated, "No."

Lucy (to herself): I don't dare ask about Danny! To Grandma he's just extraordinarily awful. How does she see herself, I wonder?

I went to visit my mother-in-law, Sally, who had stayed with us when Daniel was four and five years old. I asked her, "How do you remember Danny from then?"

"Unfriendly, stand-offish. Going his own way. But not badly behaved. I remember Oliver setting up his easel with Danny's little one next to him."

Interestingly she likes him very much now. I think he is sweet and relaxed with her because she is so uncritical of him.

Lucy's diary: There is a quality of joyful response to life, which many children have, but not all and which can be encouraged and passed on from parent to child, and from child to parent. It is a quality which Daniel sometimes has these days—open and free and joyful—some archaic memory of total acceptance of his being which is still lodged there ready to draw on, along with all the bad news.

I wrote a poem:

THIS HOUSE THIS BOY

*This house
has deep structural faults,
like the teen-age boy who lives in it.
It was built ignorantly:
a slab of heavy concrete
pressing down on insufficient foundations.*

*But the boy who lives in it,
who has added to its degradation
by smashing windows and breaking down doors,
was conceived in love—
a much wanted child.*

*So where did the pressures come from
which so crushed
the framework of his being?
Why did he
at the age of three
look at his drawing of a man
whose head was in his stomach*

like every other three-year-old's
drawing of a man,
Why did my son say:
"It's not right,"
and draw no more for six months?

My son
so finely tuned
to praise and blame
observed a sister's glowing achievements
and felt small and insignificant.

My son,
proudly assessing his father's
deep resonant voice
heard that same voice
scornfully condemn humanity's puny efforts,
and felt himself scorned.

My son,
Basking in a loving mother's
positive appreciation of him,
heard that same mother's
hysterical outbursts against him
and felt his drives denied.

My son,
coping with the senseless, lifeless
tedious requests of school-teachers
as speedily as possible
found once again
that he was considered inadequate.

So he concentrated
on what his friends wanted him to be:
daring, and fun to be with,
only to find

that when the fun failed,
his friends joined the ranks
of his critics.

Yes this boy, my son, lives still,
is not entirely crushed,
Nor has the house fallen.

Nicky phoned from the farm: "Dad is managing *so well*!"

Oliver is at Molozi with Danny, Nicky and Bob, Andrew, Michael, Paul and Steve.

Oliver says they played a "Guess the adverb" game last night. Danny had a great deal of difficulty—he guessed the emotion, "sorrow", but couldn't get to the words "sadly" or "sorrowfully" and started making wild associations.

I don't know how one can possibly separate anxiety and mental functioning, because as soon as he approaches that sort of situation he gets anxious, and the anxiety makes him function less well, which makes him more anxious.

Now that everyone is up there, Danny is staying on the fringes and playing his guitar. But he sleeps with the other guys all in one room, without any problems.

Back at home, Guy of Habilitat phoned me on Christmas Day. I told him that Danny was worried that there wouldn't be enough for him to do there. Guy laughed and said he could go on and on about all the activities there.

Guy: Is there anything else?
Lucy: Only everything!
Guy: Yea, I see.

He wished me "Merry Christmas" in Hawaiian.

For Christmas Nicola gave Danny a huge, very cuddly bear, which he loved. (Luckily the "men being sensitive" era allowed this.) Bob gave him a kite and they flew it together.

On Christmas Day Oliver smoked a joint with all of them. He said it just made him feel passive. He told Danny he was going to do it, and Danny was full of anticipation. Oliver watched him when they were all smoking and he noticed that Danny had a greater eagerness in grabbing more, more, more. Perhaps he was eager to drown his fears of the future, his awareness that he was not fitting in—and even the strangeness of his dad smoking pot. He told me much later that he had felt confused by this.

Oliver told me that Danny's friends shamed him into playing Scrabble with them. All these older friends with whom he only shared pot and music. They had not had cognitive breakdowns. Oliver said, "He wasn't much good at the Scrabble, but Michael helped him a lot. The main thing is that he *did* it! He joined in!"

Oliver and Danny came home on Tuesday 27 December and were to leave on Friday 30.

Danny proudly showed me all his Scrambler injuries. He went biking through all the thick summer weeds of Molozi. The enthusiasm he displays is probably the same as he felt for pot originally—an adventure—and him not a sissy!

"Between two roads you can always find a path," he said.

Oliver's whole tone with Danny is different. "Come on you little shit-house," he says in a comfortable way, and off they go together.

Lucy: You have been so *practical* recently!

Oliver: Well it's because of Daniel.

Lucy: You mean modelling coping?

Oliver: No. It's the feeling that I can't let myself be defeated. I used to give in too easily ... You know, Danny will never be more "intellectual" than he is now. He lives totally in his mind.

Danny wanted a going-away party. He was thrilled when I came home with "normal party things"—crisps and cokes. Before the party Nicky and Danny went round to the neighbours to invite them and apologize in advance for the noise. They congratulated Danny on "going overseas to study".

At the party all Danny's special qualities of charm and originality shone through. He looked beautiful—draped in a Kenyan cloth.

A guest said, "Someone must make a speech."

Danny said, "I just hope I survive, that's all."

I said, "Danny, if you survived the last two years you will survive until you are 80."

"YOU should make the speech," said Danny.

But we just drank to him and left it at that. Danny had a swim at 1 am, then said goodnight to everyone and went to sleep.

The next day we had a family lunch and Danny kissed them all good-bye.

Danny said to Nicky: "It's OK. I feel OK about it, but I worry that there won't be things for me to do there."

The next day he sat on the porch chatting to Bob and Nicky in a very relaxed way. He really likes Bob and has named his bear after him.

And so came Friday. It was time to leave. Danny went with Bob and Nicky to the airport and I went with Oliver. Danny now told Nicky that he was really glad to be going.

Oliver, in our car:

Oliver: I know I must look at the good things—and there have been plenty of good things—but I'm still overwhelmed by things like his running up 300 km on my car.

Lucy: Where did he go in it?

Oliver: He went to fetch Andrew at the Louis Trichardt station one night. I don't know where else they went.

Lucy: It sounds very normal adolescent behaviour to me—once you had given them your car. I'm glad I wasn't there. I'd have worried about his safety, especially at night.

Oliver: He's a good driver. I let him drive most of the way home. I told him when he was driving too fast and he slowed down.

Lucy: I'm just so glad he's physically whole after all this!

At the airport Bob and Nicola and I watched until their plane disappeared and then ran a race along the empty concourse.

Chapter Twelve

HABILITAT—THE FIRST TIME
(AGED SEVENTEEN, 1984)

It is January 3, 1984. Oliver and Danny have had their few days in Rio. I feel for them this morning. I will be glad when they are safely in America, some time this afternoon. The land of the free, but not to undesirables. Oliver has planned to get Daniel into his suit for getting through Immigration Control.

I hope in Brazil they have been seduced by sun and fun and foreignness into calming the dictatorial, problematic sides of their personalities and that everything is going reasonably smoothly.

(Nicky is glad he is going to stay on an island!)

I listen to my new and glorious recording of the Messiah, upside-down on my relaxator. I think of Danny and his strange integrity—his clutching on to his own identity and his courage in the face of all the terrors.

They got into America at New Orleans, and then spent a few days in Los Angeles. On Sunday morning, 8 January, Oliver put Danny on the plane to Honolulu—and waited.

I waited at home. I wrote my first villanelle—a French poetry form with two lines repeated in turn at the end of each triplet, and then coming together at the end:

> *Boy in an aeroplane off to Hawaii*
> *Tall, thin and blue-eyed with a bear upon his knee*
> *Mother in Johannesburg watching time go by.*
>
> *Boy will learn reality, learn the reason why*
> *he has to curb his impulses in order to be free*
> *Boy in an aeroplane off to Hawaii.*
>
> *He's imagining the girl he loves while gazing at the sky*
> *He'll change himself to please her: SHE WILL SEE!*

Mother in Johannesburg watching time go by.

Change will come if he learns how to try
Forsaking stubborn indolence, lively as a flea
Boy in an aeroplane off to Hawaii.

Tough love ahead, thinks his mother with a sigh
One among so many is what he soon will be
Mother in Johannesburg watching time go by.

"It's worth it my child—not to have to lie,"
Still she tries to reach him, offering her plea
Boy in an aeroplane off to Hawaii
Mother in Johannesburg watching time go by.

On Sunday evening, Guy from Hawaii phoned Oliver in Los Angeles, and Oliver phoned me in Johannesburg: he had arrived. Then followed many days of hope and doubt. But there were no phone calls, either from Danny or from Habilitat. The silence reminded me of the wait after he went to Grahamstown.

While I waited to hear from Habilitat and for Oliver to complete his relaxed journey home I got a standard letter from Habilitat:

Habilitat offers a unique opportunity for individuals involved in substance abuse or other anti-social behaviour. Basically, it is a "Survival School" where these individuals may learn how to redirect their lives.

Our residential treatment facility occupies a once private estate on Kaneohe Bay on the north of the island of Oahu (Honolulu is on the south). We do not employ the traditional psychiatric approaches, nor do we use mind altering drugs of any kind. Instead, our unique approach is built around the concept of an extended or substitute family (the Hawaiian word is "Ohana"). In this setting residents interact, share and learn. Through the use of group and individual counselling, seminars, academic and vocational training, residents develop new values and self-esteem.

Our programme is, intentionally, not an easy one. It is an intense two to three year, live-in experience that challenges an individual on every level. During our thirteen years of existence, our innovative methods and dramatic results have set the pace for other residential programmes around the world.

Oliver is back. He says that Danny left LA for Honolulu in a good state and that he *looks* good—all bronzed from the beaches of Rio; and to the kids he'll be a novelty. So my feeling is that the first few weeks will go well. His sociability and charm and the relief from uncertainty will be uppermost. His neurotic traits won't emerge till later.

Mark (his supportive drummer friend) says that he phoned Danny in LA and he told him to plunge into his new way of life and get the most out of it, and Danny entirely agreed. So maybe he is!

But at the end of two weeks my optimism ran out, so I phoned Habilitat and was put on to a very friendly, warm woman—Betsy. "He's adjusting very well. He asks lots of questions. He's a fighter. Of course he doesn't always understand things—but that will come. He is making friends. He plays the guitar and the piano and sings. He's in good hands."

I ran and skipped to the local park and had a swing, laughing.

On 9 February, the "Visitation Rules" came from Habilitat— revealing the tough side at last? It is as if they didn't want to put us off by telling us these things at first. Being visited is a reward for good behaviour, and there are strict rules about what you can do when you get there.

We all started writing letters.

Nicola was home now. She had finished her drama diploma at UCT and was looking for cabaret and acting work in Jo'burg. Oliver, Nicky and I floated. The reprieve was immense. Sometimes we had thought that we would be bound to Danny-the-Disturbed for the rest of our lives.

BIRTHDAY, LETTERS, ASSESSMENT

On his seventeenth birthday, January 24, Danny was allowed to phone us. He sounded fine.

Soon afterwards arrived his first letters:

Dear Mom and Da,

Hi, how the hell are ya? I'm mediocre (that is, as far as I can make out from what they say). Thanks for the cable—I really appreciated it. I had a pretty mean birthday. The kitchen crew (one of the many working forces) baked me a really outrageous heavy metal cake, and I received many well-performed "Happy Birthday"s from my friends and neighbours. Although there's a lot going on here I won't try and tell you everything, never mind absolutely everything. But I will say that I'm surviving, even though I miss home a lot, and there are a lot of rules here, I mean a hell of a lot. I get up at 6.30 every morning and work till about 6 pm apart from 9 o'clock school (which lasts one hour). Life is pretty much a tough fuck-in-the-eye in here, so I'll be expecting a lot of letters. You should be expecting my extra clothes and my tapes, magazines and photo album with my case fairly soon. I'm not allowed these things while I'm at this Treatment stage. This is a bit of a late letter but I've had very little free time. Anyhow write and tell me how you are and what's going on and give my love to any of my friends that you come across and please give my sincere affection to Sandy.

All my love,
Danny

On the back of our letter was one to Nicola:

Funky arse, How you doing big sister? Life's pretty rough in this mother fuck of therapeutics not much to talk about really. I'm in amongst a community of convicts, drug addicts and prostitutes basically. I now know a lot of people I can relate to, which is very important in this conditional structure of ball-busters. The programme is shit-strict. It is inevitable that you get into a lot of deep raps with a lot of people. I get criticized a hell of a lot and I get myself into a lot of trouble all the time. This place is a wheel of harsh generalization and fuck-all sympathy for anyone. My closest buddy is a cat called Griff—he's the son of Ryan O'Neal and he sleeps on the bunk underneath me. Me and him really get on well. He's also a hell of a jazz-pianist. We hit it off. But my action is spread, I get on well with many people. Big "Wat's-op?" to Bob [Nicola's boyfriend], but time is short, so

Gby my darling sis. Love ya lots, Write soon. IT'S NEEDED
Danny xxx

The next day came a psychological report from Habilitat. There were no doctors at Habilitat. Those whom Danny calls "doctors" in his letters are simply those in charge—and who all are in fact former residents who have completed the Habilitat course. But all residents had an initial psychiatric evaluation from a Honolulu psychiatrist, Dr Cooper. Danny was seen on January 31.

Here are some excerpts:

Daniel states that he came because of a drug problem as well as the need to do some serious thinking away from his natural environment. He gives a history of a rebellious, periodically self-destructive and confused youth.

Daniel presents as a tall and somewhat awkward youth who appears somewhat older than his stated age of seventeen. He is pale-complected, has close cropped hair and some acne, but relates in a rather mature manner with a deep, resonant voice and rather sophisticated intellectual processes that he likes to show off. He's oriented, not psychotic; there is no evidence of a thought disorder, organicity or affective disturbance. His affect is serious and somewhat superior; his mood guarded but basically friendly. He has a fair amount of intellectual insight and judgement is intact.

Though one would think that the therapy of first choice would be outpatient, individual therapy, this seems not to have worked because of this youth's strong, impulsive nature. I would certainly recommend, therefore, a "cooling off period" of some months in Habilitat while he detoxifies himself and decides what he wants to do in life.

RUNNING AWAY

Danny had asked repeatedly, "Can I come back if I don't like it?" I was uncomfortable with that question, because of course we were ambivalent. If he was in a reasonable state of mind when he was over there we wanted him to stick it out. So in answer to that question we had shrugged, or said "we'll see"—but in his mind it was a definite "Yes".

We made sure that Guy had taken his return air-ticket from him so that he couldn't easily and impulsively get home.

It was February. We thought all was well. But we were also lucky to have received Dr Cooper's report which told us that he was fine. Danny phoned us up. He had decided to come home! Luckily Oliver was there at the phone to talk to him and we took turns, listening to him, but in the end saying that we wanted him to stay. Danny got emotional, but not mad. He said that we had promised him that he could come home if he didn't like it. We said no.

Soon after this he simply walked out, but changed his mind somewhere along the road. It was a long walk to Honolulu. It would take him many hours, and when he got there he would know no one and have no money. So he turned round on the sandy road and walked back again.

I don't know how or when we heard about this, but we did get another letter from Danny:

Dear Folks,

Hello, how's everybody doing? I hope you're all doing pretty good huh? Well I hope so. I'm pretty isolated right now. Literally? Probably just as much as being far away from home, away from you and my friends and my girlfriends and my music and my life in Jo'burg as the "Sheathed guitarist" (muze with his head in a bag). I am on a dishpan. I suppose you think that's funny? Well it ain't. I'm in isolation for over 30 days, only being allowed to speak with certain people called older residents, who are in my treatment group. I can rap to about 6 of these male treatment older residents a day, for up to 20 minutes each, after which they write a resident behaviour slip on me. The dishpan, or "situation" is hard core grind, more than organized therapy. It is full time work, from when I've finished eating breakfast, attended a "morning meeting" (a mere privilege) and come out of school, the time then being 10 am, till dinner. After that I go on a "shit squad" and work till midnight. Then I dream like a mad poet till 7am. My foolish quest for freedom during the house-ban brought me a shaved head. This move rendered me a space cadet swinging on puppet strings, contemplating the eternal war of self-righteousness, as well as manic climatic conditions, like malaria of the skull. But now I'm vibing on solitary occupational therapy. Like a solid principle with no scope. It's sort of like we got nothing to look forward to, I've had all my responsibilities taken away from me. You must know what it's like. I wonder if you could try to send me my bass, my photo album and some Weather Report tapes. Even if I don't get them yet I still know that they will be there after my month has passed, because I by then I will be an older resident, and I'm entitled to some things. If in doubt, speak to my doctor, Bobby Furtado.

If you're interested, I wrote a song, but of course I cannot work on it. I can't even read it over to myself, for my "situation" is my job. It is a serious trend. I cannot smile, sing, dance, play, vibe or anything. Time is of the essence, please try and relate to that. But—write to me even if you think it sucks. Tell my friends and lovers that I love and miss them, for I hang in.

Tell Mark to hang loose for I cannot write letters to everyone, but tell him to write to me again when he can. I love him and his letter was amazing. Regards to anybody you can find. Tell Bob to feed my bear and hang loose!

Vasbyt,
Danny

P.S. I've established quite a cult singing Robbie's song, "The Spell", I even jam it for the doctors! If you're interested, here's a chant sequence done by most of the working crews for motivation in the mornings:

Shout!
Come on now
Shout!
Ev-ery-body
Shout!
Come <u>on</u> now
Shout!
Get down and
Shout!

FROM HABILITAT

February Report from Habilitat
Daniel is presently working in the Service Crew. Here, along with his crew members, he is responsible for the general upkeep of our facility. Daniel is also given the time to make some new friends who will be helpful when he is going through difficult times here.

Daniel does have a difficult time in the programme; he often thinks about the activities he used to be involved in at home and still wants to live *that type of life. Hopefully, Daniel will take the advice given him seriously so that he may return home and lead a productive life.*

Robert Furtado. Coordinator

March Report from Habilitat

Daniel is presently working in the Maintenance Crew, where he and the crew are responsible for the landscaping and the general upkeep of the facility.

Daniel has been having a difficult time getting along with a few of the residents, which is attributed to his lackadaisical attitude that he carries at times.

Robert Furtado. House Coordinator

Letter from Habilitat

Danny has made tremendous improvement in his attitude. In the beginning it was touch and go, as he felt that he had been tricked. The phone call he placed devastated him because he honestly believed that you would send him his plane fare back home. When the reality set in, he lashed out at people here; I placed him on a limited disciplinary situation which gave him time to evaluate his position and decide what he was going to do. Danny is a talented and creative young man; he has the whole world of music open to him and his only downfall at present is himself. At times, he does not relate about his inner feelings or share his thoughts. He has a very difficult time asking for help, but hopefully, with time, he will make the necessary changes in his behaviour.

The most unfortunate thing about Habilitat is that we cannot guarantee Daniel's success—it is totally up to him.

Joaquin Camacho. Facility Director

April Report from Habilitat

Daniel was recently given a job change to the Kitchen Crew, which we all affectionately refer to as the "hot spot" of the facility. With a crew of 5 to 6 other residents, not only does he have to prepare 3 meals a day for approximately 110 people, get them out on time, help with the clean up in between meals, but he must also maintain a good attitude. This is basically designed to encourage a resident to use the tools of the programme as an outlet for frustration.

It is hard for Daniel to maintain a serious attitude about what he is doing, which is not unusual at his age. In the past month, however, he has been making a conscious effort to take a look at himself and do what is expected of him. All in all, Daniel is a likeable guy and has made many friends here.

Robert Furtado. House Manager

May Report from Habilitat
During the month of May, Daniel continued as a member of the Kitchen Crew, but due to his laziness and his tendency to take his responsibilities lightly, he was placed in a limited situation. This means that he was relieved of all responsibilities and given time to think, correct his mistakes and take steps to improve in the areas that are hard for him. It is also an opportunity to strengthen his established friendships, as well as make new ones. We hope that Daniel will take full advantage of this situation so that upon the return of his regular responsibilities, his behaviour is up to par.

Edward D'Agosta. Habilitat Representative

And an undated letter from Danny:

Dear Mom, Dad and Nicky,
Basically, the story goes: My older brother in the programme, Robin, split somewhere near the end of February for various misdeeds. Robin's in jail at the moment. Anyway, Joaquin, the assistant director, became my shelter and serenity from thereon. The "isolait" I was referring to in my last letter ended a couple of weeks ago. It was 12 days long. Now I'm on a shit squad, which isn't half as bad really for it's only from 5 pm till midnight, although it's still work more/think less. This time round was for a minor thing that really didn't take anything from my role-modelship (aristocratic genius with solid community principles) because it had nothing whatsoever to do with me. I haven't been doing too badly myself. I went to see movies last weekend at Kailua—really cool. Please write and tell me if you're going to come and visit, or whatever, and send me my bass and some guitar picks whatever it takes, please, please, please—thanx!

Love you lot a whole lot,
Danny

Chapter Thirteen

HAWAII AND HOME

LUCY VISITS HAWAII

One evening in May came a glorious phone call from warm Betsy: "He's doing well enough! You can visit him in June. He's calming down a little—listening a little bit more. I think he's accepted that he has to stay. He plays guitars whenever he is allowed to."

On my way to Hawaii I visited my old friends in London. They had only known Danny before he turned three:

Gill: I remember him screaming from teething and then stopping completely when Oliver played his guitar to him.

Irene: I remember him being independent, and much less demanding than other toddlers of his age.

George: Oliver was someone who did his own thing, regardless. I rather envied him. I did not think at the time that this would be "bad" for Daniel.

After London I was far away from anyone who had even known Danny. I went to three weekend poetry-writing courses in Devon, and in between them I went to Bath and to St Ives. Disturbed Danny and disturbed South Africa were gone from my mind.

In Devon the mood was light and lively. I sat under a tree in the garden and was transfixed by the song of a blackbird, forgetting to listen to the tutor discussing a poem. That evening a student read out a poem she had written about me coming from South Africa and listening to the blackbird.

Back in London I had a phone call from Oliver. "We are all missing you so very much!" I felt guilty because I hadn't been missing home at all.

In San Francisco I stayed in a motel. I loved the town so much that I thought of postponing my visit to Hawaii by two days so as to see the re-opening of the cable-cars. But Danny had focused so long on the date of my arrival that I felt I simply couldn't delay.

The day of my departure was Thursday 21 June, which an announcer called "the first day of summer". The San Francisco people looked very happy with themselves. On my way to the airport I saw a graffito: "Eat, drink and be merry—for tomorrow you may have to go to Oakland" (an industrial town near by).

On the plane to Honolulu the huge Hawaiian sitting next to me said, "The Japanese *own* the island. I hate it now. I live in San Francisco. Japanese and Americans sell: Hawaiians remember."

Later he quoted an American professor who had said that Hawaii was "an unsinkable aircraft carrier in the middle of the Pacific".

As we were landing he pointed out Pearl Harbour.

And all the time I was thinking, "How will it be?"

At Honolulu as I walked out from the luggage area I saw the Habilitat sign being held up. I was met by giant black Nathan, the chief chef, and Bill, a three-month resident from Chicago, who had to go with Nathan everywhere. And by Danny. Danny looked open and relaxed and no longer a compulsive, driven boy.

We hugged. "You look good," I said.

"So do you. Surprisingly good in fact."

"Well I've had this little holiday."

Danny said he was getting used to things now. He was now a "concierge"—or "bell-boy". He ran messages and kept an eye on things.

They dropped me off at my hotel in Honolulu and went back over the mountains to Kaneohe Bay. I phoned Betsy at Habilitat. "He's a really nice kid," she said.

Honolulu and Habilitat are both on Oahu Island, but Honolulu is in the south and Habilitat is in the north. It is over an hour's drive from one to the other.

Friday: I'm waiting for them to fetch me to take me to Habilitat. They got lost bringing me here last night and now I think are lost again. I'm in a maze of apartment blocks—endless repetitive rectangles—all the same height—all beige-coloured. From my room I can see no mountains or sea, just more flats. This is a hotel, but it looks just like another apartment block. But on the way to breakfast I had a surprise! I walked out of the lift to find a narrow, wooden bridge to be crossed, over water with giant, exaggerated, mega-goldfish swimming along. They are big carp, but have the colour and look of tiny goldfish.

Danny wasn't with the driver who came to fetch me, so I was looking forward to simply enjoying the drive over the mountains. But these were the ugliest mountains I've ever seen: shapeless hills with nibbles taken out of them.

On the other side of the hills were scattered single-roofed houses and then a view of the sea—and then Habilitat, which is an old house with new buildings around it: it all looks pleasant enough.

When I walked into the entrance hall there was Danny answering the phone, which is his current job. It was a great joy to see him working.

When I walked into the quad I was overwhelmed by the large numbers of young men standing around, some with shaved heads; a large number of people in a small space; like a prison or perhaps a holiday camp, since they wear casual clothes. Then they all came up to me and said it was great to meet me, and I had to smile and smile and say, "Yes, the island is wonderful," and "Yes, Danny is wonderful." So I sort of accept their view that it is like one great family.

Danny comes across as self-contained, neither manic nor depressed. His thinking is clear. He doesn't spit or shout or swear, but at this stage there is a certain blandness about his goodness. Sometimes he slips into that old way of looking at me—staring in a far-away gaze, as if "thought-reading".

He said he had a headache from his job, which involves standing all day, and concentrating on getting things right.

He smokes 10 x 20 cigarettes per week—everyone's ration. Everyone smokes.

(Well that seems monstrous now! Did I get it right? 200 cigarettes a week? He now says he doesn't think it was that many. But now is 2007 and then was 1984.)

Saturday: Today was very successful. Danny was granted an outing. He and Benny arrived at about 11. Danny phoned up from reception in a clear, confident way; then we went to famous Waikiki and found an inexpensive lunch; then we all swam from a stony beach. Not that Waikiki is impressive. Could be anywhere. Beach and sea are flat and stretch for miles. No huge Hawaiian waves and surfers.

Danny does not natter on in that unrealistic way. But he does not really open up with me, so there is not much to talk about. I usually talk to the escorts—two of them have been 29 years old.

The only problem is that Danny does his "mind-reading" with me—stares at me as if hallucinating. He was not doing this before he left home. I associate it more with the first year of his breakdown.

His greatest joy today was to come back to the hotel with Benny and me and have a smoke and *hot* tea and watch some good TV.

Danny was about to take his "Grade 12" final school exams. This made very little sense to me. I could only assume that the standard was very low, and that no syllabus work was required. He had been doing only one hour a day in school. But I felt that he was getting a superb education in community living, psychology, personal development, personal organization, group organization, counselling and so on.

Sunday: I had a lovely relaxed time at Habilitat this afternoon. When I arrived they were all sitting in rows in the courtyard in the sun. Lots of shaved heads and yellow/white skins. Then the 20 school graduates arrived in their deep blue gowns and hoods. To music. Short speech by their teacher Claudia: the pleasure of working with them; what she has learnt from them. Then the mayor: "We did not have to face the world of drug-pushers; you have decided to overcome your problems; and you will be better parents for having gone through the experience."

The graduates were called up one by one. Great applause and shouts for some. Less for others. Each one was given a diploma and a hug, and then a boy (about nine years old) put a "lei" (garland) on. For the first few he tried to put the lei over the hood. The rest took their hoods off to be garlanded.

Griffin O'Neal, Danny's friend (Ryan's son, Tatum's brother), was one of the graduates. He has been here a year and has just been promoted to the next stage which is Re-entry.

Afterwards we had eats, and Danny introduced me to everyone who passed by—all with the air of being "best mates". Most had limp handshakes.

Monday: I was fetched again. At Habilitat I talked to Joaquin Comacho, the Facility Director, in his lovely office overlooking Kaneohe Bay. "Daniel is very, very lazy," said Joaquin. (My heart sank; the primary problem; long before his breakdown. But all this "work" he has been doing!) "He is gifted, an individualist—an artist. I get through to him *while* he plays his music. He's very well liked. And he's definitely not mad—just eccentric."

I said I was surprised about the "thought-reading". Joaquin felt it was LSD-connected, since he had thought like that too as an after-effect of taking LSD. He called Danny in.

Joaquin (very cool): So Danny, how does it feel, having your mother here?

Danny: OK.

Joaquin: Just "OK"? She comes all the way from South Africa ...

Danny: Oh she's been staying in London with her ex-boyfriend ...

Lucy (laughing): And his wife! Danny—d'you think you can read my thoughts?

Danny: How d'you mean?

Lucy: You used to do it, and then Jeff cured you by taking you out of the room and showing you that you couldn't in fact read my thoughts.

Joaquin: If I could read your thoughts, Danny, it would save me a lot of bother.

Danny (sheepishly grinning): I was just trying to manipulate her.

And that was that. He never did it again.

After this meeting I went for a walk, glad I didn't have to stay in the sort-of prison myself. I went to the edge of the bay and saw old boats, old cars and wooden bungalows. In this outside world I watched some all-race baseball and some all-race car-fixing. It seems the least race-

253

conscious place in the world. At Habilitat most residents seem at first to be white American males in their twenties, but then you start to see Hawaiians and African Americans, and a few women.

Danny says he is friends with a brother and sister who are younger than he is, Joby and Shay. They are there not because of drugs or crime but because they are orphans. There is also a married older couple—in their 40s, who had come off the rails because of drug use.

I stayed on into the evening. After supper Griffin and Quintin and I sat in the piano room and Danny played. Then Griffin and Danny played, Griffin telling Danny what to do. Then Danny played Griffin's synthesizer silently with head-phones.

Griffin said to me, "He goes mad when he doesn't have his music. He should come back to L.A. with me."

Griffin is dynamite. He went off to find me lava and came back with an emu stone. Then he found me flowers to smell. But he doesn't even know the year he is born—told me it was 1967, same as Danny, but in fact he was born in October 1964, so is nearly 20. Griffin thinks that South Africa is at the bottom of South America.

Danny walked out with me to say goodbye. Someone shouted, "Hullo Danny's mother! So what d'you think? Has he changed?"

That was the fiftieth time, so I just laughed and said, "Of course".

Danny asked me, "So what d'you think Ma? Do you like these changes?"

I didn't know what to say.

He was altogether more relaxed and free today. He is proud to be there and tells me things about it. The girl on the desk said, "He's a good kid—doesn't give any trouble," and Danny grinned bashfully.

The Hawaiian who took me back said his family life and youth had been perfectly normal, but he got a job as a bartender on the tourist boats which cruise between the islands. The guests were always standing him to drinks and finally that became a problem for him. "Seven days a week work and partying." He booked himself into Habilitat and is paid for by "Welfare".

Tuesday: It's a dictatorship of the older residents. I am taken out by those who have too much to lose by defecting. I can leave my bag with them knowing that they will not steal my money, whatever they have been charged with in the past.

Mike brought Danny to Honolulu today and we went again to the flat Waikiki beach. Danny and Mike swam out to the rocks. Then I swam out to the rocks and swam across a deep channel and reached the first little waves.

Danny asked me, "Did you reach the waves?"

"Yes, the first ones."

So then, not to be outdone, he and Mike had to swim out again to reach the waves! They stayed out there for a long time talking. I wondered whether they talked about drugs when they were so safely out of hearing. This is an absolute taboo at Habilitat.

Wednesday: I was fetched to Habilitat. My driver was mixed Hawaiian and American. He asked lots of questions about my home town. His brother works in the outside world as a waiter. A simple guy—yet clear about "the programme" and the issues. He said that Danny has a short attention span and can't always concentrate. I was sad, but on reflection I thought that this guy was the only one who had registered Danny's cognitive weakness. (And Habilitat later gave him unmanageable tasks because they had not.)

We arrived and ate. I was ravenous. Chicken and veg and salad and canned peaches. The food is basically good. White flour products and white rice of course—but lots else besides.

Griffin came to sit with us. Griffin told Danny to tell me what was worrying him.

Danny hesitated and then mumbled, "… not sure you love me."

"Danny. How can you not be sure? Of course we do!"

"Let's go somewhere private to discuss all this," said Griffin.

We went to the piano room but there were others there. Paddy took me up to see the girls' dorms. She was 32 and very articulate; she had been at Habilitat two months. She showed me three dorms:

> Treatment: nothing at all on the drawers
> Re-entry: drawer tops half full (with photos and ornaments and personal things).
> Post-re-entry: drawer tops completely full.

We watched a movie on TV—Griffin and Danny and I. Danny restless—without cigs. He got a cigar from Front Desk. He has finished his weekly supply of cigs two days early.

Griffin felt that Danny was in a bad state. Well, if this is *bad*!

The three of us went outside by the low wall overlooking Kaneohe Bay. I tried to do a gumboot dance for Griffin. Danny remembered a few Zulu words. Danny and I sang Nkosi Sikelel'i—well I sang it and Danny pretended to.

Griffin said that Re-entry was actually more difficult than Treatment. More was expected of you.

Somehow the "issue" starts up:

"You can't deny that you said I could come back after three weeks!" said Danny, bitterly.

"Danny, listen to me a moment," said Griffin. Danny keeps interrupting, but Griffin holds his ground. "*My* mother just pretended she was taking me out to buy something and then she took me to the mental home!"

Danny got very excited—swore at me a lot. Griffin protested. I worried lest Danny jump or fall off the low wall into the sea. But he calmed down.

Griffin introduced me to his two "younger brothers". He was a "role model" to them. Then he explained to me about "The Game": it can be announced at any time. One person is the victim and the others say what they think of him. But only the bad things!

We sat down near the wall. I talked about the "too good" upbringing Danny had.

"Well I'm very glad you made everything good for me in my childhood," said Danny. "It's remembering my childhood that keeps me going. After all some people did think I was OK then (looking at me for reassurance)—I mean—Terry and so on."

"But I wouldn't leave now you know," Danny continued. "I've got my buddies here and everything. And I know you love me or you wouldn't be visiting me. There's no *reason* why I think you don't love me. It's just a frightening dream."

All except Griffin seem sexless. Because of the shaved heads a lot of them do look a bit like prison inmates. The girls keep completely separate.

During the week they acquire good points. If they have enough of them then they can have a Saturday treat. For Danny it's a difficult choice between sushi, which he has come to love, and playing a guitar for the evening.

It is evening food time—cake and fruit and tea. People put on pounds of weight here. Many need to. But there is also a club for "fatties".

This was "goodbye" to Habilitat, since Danny is coming out with me tomorrow. Griffin gives me a big hug and kiss at the entrance. He has also rounded up about 20 residents whom he leads in "Aloa—ay" which I join in. Like floral jacket shirts, this is an international aspect of Hawaiian culture.

Thursday outing: After all Betsy's worries—that Danny was very restless and might run away—he was completely relaxed and happy. We had no arguments. Neither did we talk, except right at the end.

Keo the Mexican, and Frank the American, were thrilled to be on an outing. As usual they seemed balanced, articulate and grown-up compared with Danny. Frank saw someone he knew on the streets and successfully indicated—by open arms—that he could not talk. Then he met an old girlfriend in the Pagoda, and could not resist talking to her. Keo scolded him.

"But I didn't know how not to. This is a girl for whom I have warm feelings."

Keo shrugged—Frank will get points off.

We struggled to find parking—parked high up in a parking building. When we came to fetch the car I voted to stay on the pavement with Danny—but this was not allowed.

At the hotel Danny had to be "covered" by Keo, even when he went to the toilet. He accepts these rules absolutely. I think he feels very secure at Habilitat.

We found a film we all liked the sound of, which started at just the right time. The film was *The Pope of Greenwich Village*. Warm and funny. It had a young, charming inconsequent Latin boy—had Danny gestures and looked at himself in mirrors as Danny does. I wondered whether Danny identified with him. His cousin, the "Pope", was a worrier.

We got take-aways at Nicks and took them to my hotel room. I phoned Habilitat and got some extra time—they are generous with this.

Frank referred to the *People* article, which all his relatives had seen, and was astounded that I could produce it. This article is recent and is about Griffin's life and about Habilitat. Here is an extract:

> *When Griffin arrived he had to contend with the induction interview—
> an exercise in ego demolition calculated to shake up the newcomer. Says
> Vincent Marino, 45, founder and director of Habilitat, which has 115
> residents (27 female) and a staff of 41 (almost all ex-users): "That's
> where my shocker came, because I thought I had all the answers for
> everybody, as with most of the people that come here." At the end of the
> interview, Griffin was told, "This place is not a democracy. Your only
> right is to walk out of the gate you came in." (Which Griffin had done
> once—and got shaved on return, just like Danny.)*

Danny loves my hotel—wanted to eat here, but accepted that it was too expensive. He does not push for things—seems to have two personalities—the wildly driving one, and the passive one.

In the room he smilingly found a radio programme, lay back on the bed, smoked and drank tea.

I walked to the car with them. Hugs all round. Keo gave me and Danny permission to walk to the entrance with me and we had a lovely alone chat.

"Tell them I love them all very much," said Danny.

"Yes—and I'll tell them how well you are doing."

"Tell them I've got lots of buddies."

And then it was all over. I sat back in the plane, very contented, and allowed myself to be taken home like a parcel.

LUCY'S THREE CAPTIVE MEN

In the time between when I left Habilitat in June, and Nicola's visit there in November, everything seemed fine with Daniel. In the Treatment part of the programme, which was clearly structured and monitored, we had been sent monthly reports. That stage was over. Daniel was in Re-entry, when reports were no longer thought necessary. Nor did Danny write us letters. I remembered Griffin telling me that Re-entry was worse than Treatment because of the concentration and responsibility required. So I worried a bit that Danny would not be able to cope.

From time to time I phoned, and he was allowed my phone calls. From my diary:

August: My Danny is a "facilitator"—really helping out with the newer residents. I'm so proud of him for this. And so happy for him. He says he has fallen in love with one of the new residents, and she with him!
September: I phoned Danny and he sounded terrific. He says Re-entry is great. He has been working in the cookie factory. He is responsible for boxing and labelling all orders to be shipped.
October: They are getting all geared up for Christmas—practising songs and making decorations. Danny has been selling Christmas trees. He is very happy about his bass guitar coming next month with Nicola. Then he'll be able to get a real band going over there.

Meanwhile back at home my life was quite dizzily satisfactory. I was a published writer for the first time. My poems and stories were being published in Lionel Abraham's magazine, *Sesame.* Lionel was a poet, a guru and an editor and we became great friends. He longed to see each new poem I wrote.

Lionel was spastic. Ordinary life was extremely difficult for him. Getting up in the morning was an ordeal. But by the time I arrived on my bicycle with my next poem, he was a quizzical wizard, neat and eager. He lived in a small flat at the end of a quiet dead-end road. As I arrived on my bicycle I could see him sitting there through the open door.

So Danny was captive in Hawaii, and Lionel was captive in Cheltondale. What about Oliver? Oliver rushed in and out, noisy and busy with pupils and pupils' concerts. He was good-humoured because things were going so well with Danny.

I thought: Oliver is very loveable in his enthusiasm and his new freedom from defensiveness. He is now composing pieces for his pupils so we are giving support to each other's creativity. He was critical and dismissive of my poems at first, but now likes them.

Then into this merry life came a shock phone call. Oliver had broken the tendons of his knee in a school accident in which the Standard Six pupils tried to keep him out of their classroom—as a joke. This was at the Afrikaans Arts School, *Die Kruin*, where these kids (the thirteen-year-olds) adored Oliver for being such fun. Oliver was in flip-flops instead of proper schoolteacher shoes, defying convention and twisting his knee.

He went straight to the Milpark Hospital for an operation. I was waiting in his ward when he was wheeled back in, but he had difficulty coming round. I coaxed and rubbed him back to consciousness and got him to sing through his oxygen mask, until finally he said, "Give me a kiss,"—a most unusual thing for him to say!

I enjoyed looking after him back home. He was my third captive man. He had never been ill before so I had never had the pleasurable feeling of looking after him. It had always been me who was poorly—and him putting me to bed and making me omelettes and looking after the kids.

Oliver said to some visiting friends, "She's a bloody miracle—she cleans and cooks and deals with urine and ..." I interrupted him, "Keep talking and I might do it for another two days!"

Lionel's poetry book came out: *Journal of a New Man*. Oliver and I both read it:

Oliver said, "He has tremendous spirit. I will take him for my model."

I was doing First Year English through Unisa (our correspondence university). I had decided that if I was going to be a writer I had better catch up on what others had written. I was behind with my studies, what with the overseas trip and other distractions. But Oliver, stuck in bed with his leg in plaster from foot to hip, was marvellous. He understood the poems I didn't, and he read right through Shaw's *The Applecart*, which I couldn't see the point of at all. He said, "I can see that it's not subtle enough for you, but I'm just an ordinary bloke you see, so I can appreciate it."

And then, with no warning, all the euphoria vanished. Lionel went off to Europe with his wife-to-be. Oliver was suddenly in great pain and had to go back to hospital. And there was bad news from Hawaii, where Nicola had just arrived.

I felt very lonely.

THE CULT OF NON-CONFORMITY

Both children had fallen in love with the cult of non-conformity. Anything lucid or sensible or predictable or honest or considerate was labelled "conformist". But what happens when no one is "conforming"? When everyone lets everyone else down?

Conforming to non-conformity lead to chaos, drugs and madness; to heavy criticism leading to massive defensiveness; to accidents and misery and depression.

Nicola had been through all this in her adolescence. In Cape Town at the end of her first university year, her boyfriend had told her not to write her exams. She dumped him and wrote her exams, but still went on believing in impulsiveness and spontaneity.

By 1984, when Daniel was in Habilitat, Nicola had calmed down, although a part of her still wanted to "go mad". She wrote this song:

Other People's music
Other People telling me what's good.
Other People's words
What's bad what's good what's good what's bad
Listen to them and you'll never go mad
Then you'll never go mad.

Once I had a vision what a very dark vision
A vision of death on a swing.
But they pulled me out and they told me "no"
And I couldn't help, couldn't help listening
I couldn't help listening.

Now my life is sweet and sane.
And the clothes that I wear are neat and plain
I never wear crystal or cellophane
And I know that I'm not the same any more
I know that I'm not the same.

Now I have a brother what a very sad brother
He's far away on his own.
Cos he followed his vision and got lost inside,

And I don't think he'll ever come home again,
He's out there all alone.

Well his life isn't sweet or sane
And the clothes that he wears aren't sweet or sane.
And he lives in a palace of cellophane.
And they frequently call him "insane", yes they do,
They secretly call him "insane".

He wouldn't listen to:
Other People's words
Other People's music
Other People telling him what's good what's bad.
Listen to them you'll never go mad,
Then you'll never go mad.

DANNY'S DESPAIR

Nicola, now 22, started her trip in great spirits. She had an exciting week in New York staying with her uncle and aunt. Then she went on to Honolulu and spent a morning at Waikiki before being fetched by two residents who took her to Habilitat, where she was to live for a week, in the girls' dorm.

But meanwhile, unbeknown to us, something had happened to Danny, who at first just seemed not to be working as well as he should be. One of the staff said he was "acting", but another staff member thought he should be seen again by Dr Cooper, the psychiatrist they sometimes resorted to. Habilitat rejected psychiatric labels and medication but sometimes even they were pushed into doing something.

What had happened? It is difficult to be exactly sure, but one thing that had happened was his public exam. He had passed well in the mock exam given to him at Habilitat. But when he looked at the paper for the public exam nothing made sense. He got into a panic state and simply had to walk out. Once his mind started to "go funny" he would have been less able to keep up with the programme, and would have been criticized and put on "dishpans", and even, it seems from Nicola's letter, had his hair shaved again. And slipped even further into despair and out of gear.

While writing this part of the book in 2007 I asked Nicola what she remembered of her trip and here is the letter she wrote to me.

I find that it is distressing and painful to think about this time. My chest goes so tight I find it hard to breathe. I have blocked a fair bit of it out and so I am not even sure that my memories are correct. This is what I think I remember:

Hawaii was boiling. The famous Waikiki beach was literally crawling with drug pushers. I think I was offered dope at least three times in an hour. I travelled over the mountains to Habilitat. I was looking forward to seeing Danny and hoping he was well. When I got there, he was outside. He was terribly thin and his head was shaved. I think he was smoking a lot (cigs). I was utterly shocked at his condition. He was unable to make eye contact. He kept laughing inappropriately. He couldn't communicate with me or initiate any conversation although he seemed pleased to see me. He had told the other inmates I was coming because they knew who I was and seemed friendly. I also remember that they knew his name and called out to him every now and then. He seemed to have quite a few people who liked him. So he must have been functional enough for some of the time. He told me about "dishpans" which I think was some sort of punishment. He was talking to himself and muttering intensely at this time. How the authorities there didn't put him under medical supervision is completely beyond me when he was so obviously ill.

They let me take him to see a Prince movie called Purple Rain (High profile guitarist/musician) and I seem to remember that he enjoyed it and laughed a lot to himself. In retrospect perhaps it was a bad choice but at the time the only thing I felt I could relate to him about was music, as that was his soul.

I don't remember anything else except the journey home on the plane where he put the blanket over his head and talked to himself so loudly that people started asking me if I needed help and what should they do? I was completely out of my depth. I had no idea what to do or how to help him. He was obviously in terrible pain and distress and nothing I could do or say helped him to calm down. I felt so sorry for him but had so little understanding of why he was like this.

Just before Nicola arrived, Danny had seen Dr Cooper again—the psychiatrist who had first evaluated him and had then said that Danny was "oriented, not psychotic and no evidence of a thought disorder". Here is his second report:

This individual is being seen at the request of the staff because of his increasingly bizarre activity. He came to Habilitat as the result of a supposed drug problem.

Over the past 9 months he seems to have been fairly stable until more recently, at which time he was observed to exhibit bizarre behaviour, such as talking to non-existent persons and rambling incoherently. He's under no court pressure and when seen today states that he feels overly stressed; that he really feels that he needs at least some days to be relieved of Habilitat's responsibilities and, hopefully, to return to a more centered position.

He has maintained contact with his family via the phone over the past month and states that his family, though supportive, still exert pressure on him to finish the Habilitat programme.

When seen today, Daniel seems to be a seriously disturbed individual trying desperately to hold on to reality. He makes evasive, intermittent eye contact and rambles off, manifesting pressured speech, loosening of associations and appearing generally incoherent.

We had not seen this report when Nicola was in Hawaii, and she herself did not know about it. But she was worried not only about Danny's mental state but also that he had large lumps under his left upper arm. Had Danny himself not noticed these? He was probably so living in his head that these lumps, like the rest of the outside world, were scarcely noticed by him. There was a weekly clinic at Habilitat with a qualified nurse, but Danny told us later that there was always a long queue which he seldom thought was worthwhile enduring for the sake of an aspirin.

Nicola wanted to bring him home, and we agreed with her. Habilitat gave her his return ticket and home they came.

While Nicola and Danny were making their way back we received Dr Cooper's report and I phoned him and had a chat. Then he wrote us this letter in November:

I am writing to pass on a few thoughts about Daniel that I wished to convey. I was pressured during our phonecall and later realized I may have seemed abrupt.

Firstly, I would strongly support treatment with lithium and only lithium initially. When it works it is truly miraculous.

Diagnostically, there is some question as to what Daniel is suffering from: some psychiatrists would diagnose schizophrenia and others manic depressive illness. Because the cause of both illnesses is not known one must rely on clinical experience and sometimes try medication empirically to see what works.

Though recognizing that Daniel has been diagnosed as schizophrenic, I personally would see him as more manic depressive, which carries a less bleak prognosis. Therefore find someone who will try lithium in low to moderate doses <u>for months</u> and be guardedly optimistic.

Secondly, don't feel that the months at Habilitat were a total waste. Illegal drugs often complicate the picture so much that it is worth placing adolescents in drug-free environments (and if anything, Habilitat is that!) for months to rule out the possibility of contamination from the outside.

Lastly, though I do feel Daniel has a serious problem, it has been my experience that adolescents, particularly bright and sensitive ones, not infrequently fall apart at Daniel's age, even to the point of becoming psychotic for a while. I have seen such individuals later go on to become totally normal and highly productive people.

My best hopes go out to you both and to Daniel.
Sincerely,
Douglas Cooper

NOVEMBER/DECEMBER

My first diary entry after they returned was as despairing as he was: Poor, poor child. Not delinquent, not on drugs. Yet cannot concentrate, follow through or attend unless helped to. Everything is immediately chaotic here—wads of paper in the loo, hyperactive moving around, strange talking to himself. As soon as I see him, and I hear from Nicky about how he wandered off and got lost at airports when she was seeing to tickets and luggage, I realize with horror and grief that the schizophrenic diagnosis may be right after all. A real mental problem, rather than the manic/depressive situation with its good prognosis. Either way his mind is disorganized.

From the second day back he was on lithium, and stayed on it for the next six months. He was roaring and raging a lot, but not directly at me.

> Diary: We have been interacting for about an hour—me quite bossy—making plans, getting him to help with the rubbish—just keeping him in the world. He is not spitting any more, but has a new and very irritating habit: talking aloud to himself—incessantly. His cousin Hector thinks it's from the dishpans, when he was prevented from talking to most of the inmates, and in particular to his buddies. He could work and he could eat and he was not physically isolated—just conversationally. Now he sits in front of the mirror saying, "You are Daniel; you are Daniel."

He went back to his nice therapist, Sandy, who tried to get him to focus on one task at a time. He has fallen in love with Lisa at Habilitat, a newer resident whom he helped to settle in. Sandy has given him the task of writing her a letter.

"Can you explain that again please," he has been saying to me, instead of pretending to know what I said. His concentration is poor, but he *wants* to think clearly. I suppose he got into trouble at Habilitat for not knowing what he was supposed to do—and that was because he had not focused on the speaker.

I told him I would get him an amplifier as soon as the garage was cleared up. He was astonished by this, having always wanted one but thought we would require much more from him in order to get it. He cleared up well and I gave him the amp.

He had only been back a few days, yet now I was able to write: All joy this morning—dancing around and around. What vitality and magnetism! A born entertainer. He is ecstatic about his "first amp". Gave me a big kiss and said, "I've wanted one since I was six!"

He went to his next Sandy session having done nothing about the "letter to Lisa".

"Sandy says I must go home and force myself to write the letter. She asked me what I had learnt at Habilitat and I said: 'Patience!'"

After three weeks at home and on lithium and seeing Sandy once a week he had finished his letter to Lisa and he asked me for stamps and went off to post it.

Then his cousin Hector came to stay. They would be sharing Danny's room; and in preparation Danny spring-cleaned his room without being told to do it.

My diary: It seems that if everyone is being totally supportive and loving he *can* be perfect. But criticism launches him into disaster. I was talking about the band he walked out of two years ago and whoops, all of a sudden, he was in a complete violent hostile rage against me.

Four weeks after coming home Danny was so OK that when Terry, his old Saheti teacher, phoned and asked if Danny would agree to being interviewed on a television programme about adolescents, I said I'd ask him, and he said yes.

Danny was marvellous on this live TV interview. Terry asked him questions and he replied lucidly and intelligently. He looked ravishing, and was very expressive and alert. He told Terry and South Africa about Esmé and Daphne and Lisa.

Terry: Where do you expect to be in five years time?
Danny: Probably married to Lisa.
Terry: What do you feel about sex?
Danny: Ja well—you know at Habilitat these guys said, "If you want some sex you have to do this and that to earn the right," and I had to explain to them that I was in *love.*
Terry: What about drugs?
Danny: Drugs make you feel powerful and strong and happy. I would like to smoke pot the way my sister does—when she has finished a play.

(Sex at Habilitat: Couples who had proved themselves steady were allowed to have nights out at another Habilitat building where there were empty rooms with mattresses.)

One day he walked out of Sandy's house and came thoughtfully down the path and climbed into my car, saying, "She really helps me clear my mind. I was talking to her about getting Lisa out of Habilitat."

"It's lovely to hear you showing such concern for another human being."

"Ma, that's a wonderful compliment!"

But that night Mark and Hector wouldn't give him pot, and he came home in a manic rage again. I sat next to his bed for a while and his raging quieted a little. It was 1.30 and I realized that it was my birthday. I made us both Milo and went back to his room. I told him it was my birthday and he came and hugged me and we talked for a while. I was 53. He was still 17.

The next day I talked to Hector who said, "I used to have rages just like Danny."

"Why?"

"I just used to feel massive resentment against anyone who prevented me having immediate pleasure."

"So how did you change?"

"Gradually. I gradually realized that I had to take control over my own life."

Hector was 20. He came from an unhappy marriage. He had run away from home and school. But now he seemed centred.

Oliver and I realized that in April we would have been happily married for 25 years. We decided to have a Silver Wedding party. Danny said, "It's a knock-out idea! I'll play with Robbie's band!"

He wanted to phone Habilitat and wish Lisa "Happy Christmas". We said he could but would probably not be allowed to talk to Lisa, who was still in Treatment.

He sounded very lively and strong on the phone to Habilitat. They haven't given his letter to Lisa, but have read it and say it is "very dynamic" and she'll get it in Re-entry. The only thing I feel sad about is Lisa singing carols at a hospital and Danny missing Christmas there.

Meanwhile, he had seen our doctor and a neuro-surgeon for the nerve lumps: they had to come out; and they might be cancerous, but Danny wasn't told this.

He went to the Kenridge Hospital for a few days. While he was there his hero, Robbie Robb, visited him and invited him to come to

Cape Town with the band and be a "roadie". Danny was overwhelmed! "I just couldn't believe that Robbie would come into a hospital and that it was Robbie sitting there and saying these things."

When he came out of hospital I took him Christmas shopping at Pick & Pay. I sat having coffee and he wandered back and forth with presents, playing games with his feet on the squares, or gazing ahead, saint-like.

At home he wrapped the presents and wrote the names in a beautiful script.

"You are a very dutiful mother."

"You've never given so many presents."

"I've never thought so hard about present-giving."

"There must be at least a million people wrapping Xmas presents this afternoon ... Which part of your arm hurts?"

"All of it."

"That's because it was on the nerve. It must be quite rare. I've never heard of it before."

"The Habilitat people say it's because of all the nervous strain. But I feel much happier now. I feel much happier about life in general."

"You're getting tired, my love. Never mind. In the Karoo you can rest and dream."

"I want that so intensely! I want the time to think and think."

The next day he came to me pulling a horrified face: "My bandage slipped and I saw the terrible black and blue wound. Ugh! I never want to see such a thing again."

"Better let me look."

"You'll never stand it!"

I looked. "Imagine Nicky's making a big doll ... and she threads this needle with black thread and makes these stitches."

He smiled and calmed down and looked at it himself.

And the next day he was in the Karoo in the train, all alone, the others having gone ahead.

He had been in real-life situations but with plenty of support. And not too much had been asked of him.

Both children were gone to Cape Town. Oliver was still in plaster but was limping around on crutches for a while every day. His Christmas Day treat was to spend the day in bed. I bought pizzas and we played

Trivial Pursuit. Danny's medical results were taking a long time because of the Christmas season. So we were not jolly.

Danny was in Cape Town being a "roadie" with Robbie's band. Roadies are supposed to carry heavy equipment around, but Robbie knew about Danny's arm, so gave him lighter tasks. However, Robbie did now have to get on with his work so he came across to Daniel as "controlling" and Danny got hostile.

When they returned, Robbie phoned me: "Bruce gave him a slap when he was 'carrying on', and after that his behaviour was perfect. Except that he was lazy about his jobs, and also he talked to himself all night. We called him 'All-Night-Radio'."

One day they had left him to clean up the house. They were angry when they got back that he had done so little. But he said he had spent one-and-a-half hours doing the kitchen and felt he had done a good job.

One of the young women had some nursing skills and she successfully took out his stitches when the date was due.

And back home we got the lab results: clear! And so ended 1984.

Chapter Fourteen

DANNY AT HOME
(AGED EIGHTEEN, 1985)

"I MUST HAVE HOPE"

After the excitement of the arm operation and being a roadie with Robbie's band, Danny was at home with nothing to do—except dream of Lisa. He came to my room and flopped down, looking a bit miserable. "What's going to happen Ma?"

"You are feeling a bit depressed? Well, it shows you are healthy—more in touch."

"There's such a very thin, thin line holding me and Lisa together."

"That's the reality of it. I'm afraid in the end it may not work out."

"How can you *say* that Ma! How can you be so insensitive? I must have *hope*." He continued, "I was on a black wheel. The black wheel was nothingness. The white wheel is love. But I have to be very strong and *defend* myself. If I have no hope I come down through the levels and then suddenly there's nothing."

"You could go back to Habilitat." I said, very mildly.

"They would shave my head and shout at me. There was this guy on 60 days of punishment. But thank you for suggesting it. I do appreciate that very much."

And then suddenly he *wanted* quite overwhelmingly to go back. Oliver and I didn't push him—we didn't even encourage him. We simply listened.

At supper he said, "It's my aim. To become normal and get out of all my mess. You can't help escalating at Habilitat. It's a growth situation. The first time was like jumping out of the frying-pan into the fire. Now it would be like out of the frying-pan on to dry ground." To Oliver he said, "Will you be proud of me if I graduate Dad?"

"Oh boy will I!"

We didn't know how much his calm mood and lucid thinking was due to lithium. Habilitat didn't accept any medication for mental problems.

I phoned Betsy at Habilitat. I tried to persuade her that lithium is a salt and different from a drug but she was not convinced. Then we talked about Lisa. Betsy said, "It may break his heart you know. She has lots of admirers."

I took him to Sandy. Afterwards he said, "She thinks it's an *excellent* idea!"

"What does Lisa look like?"

Danny said enthusiastically, "She looks like you. Like you when you were younger and your hair hung onto your shoulders."

"She's tall then?"

"Yes."

I went to Dr L, the lithium psychiatrist, to ask about other places in case Habilitat won't take him. He said, "You are giving me a double message. You say he is better and yet you want to send him away!"

"Well there doesn't seem to be anything workable for him to do here."

"He could do a correspondence course."

"I don't think he is focused enough to do that."

"*Thousands* do it. Young men in the army do it."

"Yes, but they are very organized types."

"You are full of 'Yes buts'. I don't know who is more in need of treatment, you or your son."

I drove home angry, thinking: There are *gradations* of "betterness" Surely a "behaviour expert" should know that!

At home I phoned Jeff, who had once been our family therapist, but now worked in a residential centre. He had not seen Danny for nearly two years. I often phoned him to tell him about the good things. But this time his approach had totally changed. He had decided that schizophrenia was a biochemical, genetic disorder which could not be cured. Danny had this disorder and we should accept it.

I phoned Sandy, having so far only had Danny's view on what she thought about going back to Habilitat. "Well Lucy," she replied. "It seems to me that he is very positive about this idea. Some of the things about Habilitat he now sees in a new light. And as he says, there is absolutely nothing for him in this town. He is hating lying around doing nothing."

"And Lisa?" I asked her.

"I will try and prepare him for possible disappointment over the next few weeks."

Meanwhile, Oliver and I were enjoying him so much that we hated the idea of him going. I thought: He has a richness of personality, a warmth, an honesty, that gives me strength after I have been with him.

Oliver said, "I think to myself: What would we do if we didn't have Granddad's money? We would just have to do something second-best—send him to a farm or something."

"But a farm in South Africa would be wonderful!" I protested. "You do know that I tried and tried to find something suitable here. Imagine a farm where the kids have structure and no drugs, and instead of dishpans they have animals!"

And singing and dancing, I thought.

Danny found a few things to do at home. He found things stored away:

1. His coin collection. He is amazed at the beautiful coins he has. He is sticking them on his belts.

2. His skateboard

3. His punch bag, which he has attached to the branch of a tree

And I gave him his "Dear Engelbert" diary which he had written at Saheti when he was eleven. "It's excellent!" he said.

I asked him if he minded me telling Hector stories about when he was young. "No," he replied. "No—I don't mind those stories at all. In fact I *like* them. They are so sweet! It's somehow part of my tradition."

Sometimes when we were talking about something he switched to Afrikaans. He seemed happy and relaxed when doing this. He never talked Afrikaans when he was talking to himself or upset.

On a medical aid form our doctor called him "schizoid" and Sandy called him "schizophrenic". I was reading Erikson on adolescence and I thought he just had an adolescent identity problem.

I asked Danny what was the silliest thing he had ever done. He replied, "Oh definitely it was stabbing my leg! I can't believe I actually did that. I was truly fucked up then."

And another day he said, "At Habilitat you just *have* to do things, and you hate it but you get used to it." He added, "I think I'm getting on wonderfully well."

"I think so too. All this doing nothing—and you don't even smoke pot."

"It's self-discipline."

In front of Hector and Toby I said, lightly, "Well it seems that Lisa is a pretty chick—and there are so few women at Habilitat. She may just prefer someone else."

Danny didn't go crazy, simply said, calmly, "It's all experience."

He played at a club, Rumours, as a guest for one night. He got very over-excited before he went but once there he played well.

The next day he did a double tape with himself on guitar and guitar. A duet with himself. He is full of confidence.

Of Lisa he said, "The only thing that can get between me and Lisa is drugs."

One evening Oliver made Chinese and we ate on the porch with Hector's girlfriend, Chantal. I said, "Tell us about dishpans Danny. Are they the only punishments?"

"No, there are contracts. Contracts are *bad*! They have to scrub concrete all day."

"Did you ever have one?" asked Chantal.

"No. I haven't been back to prison. Well, I haven't even been to prison! But people come back from prison two or three times and then there's a general meeting and everyone says what they think this person should have: a contract or two."

When the guests had gone he said to me, softly, "I was scared for ten months. But I won't be scared this time because of Lisa. And Keo is my father—he knows what love is."

Chantal talked to me about a band he had played in with her long ago. "If it was *his* idea and he took the lead, then everything went very well."

Of this same band Danny said: "We were so tight then—and then my life fell apart."

The worst thing for us was when he talked to himself during supper. We tried to control him, and sometimes succeeded. One day he was in a very excited state before dinner. I said to him, "If you want the film money then you must not talk to yourself during supper."

He went outside with a cigarette, then came in and sat quietly. Halfway through the meal he made a slight noise.

"Careful Danny!" I said, cheerfully.

"Thanks for reminding me!"

The next day I was lying on my bed and he came in for a chat. He sat at my desk. He asked, "Why d'you think I controlled my self-talk last night?"

"Because you wanted to go to the movies?"

"Why else?"

"Because you've got a lot of goodwill and you want to try and get completely well."

"Why else?"

I sighed. "I don't know. Listen Danny. Nicky is coming back next Friday and she thinks you have not improved at all. I say, but he doesn't spit or steal money ...' but because of the talking to yourself she thinks you are still mad."

He sat silent at my desk for a long time. I shut my eyes. The rain rained. I realized that the answer to the other "Why else?" was of course "Lisa".

Oliver said to me, "Basically he's winning. He returned my tools all neatly, and he apologized for leaving his things in the studio."

One night I put my arm round him and read poetry.

Danny said, "I'm interested. Please read me more."

"Do you do any literature at Habilitat?"

"I can't remember. On Friday *ons sit in die groot kamer* (we sit in the living room, and we do projects—he explains—all in Afrikaans)."

Nicky came home. She talked alone to him. To me she said, "He is *amazing*! We had a two-hour completely lucid chat."

But two days later she was fed up. "When he made an *effort* on Sunday he was wonderful. Now he's just a brat."

Lucy's diary: Danny thrives in a one-to-one situation with a dynamic person and clear goals and lots of warmth and encouragement. Without this he easily slips into a state where he is not in touch with the world.

He resents tasks imposed on him, but seems unable to think through the steps needed to carry through a task of his own.

If he is caught up in a fever of excitement he can for a few days work on his own goals—like the time he taught himself bass guitar when he was still only fifteen and it was after his breakdown.

This was written at the end of February. We decided to have our Silver Wedding at the end of March and then send him back to Habilitat in April.

WALLA WALLA WALLA

Following "Doing Nothing" in February, what would he do in March? Everyone was getting nervous. Then Nicky found a place for herself and a group to play and sing at the end of March. She invited Danny to join her band.

The question now was would he be able to play simple music with Nicky's band? Hector described how in the past Danny had played a most complex piece with Mark's band, but got bored when asked to do something simple.

Nicky said, "I know what happened to Danny. He modelled himself on Robbie. Robbie was his god. I fell in love with Robbie and didn't take any notice of Danny, but Danny always wanted to be in my room." (This was when she was fifteen and he was ten.) "I showed Danny off to my friends."

Hector said, "Yes, I did that too."

I decided to prepare Danny for this new situation of simple music and fitting in—that's all. So I said to him, "You won't be any sort of star with Nicky's band."

"I know that. I'm doing it to help Nicky out and to get some money."

So far so good. I hear Danny's energetic plucking and Nicky's whoops!

Nicky's friend Natalie came. She was singing with Nicky in this band. Of Danny she said: "Such energy! I'm going to start creative workshops to channel people like Daniel."

Apart from the emotional hurdle of playing simple music, there was the more mundane problem of whether he would be able to concentrate—to keep focused?

Danny said, "I've got it all sussed out how I'm going to concentrate (and he mimed holding his bass and focusing). And I know how I'll dress up."

He had a good rehearsal with them. We breathed again.

"Are you proud of me?"

"Yes, very!" I replied.

"Will you come and see me?"

"Of course!"

He watched me doing the census at the kitchen table.

"What's this—oh, the census."

"Ja. What shall I say you are?"

"Just say: temporary musician and indirect scholar."

Too much casual criticism could throw Danny immediately out of focus. I told Oliver to be an arch-diplomat over the electric equipment—show him how to handle it as if he was five and Oliver his adoring dad. Now Danny is sitting on the steps and soldering his leads. Doing a careful, delicate job.

But something went wrong in the next rehearsal and Nicky said she couldn't use him. Danny accepted it calmly from her—but later I heard him raging in his room.

"Are you disappointed?" I asked him.

"I'm not disappointed. I just want to cry."

He took it out on his punchbag—jumping and back-kicking it. Then he walked in a straight line, head down, along a row of bricks, flattening each foot and then leaning on the outside of it, then back again in the same way. Then running from a distance to punch the bag. The punches were sometimes weak and accompanied by quick hugs—then strong—then spinning it round on its metal chain. I watched from the kitchen where I was clearing up.

Nicky relented and said he could play in four numbers, but that he must practise his part. This he seemed unable to do.

Then the first night: We arrived at "Quavers", the venue. Danny was standing at the entrance talking to two old friends. He looked very good—in a hat and a bow tie and three metal belts. He also looked very pale. Then I saw Nicky: "You can take him back with you," she said, and then they played a set without him and I thought he was out of it again.

Then I saw him walking up. He played the second set with them—beautifully strong and controlled. It sounded good and he looked good. Afterwards he was congratulated by everyone.

In the car he said: "I worked out how I could do a few little things within Nicky's framework."

"Well I think you kept it well under control and made things more interesting."

But the next time he played with them Nicky said he had friends there who encouraged him and it got a little out of hand, as when he played his little personal bits *while* Nicky was singing.

Danny said to me, "It's different for me. It's not my group. I'm ashamed to play that pop stuff. You know I always hated cover numbers."

His identity was tied up with his friends and with pot and with his own freely improvising style of music.

Danny and I had started having sessions together to air difficult issues. I'll explain this more fully in the next section.

We explored the problems of playing with Nicky:

"At Quavers while I was waiting I met a couple of buddies and we went outside to smoke. Then Nicky came and accused me and we had an argument."

"Just to clarify: By "smoke" do you mean dope?"

"Ja"

"So what was wrong with that?"

"I smoked knowing that Nicky would freak out."

Nicky had to handle his not conforming to what she needed him to play and now there was this dope-smoking as well. Danny and I went on with our session:

"I was a little boy with a locked body. I needed to be comforted. It can't be sorted out. It can't be helped. Until that emotion goes I'm like a little child hit by an electric storm. I really had very little dope. But I know it's too much for Nicky. She gets tense and hostile. But I would have handled her hostility better if I hadn't smoked dope. I can't play for Nicky any more. I'm just too much worry for her."

So that was that. He stopped playing with her.

Nicky and I had a chat about it. She said, "When he was five he was our musician at the Brewers (neighbours). We asked him to play flamenco and he would start—and then he would change to 'Walla Walla Walla' soon afterwards. So he couldn't listen even then."

"SESSIONS"

Sandy, his therapist, had always been supportive to Danny by focusing on him in the present, which had worked well. But now she had a theoretical idea that she should take him back to his childhood, "when he made all those wrong decisions". Danny started to find the Sandy sessions heavy-going. Instead of working with his life-affirming elements in the now, he had to go backwards.

"I don't know what's got into Sandy," he complained.

"Well her idea now is that you have to face the pain of the past."

"But why should I do that? It's very dangerous. I was very confused!"

And I, having been in empathy with him in his paranoiac phases, would also not like to go through those times again.

Sandy said this form of therapy would take five years! So we said we would rather leave that method for the moment. We had the excuse that he was soon going back to Habilitat, but we also thought it an unlikely road to full functioning. I thought it was doing small good steps in the present and having them acknowledged which built up his confidence. Certainly he needed to be treated as younger than he was—but in a positive way. He still went to Sandy once a week but just for friendly support and facing up to the fact that Lisa might not want him.

At home he would slip into a defence/attack mood if any emotionally difficult material was brought up, even if in a non-critical way. So I thought of an answer:

Lucy: I'll motivate you to have a non-aggressive session with me.
Danny: How?
Lucy: Ten rand.
Danny (immediately eager): OK!
Lucy: The rules are no attack, no defence, and no talking to yourself.

We had a lucid chat about the Ten Commandments and then I gave him his ten rand.

In another session we talked about why he worked at Habilitat and tried to avoid it at home.

Lucy: Why do you work at Habilitat?

Danny: We discussed that last time.

Lucy: You said it's because there's this massive force?

Danny: Ja.

Lucy: What was different from working for Robbie in Cape Town. when they criticized you?

Danny: Oh Habilitat's quite different. There's no fear. For instance if I was on a Dishpan and then Keo told me to go round to the garden at the back and work out a project—and I dug a hole—and then Keo came and said, "That's not what I meant by a project!" and then he put me on a dishpan for another week.

Lucy: Nicky says, "Why doesn't he just ask?" See if you can't get more idea what they expect you to do.

Danny: On mostly I just do work at Habilitat because it's a completely different world.

A lot of our chats were to help him be more organized and reliable. He wrote notes to himself for the next day, and even set his alarm clock on one occasion.

Lucy: What will you actually do this evening?

Danny: Come in late—the house will be empty—I will be aware of vague shadows entwining my path to my ultimate destiny. Organizing yourself can make you a happier person. It can mean that you're the most innovative guy in town. I can see Jimmi Hendrix at his writing desk with lamplight, with his black ink feather pen. He's an original guy and he's organizing his own life.

Lucy's diary: He still lives in his head unless he has a strong motive not to.

On the problem of not working when there were things to get done:

Lucy: What would you say to a ten-year-old to get him to do some work?
Danny: "Just do it! You know you can summon up the incentive."
Lucy: What is going on when you don't listen to Nathan the chef at Habilitat?
Danny: I'm in a dream world.
Lucy: What's happening to your dream world?
Danny: It can be saved for when I'm out of Habilitat with Lisa.

In none of these sessions we were having was he "half-asleep" or "not there". He said he liked the sessions and often asked for them. In one of them he said, "I must not do things which would make me less available to my own control."

Another day there was another summing up. He said, astonished, "It's about insights!"

I didn't at first mention these sessions to Oliver. Paying Danny was of course embarrassing to mention!

Danny: Hey Dad! I earned R10
Oliver: How?
Danny (looking at me): What must I say?
Lucy: Well leave it for now. Let's say it's a secret.
Oliver: Now you've really got me curious!

I told my therapist friend about these paid sessions:

Friend: Only don't think it's "therapy", that's all.
Lucy: Oh well, I shall think it what I choose.

Uncooperative behaviour still happened:

Lucy's diary: Nicky's car stuck at Raedene. I asked Danny to come with me. He stood in the kitchen giving every sort of glib reason why he couldn't. I went off feeling pure hate. A foreigner and his two young sons pushed me. I felt great goodwill towards them. When I came in again, Danny said, "Sorry Ma."

The money he earned from the sessions he spent on records. For the first time since being back he did some reading—of the backs of the record covers. One day when the post came he said, "Are there any magazines?" There weren't any in the post but I fetched some old ones.

"Hey!" shouted Danny, "This is the magazine we weren't allowed to read! (About Griffin and Habilitat)."

He took it into the garden and read it.

Another activity outside his head was sewing. He was sewing designs on his jeans.

Planning for Habilitat and the Silver Wedding plus these sessions brought out the best in him. He did chores more willingly.

Lucy: Your helpfulness is escalating.
Danny: I'm co-operating more.
Lucy: Ja!

SILVER WEDDING

We had married with two friends and two family members at Hampstead Registry Office, London, on April 8, 1960—right at the beginning of the sixties era. We now celebrated 25 years of a good marriage: plenty of arguments but never a hint of breaking-up, whatever the problems.

Over there, then, it was early springtime. Now, here, it was a lovely Transvaal early autumn evening. Nicky was 23, Danny 18. About 50 people came. There was a marquee but mostly we were under the clear sky. Oliver played solo flute: Syrinx by Debussy and a piece by CPE Bach. Nicola and I made speeches and then Nicky played her guitar and sang: "Once I lived the life of a millionaire" and "Trouble in mind." Then as a surprise for me: "A Farmer's Wife"—a folksong which I had sung at a Xmas concert. Both she and I changed the last line to "It's a musician's wife I'd be".

Danny played his guitar in the background—but not during the speeches or the performances!

Lucy's diary: Danny was dressed all in black with a peaked cap and a feather ear-ring. He played beautiful jazz guitar in the background. He was pleasant with guests. Introduced G (bad influence) to K (sometimes insane relative). When he felt left out he went back and played the guitar instead of talking to himself. The night before, he had decided against going to the club called Deviate, perhaps to prepare himself for this occasion. (A club called "Deviate" would not have existed in the fifties for our generation to decide not to go to.)

At the Silver Wedding I asked him how he liked it:

Danny: "Very, very much. It's wonderful!"

After our prepared ceremony Nicky's cabaret friend Natalie jumped up and sang a song and then famous Robbie Robb jumped up and sang a song. And then Oliver called up Monty, his childhood friend, who told a funny story about Lufthansa.

Afterwards everyone chatted and ate, and Danny went on playing his guitar.

Jeff, our family therapist, said, "If I'd known how informal it was going to be I'd have brought my daughter. What an excellent idea to let Danny play his guitar by himself like that."

Piers, a young cousin, said, "It was such an honour to meet Robbie Robb!"

An older cousin of Oliver's said to me, "It is extraordinary the way you can be so open and honest. You just look us straight in the eye."

And Lionel, my writing guru, said, "I enjoyed filling in the gaps. You have beautiful children! And the Debussy was marvellous. A unique occasion."

The next day came a letter for us both from Robbie Robb:

What can "I" say? You have been the example of the most "modern philosophy" of "Man and Woman Married" to me anyway.
Well done—ek se.
Love you both,
Robbie

Chapter Fifteen

HABILITAT—THE SECOND TIME
(AGED EIGHTEEN, 1985)

The morning after the silver wedding Oliver said, crossly, "He'll jolly well have to fetch his own amp (from under the marquee)."

"Can you think of anything *good* he has done lately?"

"Well he did put the amp in the marquee on his own initiative, and well in advance." This thought changed Oliver's mood and they moved it together that evening in a friendly way.

Danny said, "It's as if there is a machine. You do not know how the machine works, but that does not mean it is hostile. Life just exists. Things just exist."

At our first session after the silver wedding, I told him all the good things he had done. He smiled happily, "I really liked that session!"

The next day he told me about a guy called Cuddles who tried to seduce him. This was before his breakdown but he just felt like sharing it with me.

I asked him, "Did you mind?"

"No I didn't—because I knew him already. He didn't persist. He said, 'Oh you are such a beautiful boy.'"

"Since you are in such a good state let's tackle something heavy."

"OK."

"What if Lisa *really* isn't interested?"

"I could come back and join Robbie's band."

"Wouldn't it be worth getting your High School Diploma over there?"

Danny grinned, "Yes it would, and then maybe I could find another girlfriend and stay even longer."

He had been off lithium for a few weeks. It made no difference. With hope and a plan he stayed stable.

A happy Danny walked into the kitchen the next day: "Now these are all the things I have to do today."

I hugged him. "It's marvellous the way you are taking over."

At supper I said, "Danny says we should tell him if he talks to himself."

"In training hey?" said Oliver. Danny grinned.

"But I haven't had to tell him once all afternoon."

He's like a normal, charming ten-year-old. We can speak to the child Danny, give that child support—get him back to the point where his mind started functioning at a falsely adult level—and where he started playing the "genius" role.

We told him we would be perfectly content for him to be a happy plumber. He was surprised and interested. Our expectations had changed. But really it was his peers who had given him "star status", not us.

As I went through the kitchen he said, while doing the clearing up—with a wistful smile, "Why can't you make everything right?"

I wrote a summary of him in my diary:

A child with an extremely definite personality, living in a very organized world where he was able to feel free and creative. He had a mother who was supremely able to explain things to him at his level. Then this childlike self was thrown into an adult community without having the necessary inner restraints.

Now he is starting to understand the need for him to take control, and little by little is behaving in a way which indicates self-discipline.

The next session:

Danny: There's no reason why I shouldn't be doing something today for myself because tomorrow I'll be a better person. If I'm five and I want a dinky car and I want it so badly that I think about it day and night ...

Lucy: Now you think about Lisa day and night. Can you link it up to these other things?

Danny: It's the way you handle things. I have to improve my character.

Lucy: What can you take from Dad?

Danny: His manners—and his coolness.

The next morning we had another good session:

Lucy: It's like workers who have to be watched all the time. If Keo goes to town and doesn't know whether you are working ...
Danny: So I should work even then—at least a little bit. It's like I should buy these presents anyway, even though Hilary and Michael wouldn't know if I didn't (people he would be seeing on his journey).

He had money for these gifts, but was putting off going to buy them. Then he went off to buy the gift for Hilary, his aunt, whom he would be staying with on the way to Hawaii, but when he came home he wouldn't show me what he had bought, and I didn't know if he was telling the truth and he got angry.

In the next session I made him paraphrase "why he should work". The result was:

1. DON'T WORK
2. PEOPLE CRITICIZE ME
3. I DEFEND MYSELF
4. PEOPLE GET ANGRY
5. I GO MAD

In the next session I asked him what we should do. He replied, "Well can we go through what I do on my trip? I'll ask you questions."

So the days passed, and then he was on the plane and off to Hawaii again. He stayed for a few days with my sister Hilary in Connecticut. Unlike the time he stayed with my sister Jenny in Toronto, this time he was co-operative about smoking and never smoked inside. He and Hilary were there alone together and he helped her plant a tree.

In a letter to me Hilary said:

He is very charming, very dreamy—quite content to be around the house and play the piano. He's no trouble. And he goes outside to smoke. I was very touched by his gift of the two pens.

PHONE CALLS

Lisa, Danny's Habilitat dreamgirl, did have someone else by the time Danny got back, but he seems to have handled that with no difficulty. He was glad to be back and he threw himself into the work.

My May phone call: I spoke to Betsy: "He's doing very good—there's no need to worry right now. He's on the service crew."

My June phone call: I spoke to Bobby: "How's he doing?"
"Well you know Danny! Danny is Danny."
"Well is he better than last year?"
"Oh yes! He hasn't given us any real trouble. He goes off on his own sometimes and that's not something we approve of here. But he's doing everything willingly now: school, work, social activities."

My July phone call: I spoke to Bobby again. He said, "Danny is not the same boy he was last year. He's got his feet on the ground. He knows he's doing it for the second time. He doesn't go off on his own like he did last year. He's doing very well."
"Is he still on Maintenance?"
"Let me just see—yes—but he'll be moving on soon."
"Well he mustn't go too fast."
"No, we do know that."

But did they?

My August phone call: I spoke to Keo (the Mexican whom I had met last time). He said, "We think he gets bored easily, and we want him to move faster, so we are putting him into Admin."
"But he's never done any!" I protested. "It may just be too much for him."
"He will learn easily."

Then a letter from Danny, written just before this move to Admin:

I've gained a hell-of-a-lot. I'm becoming motivated. I'm becoming real again. The Re-Entry people were put on a houseban. We got so close. 19

287

people talking about life. Rap sessions at night. I gave so much. I felt so clear-headed, I felt better. I do want to finish school, I do want to stay here. I feel very steady.

This letter made us at home feel happy and optimistic.

My September phone call: I spoke to Keo again. He said, "We are working at giving him more and more responsibility in his admin job. Danny never did cause problems. He just can't motivate himself. I have to constantly tell him to pull himself up. He goes off and I have to tell him to make friends. But of course if it was his <u>music</u>!"

"Perhaps he needs more encouragement?"

"Oh no—that would be babying—we don't believe in that. He knows that if we don't pull him up he is doing his job."

I felt uneasy about this phone call. It sounded like too much pressure on him. The minute-by-minute focus on administration tasks sounded wrong for him. His concentration wasn't up to it. His arousal was too uneven. There was too much competing stuff going on in his head.

And then in mid-September came a phone call to say they had sent him to the Kahi Mohala Psychiatric Hospital. He had fallen off the world again.

LUCY'S JOURNEY

Kahi Mohala Psychiatric Hospital told us that if we left him there for six weeks they could come up with a definite diagnosis. Habilitat told us that the hospital had an excellent reputation. It was just outside Honolulu, beyond Pearl Harbour.

We were worried about the expense, but amazingly, Oliver's medical aid said they would pay. It fell within some category that they accepted.

By the time I spoke to Danny he had calmed down and said that the place was a real luxury for him and he could have a good rest there. I gave him all our love and wished him vasbyt (hang in there) and told him I was coming to visit him.

I had a long phone chat to his main doctor—a small Chinese woman, whom I will call Dr S. I told her that if I said, "If you don't

talk to yourself during supper you can go to a movie, then he didn't."
She was very surprised. "Now that really is interesting! That will help
us a lot."

I left Johannesburg three weeks before the end of his six-week
stay. I stayed in London for a week. In Harley Street I had an hour's
appointment with the world authority on schizophrenia. I told him all
the aspects of Danny's breakdown. He said that there was no doubt
that Danny had schizophrenia. He said that the best thing for me to
do was to drop Danny off in England on my way back. Since he was
British the state would then have to deal with him. He would be put on
permanent medication and would live in a protected residence. Then I
could live a happy life with my husband and daughter back home. He
was a very cold man. I was shocked—and didn't contemplate that route
for one moment.

My plane trip from New York to San Francisco was memorable.
A few daytime hours sitting next to a woman about my age (fifties)
travelling alone. I think we must have moved from social chat to our
common topic very quickly. I learnt that she was the head of the main
public psychiatric hospital in San Francisco. She listened intently to
my story of Danny, then she said, "Our hospital is huge. We have
large wards for schizophrenic patients—20 or 30 in a ward. We often
find them on the pavements of the city. Each patient has a one-on-one
interview with a psychologist or doctor about once a month. How can
that compare with your hour-by-hour bond with your son when he is
at home?"

"So schizophrenia is 'permanent' or not depending on the type of
help?"

"Many types, many outcomes. But yes I think that some psychotic
breakdowns would only become permanent if the patient goes on
experiencing failure and neglect."

In San Francisco I stayed with friends. Danny had now been at
Kahi Mohala for nearly five weeks. I phoned him up. He was strong and
warm and open. His communication seemed quite different. I waited
for him to initiate things—and that's exactly what he did.

"I've been doing marvellous things in Occupational Therapy. I feel
very proud of myself. I wanted to ask you. Do you think you could take
these things back? I've dedicated this cross to Robbie."

"Sure I could."

"Could you really! I'd be very grateful. I've been worrying about what to do with them. I didn't want just to leave them here."

Then he asked, "Did you see Hector in London?"

"Yes of course! He's crazy to get a copy of that tape you made."

"Well I'm very flattered. I feel very confident about my music. I've played often to the people here."

"Are you on medication?"

"Yes—a tiny pill."

"Will Habilitat let you take it?"

"I don't know. Shall I ask my doctor? She's right here."

"No, that's not necessary. You can ask her later. So you are happy to go back to Habilitat?"

"Yes, of course. "

"But what happened there?"

"I just needed a rest from the pressure. But now I think I can handle that. And I miss my friends terribly."

Much later he said to me: "I so much wanted the storeroom job—just two or three people quietly sorting out and stacking the groceries and stuff." He knew what he could manage.

And another time he said, "I remember deep disappointment with a young woman. One day I was in charge of showing this woman round Habilitat and telling her about the programme. I fell for her and I thought she had fallen for me. I went to bed glowing. The next morning I came downstairs and found her sitting in the foyer with all her suitcases. She was leaving!"

It may have been the last straw. He had been given a job in Admin which he simply couldn't manage. His concentration was still too weak. Habilitat wanted to "push him to the next level" and constantly criticized him. But since he had been trying already, he simply felt a failure.

DANNY AT KAHI MOHALA

The Kahi Mohala Hospital had six weeks in which to diagnose him. But first they had to calm him down. He raged and shouted and was put in a padded cell for a while.

The next day he said he did not want to be tested. He was of course anxious about what the tests would show.

Report on admission: Daniel was sent here because of his bizarre, inappropriate behaviour. They observed him crying for little or no apparent reason. He was also described as having a very low stress tolerance and poor concentration.

His differential diagnosis at the time of admission included the possibility of chronic organic brain syndrome secondary to his history of heavy polysubstance abuse, psychotic disorder, first break schizophrenia versus schizotypal personality disorder versus an affective disorder, bipolar or major depressive episode with psychotic features.

In his crazy initial state he was given an IQ test. His estimated IQ score of 86 was in the low average range.

The first Kahi Mohala report continues like this:

Daniel presented here as oppositional, distractible and flippant. His verbal expression was odd at times. For example he indicated that a fly and a tree are alike in that they are "natural offsprings of biology". When asked the meaning of proverbs he said of "spilled milk": "just forget it and go on with it", and to "birds of a feather" he said, "birds flying together for a purpose".

The patient was initially uncooperative and defiant, refusing to comply to the treatment programme. However, after firm confrontation by the male co-therapist we were successful in breaking through his resistance. At this point behavioural modification included firm limit settings to curb inappropriate behaviour, i.e. acting out, assaultiveness and threatening behaviour. Restraints and seclusion room were ordered if patient became inappropriate and uncooperative. However, during the entire course of his hospitalization the patient did not require institution of these firm limit settings. The patient responded very well to positive reinforcements, and praise for mature behaviour and adaptive coping mechanisms.

Recommendation for treatment: Provide structured activities that are task and goal oriented. Encourage music activity such as guitar and piano to help channel his aggressive impulses appropriately and increase his self-esteem by providing him with praise and positive reinforcement. Encourage initiative and independent activity to increase his sense of mastery and autonomy.

In the fourth week, by which time Danny was much more relaxed, he was given a neuropsychological test. He was more or less normal on all scores but the tester felt that he might have "mild prefrontal damage"— probably from "polysubstance abuse". Danny seems to have exaggerated his drug use. Cannabis alone was not then considered "bad enough" to have caused what had happened to him. "Prefrontal damage" would mean that the organizing part of his brain had been damaged.

It was noted that he was able to function at a much higher level at times, "with the problems he experiences hardly noticeable. At other times interference in attention due to preoccupation with internal thought processes could account for the pattern seen in some of these results." This reminds me of Danny aged nine when the teacher said, "Why can't he perform like that all the time?"

In a family history interview Danny said:

My mother was really concerned about my future. She was a kind, gentle and caring person. She was really into health food. She tried to prepare me for the unexpected. She liked everyone and got along with all sorts of people. She was easy-going. She had a little bad temper and got aggressive at times.

My father was extremely easy-going. He got aggressive only when he couldn't handle us for some reason. He was very happy and jolly. He got along with others and they got along with him. He joked with others. He was concerned about my happiness and gave me a lot of solutions to problems.

My parents' relationship is excellent. They handle their problems very well. They have been married for 25 years and are really happy.

He stated that his own ambition was to be a lead rock musician with a band that played the music he had composed.

HAWAII AND HOME

In Honolulu this time I stayed in a pretty place, far from the built-up part, up a hill at the YWCA where I shared a room and looked out on a view and vegetation.

Every day I took a taxi to Kahi Mohala, which was just out of the town. The first day Danny and I were left alone to chat:

Lucy: So you don't know yet about Habilitat?
Danny: No, but Keo has phoned me twice to see how I was getting on, so they must really care for me.
Lucy: What do you think of Dr S?
Danny: She talks so much! I've never known a woman talk as much as that! She even disturbs me when I'm trying to do my homework.

Later I read in one of the reports that Dr S had been assigned to check up on Danny every half-hour, whatever his activity. The idea was to keep him in the world and check on his symptoms. His talking to himself outlasted all other symptoms but he was trying to control it.

After seeing Danny alone I saw Dr S alone (the small Chinese doctor/therapist). She went through the history of his time with them: When he came he was listless and shutting out, and didn't answer in a goal-directed fashion. But his improvement had been dramatic. Dr S said, "But the problem is that as soon as he feels better he wants to challenge our expertise. He needs to practise humility." I wanted to laugh.

She already knew that Habilitat wouldn't take him back, but was waiting for my visit before telling him so as not to overload him. The next day she told him, but at the same time she said that Habilitat had agreed that he could come and visit them and say goodbye.

The day after that I visited Kahi Mohala again. I found Danny looking black, sitting by himself in the dining area. He was mumbling. I put my arm around him.

Lucy: What's up? What are you feeling?"
Danny: Angry!
Lucy: What happened at Habilitat?

Danny: They said they knew nothing about my visit. No one took any
    notice of me.
Lucy: The lousy bastards! No wonder you're angry. I'm angry too.

We talked a while to a black patient who had worked in mental
health. He ran down Habilitat.

"Good riddance to bad rubbish," said Danny.

The next day Danny and I and Dr S had a quiet time in the sitting
room. The only other person there was a patient who was frightened
to be alone and who sat quietly in the corner. Pretty, serious, talkative
Dr S, with her huge tome of pharmacopoeia reading about contra-
indications.

We talked about the time that Danny had stabbed his leg, but he
was in a good mood, joyful to be going home with me, and he managed
to make even the leg-stabbing incident seem sane. He leapt up and
illustrated how he had done it—the excitement of dancing in the rain
with his knife building up, and then the challenge and the wondering
if he dared—and then the plunge.

Danny and I were going home the next day. He had no "definite
diagnosis", just his own unique self.

It was Saturday. We were going home. The Kahi Mohala driver brought
Danny and his reports to the Honolulu airport.

From Dr S's discharge report:

During his first three weeks of behavioural modification therapy,
much of his inappropriate behaviour, i.e. mumbling and bizarre posturing
diminished, although it occasionally became prominent when he was under
moderate stress due to the intensity of group or school work. The patient
showed significant improvement when given highly structured activities and
intensive staff contact, i.e. frequent 30-minute checks, giving him positive
feedback, encouragement and support for appropriate behaviour. It was
noted that the patient's motivation to complete projects improved. Initially
Occupational Therapy reported that it took patient two weeks to complete
one very simple task, however, in the latter part of his hospitalization the
patient began to finish projects in a reasonable amount of time.

A problem Daniel has is his tendency towards creating high expectations
for himself and impatience in achieving his career goals.

I believe the patient is not quite adequately equipped emotionally or cognitively to handle the demands and stresses of a less structured environment in the outside world.

DISCHARGE CONDITION: Daniel is stable for discharge. Thought process: no loose association. Speech: goal oriented and coherent. Since his mother's arrival a week ago, Daniel has shown himself to be warm, pleasant and engaging with her. He has also shown to have improved his socialization skills and was able to terminate with his friends, staff and therapist appropriately. He no longer expressed desire to return to Habilitat, especially after being given a four hour pass to Habilitat and was rejected when visiting his friends. The patient expressed his anger appropriately to the whole situation and was able to accept the rejection maturely.

PROGNOSIS: Fair, provided the patient continues with our strong recommendation for continued residential treatment.

(Although they did not achieve their goal of a diagnosis their reports did get Danny out of the South African army for ever.)

Lucy: Are you all set for the journey?
Danny: Yes. I'm not looking forward to it—but it just has to be done—right?
Lucy: Right.

Danny was OK until the trip to London. Then tiredness made him anxious and he started hyper-ventilating. I gave him a pill, and he breathed into a paper bag.

When we arrived at the YMCA (near the British Museum), I changed my booking to one room with two beds instead of two rooms, so that I could be nearby if he woke up frightened and alone in a strange place. It was late at night. We stood there like zombies. I signed and then Daniel stepped forward to sign. The receptionist said to Daniel, "You're not really her son, are you—but you can just put the same name—that'll do."

Danny was unaware of this small comedy. He fell asleep as soon as he got into bed. I wrote my diary.

The next day we sat well rested but very cold in a boat on the Thames. It was now November. Danny (suddenly taking note) said, "What did you say that is called?"

"Cleopatra's needle."

We listened to the cool, humorous British commentator.

"The British are nice, aren't they!" said Danny.

LEAD GUITAR AGAIN

Two days after we got back from Hawaii Danny said to me in an agonized voice, "But please tell me this, Ma: will I *ever* get a girlfriend?"

It had not been mentioned on his reports, yet was one of his major frustrations.

Nevertheless, there was suddenly something else, almost better than a girlfriend. An old friend, Anthony, had moved to Midrand with his family. He invited Danny round. Danny got instructions and I, wanting him to be successful in finding a friend, took him in the car. (Mostly he went everywhere on his old motorbike.) But Anthony's instructions didn't work. We kept good-humoured above some underlying desperation: he had spent days trying to locate a band friend without success. Eventually we asked—and found we were on the right road but pointing the wrong way. At last we found Anthony's "sandy road" but were not sure of his house. Danny went into one he thought was right—then whistled for me. I heard a great shout—as Mark, Anthony and Joe saw him. Anthony said he would give him a lift home, and off I went.

That night when he came home he said he had a job with them: "You'll never believe this Ma: they just needed a lead guitar!"

Mark visited us the next day and said: "What d'you think of Daniel just happening to arrive at the moment we needed him?"

Mark was his long-ago drummer friend from his successful childhood band, who had tried to help him during his breakdown. He was spending five years in the army band in Pretoria.

Back to band music meant back to pot. I asked Mark about it and he said, "I can guarantee that he won't smoke pot in the band-room."

His long-ago teacher from Saheti, Terry, came to visit us. Danny told her, "Apparently they had auditioned all sorts of people for lead guitar and not found anyone! I can't believe how well everything is going in my band!"

Oliver said to me, "Danny has got all sorts of pizzazz—even though he may be playing on a different planet from everyone else."

Nicola visited and looked at the many songs he had written since being home. I didn't understand his song words, but she said they were fine.

After she went, Danny said to me, "Hey, Ma, d'you know what? They say *I* am the leader—because I have the ideas. And Anthony gave me a foot-pedal because he forgot my birthday."

I thought: Danny's emotions come in an unpackaged form until he can focus on a creative act.

One day we fetched Anthony and his girlfriend. In the car Danny discussed with Anthony what he wanted done in the band, in a confident and clear way. "Such a tough masculine streak he is developing!" said my diary.

Oliver's term was ending and he was at home a lot and taking a lot of notice of Danny.

"Danny is in a lovely state," said my diary. I hugged him and said: "Don't get worked up about the concert. Don't think that because you have been such a failure that now you've *got* to succeed. You've done the work—so enjoy yourself."

"Ja, you're right. I will," said Danny warmly.

(I had been remembering the concerts when Danny got out of control, when he forgot where he was and simply went on playing and playing his guitar when this was inappropriate.)

Danny: Look at my new studs (ear-rings). Joe gave them to me. He said he would give them to me when I deserved them.
Lucy: How d'you mean?
Danny: Well when I have been calm and co-operative. And now I have! Joe looks after me. He's like a father to me.

Lucy's report on the first concert: He played like an angel. Total control—stayed behind the synthesizer doing myriad things and then came out to play his guitar and ended his part appropriately.

I had a chat to Carol who is singing with the band. She told me that she, Mark and Danny do not smoke pot. Joe P and Anthony do.

I wrote to the doctors at Kahi Mohala:

This Christmas Eve I would like to tell you that Daniel is completely free of all his odd symptoms. He is lead guitar with a band which is giving its third public performance tonight. Most of the pieces they play—both the words and the music—have been written by Daniel. I think you would be astonished at the calm way he handles all the complications involved in his band—moving from keyboard to guitar—and coming to the mike and singing etc.etc. If I could summarize the change in one word I would say: Confidence!

I talked to Dr S on the phone—his chatterbox doctor. She said, "I'm overwhelmed and delighted. Tell him I am waiting for his first record. I stressed the building of character. For intellectual or artistic success the building of character is crucial. You were not the person we were expecting you know. You are humble—no airs and distance. I really do miss Danny!"

Chapter Sixteen

KAWASAKI AND KARATE
(AGED NINETEEN, 1986)

PAIN AND RAGE

The triumphant band was unfortunately just for the Xmas holidays. Mark went back to the Police Band in Pretoria, Anthony went back to university and Jan K went back to working with his dad. Danny was offered a job for six months with a band in Durban, but neither he nor we felt he was ready to move away from home at this stage. "It's just such a relief to be home again," Danny said to me as we sat relaxed in the garden.

This year of 1986, when Danny was nineteen, was a year of horror and success, out-of-control rage and delightful behaviour, ups and downs. Danny had extreme rages which seemed to come from nowhere. One January morning, when Oliver was still on holiday, Danny had said he was going to town to get some band equipment. But he had not gone.

I criticized him for not carrying through his plan. Suddenly he ran from the gate and pushed his fist through the back window of my car. The whole window was smashed: a gaping hole on one side and shattered glass on the other side, with jagged splintered pieces projecting into the space.

Oliver rushed him to our doctor for stitches.

He lay in bed being nursed and mothered by me. While I was dressing his wound I said:

Lucy: There are inner stitches as well.

Danny: That's heavy hey!

Lucy: Yes. That's why we don't want it to happen again.

In the evening he was in great pain. "Can you stroke my shoulder again? That relieves the strange feeling in my arm. In the fridge you will find a box of cherry chocs—they come from one of Dad's pupils. You can have one too!"

Part of me queried the coziness of all this after the outrageousness of the act. Why had he done it? He had been on an anti-depressant— "Amilent"—which I had stopped the week before because his behaviour had been so marvellous. Then he had smoked pot on the Saturday night and this violent act was on the Tuesday. I had noticed that rages following pot often happened not the day afterwards but two or three days afterwards.

But his black rages were not always associated with pot. He had after all been raging went he went to Kahi Mohala—after months of no pot. I think in his mind he had mountains of failure—insults, humiliations, not making it. His friend Toby, who had owned the Orange Grove drug house—and who had sold all types of drugs to others—now had a B. Mus from Wits. Of this Danny said, "It's too painful to talk about."

Oliver and I had a breakthrough session with him. I started by saying we couldn't live with this acting-out. He said it was worse for him and we acknowledged this.

Lucy: Yes Danny, we do know this: however much Dad and I have suffered in our lives—from bouts of depression and frustration— what *you* have suffered is unimaginably worse.
Danny: Well I'm glad you appreciate that.
Oliver: We are behind you all the way. And we very much appreciate the changes in you—I enjoy very much having you at home now.
Danny: This thing that has happened to me is very very good—but it is still a *change*.
Lucy: Yes, that's true—even *good* changes can be stressful.
Oliver: So you have to find a way of dealing with your bad feelings without the rages.
Danny: OK, when I come in tonight I'll watch something on telly.

We also decided to notice and to stop negative behaviour sooner when that was possible. Some days later I told Danny firmly that his shouting at Oliver (who had told him to turn the music down) was not acceptable. He protested a bit—talked about "misunderstandings". I just walked out and that was that.

Nicola was not living at home any more, but she came across Danny's rages often enough to be disturbed by them. "People are frightened by him," she said.

She and I both had nightmares about him.

Nicola's dream:

I was on a bus travelling north in England. We were touring with a play. I gave birth to twin boys—fair-haired Sean was the father. I was breast-feeding. They were identical to look at. But one was peaceful and gentle and lovable, and the other was angry and bit my breasts and I hated him.

Lucy's dream:

Last night I dreamt he was arrested for murder and about to be executed. No court case. I thought "perhaps it's best", but then couldn't bear it and went looking for lawyers. Then I woke up and was relieved. Then I went to sleep again and was back in the same situation—visiting him in jail.

The trouble with Western liberal society is that it waits until too late before exercising intelligent adult control. We are so busy being loving and understanding.

POT

Danny's two periods at Habilitat had not really changed his attitude to pot. Even before he went there he had realized that smoking a lot was bad for him. But what about smoking a little—sometimes"?

The first time he smoked after Kahi Mohala he told us quite openly: "It gave me such a good feeling!"

One of the problems was that the Western liberal world still thought pot was harmless. Have they changed? I read last week (2007) that the British government was about to legalize pot when it received a damning report from researchers, so they changed their minds.

But most people go on saying "It's no worse than alcohol". But in my experience—and not only because of Danny—"a little alcohol is good: a little pot is bad". One difference between them is that alcohol is out of the blood in a couple of hours, whereas pot can still be found in the urine two weeks later, and in the fat cells six months later.

This was the year (1986) that Nicola, now aged 24, gave it up completely, for ever.

In February, after the black rages and his putting his arm through the car window, we simply said that going to Sanca was now compulsory. He accepted this, knowing that he could not pay for the window, although not really thinking there was a connection between pot and rage.

Lucy's diary: The hectic phase is over. We are all calm and cheerful again. Danny bathed, rode his bike in the rain to Midrand and then to a movie. In the morning he had attended his first session with Mavis, the Sanca therapist.

Another day we were chatting idly in the car. I asked him, "Was St Martin's a complete waste of time?"

"No, not at all." He said, reassuringly. "Me and my mates were real drug addicts and had a very good time."

But a few days later he said:

Danny: It makes me shiver to think of it. I used to be so reckless. It was only about 10 months ago—when I went back to Habilitat—that I started to quieten down.

Lucy: Who do you think has helped you most?

Danny: Sandy. She gave me the confidence that I could do things. She made me go so deeply into my life.

But he didn't want to go back to Sandy now. He felt he had had enough of that kind of therapy. And Kahi Mohala had saved him at a bad time but now he saw it as a battering, intrusive experience.

In addition to his personal sessions with Mavis at Sanca, he also went to NA (Narcotics Anonymous). He was very pleased with this group. He told me, "They are such nice people. Shame—there was this oke there who has to do his army training, and he feels it's such a waste of time. I told him just not to think about it."

Another day he said, "Mavis says she is not interested in my giving up pot—just in being a third person I can talk to."

"That doesn't sound right to me. I need to know what your intentions are."

"My intention is to become the best human being I can possibly become."

"Yes, that's very good. But do you think you can become that person and still smoke pot?"

"Yes."

Another day, I said, "I think from the sniffing that you have been smoking."

"Well I'm trying to cut it down. I really am."

Oliver took the "All about Dagga" pamphlet out to Danny in the garage for him to learn. Oliver said to me, "He says they recite it every Tuesday. But he didn't know what 'chromosome' meant."

Everything was going so well that I decided to go up to the Molozi farm to write a story. Oliver was nominally in charge, but working most of the time. He reported to me that Danny had hurt his foot by riding barefoot on his bicycle and therefore did not get to Mavis. I said, bitterly, in my diary, "As of course he would not, because he cannot take charge of his life." Oliver's next report said Danny had been completely passive. I wrote in my diary: "He slips back into the basic problem of passivity as soon as I am not there."

Lucy's diary: I came back yesterday from Molozi at 1 pm to find Danny zonked—there had been crazy shouting the night before—and only half of his pills taken. I found him asleep on the couch and he slept through until 8 this morning. I was exhausted and mentally frantic, thinking of schemes to get him somewhere else.

The next day I woke up with shingles and for a few days hardly noticed Danny. Eventually I went to the garage and found two broken bottles, indicating "white pipes"—dagga plus Mandrax. We locked the garage and took away his bike key. He had calmed down by now and settled to a quiet life sewing and writing songs in the house.

Some of his going back to drugs was due to the Mean Machine—a place on Louis Botha Avenue—where he played pool, but also where he met drug-takers. He said he felt at home there. "They are all Standard 7 drop-outs like me."

I thought: It is really only now, when he is so sane most of the time, that the clear effects of pot can be seen.

ONE SATURDAY AFTERNOON

Danny's plan of putting his own band together and smoking pot occasionally was not working. He put notices in shop windows for musicians. They phoned him up and came round. Some of them could play, but none of them proved reliable. They were drug addicts and drop-outs.

One Saturday morning Danny was sleeping late. I was going to lunch with my mother. I walked round the house. In the studio, Oliver was teaching a pupil. I heard her practising a phrase over and over until she got it right. In the garden Moses, an elderly gardener, was pottering around. I sometimes suggested things to him that I thought needed doing, but mostly I left him to decide what to do.

All was peaceful. I was not needed. I drove off to have lunch with my mother.

At three o'clock I returned. As I got out of the car the sound of Danny's rage doubled my pulse rate. I stood there, paralysed. It was as if all the windows and doors of the house had been closed, and so much air had been pumped in that the walls had to fight to stay steady. I walked to the garden studio, but the door was locked. The pupils had gone home. Moses came to me, "I told Danny to put down the knife. I told him he would hurt himself with that knife."

"Has he got the knife now?" He shrugged.

I went to Danny's window. I saw him in an attitude of extreme violence in front of his mirror, holding his knife. I went to Oliver's window. He was lying on his bed. He had a migraine. "I'm outside here," I said, "Giving you support."

"Best to leave him alone, I think."

"Ja, OK."

Moses came to me again. He talked very fast. "It's not right—that small boy—I see him giving Danny matchbox through the window."

"What small boy?"

"That one he come. Then they say all the black people is bad."

I went back to Oliver's window. "What does Moses mean?"

"Phineas' son came round."

"But he wouldn't give Danny pot!"

"Who knows?"

I sat down and leaned against the wall for support. In my mind I was running here there and everywhere seeking and rejecting solutions. Perhaps Sandy would have some suggestions. The last time I spoke to her she said his rages were "good". "Write that on my tombstone," said Oliver.

I got the studio key from Oliver through his window and went to phone Sandy. "But I haven't seen him for so long. I don't know whether he would accept me."

"Can I say you are on the phone?" She agreed.

"Hi Danny!" I shouted merrily through his window. "Sandy's on the phone. She'd love to say hello!" He hears me, thank God. "I can't talk to her now," he shouts, as if working on something vital. He went back to swearing at his image in the mirror. I talk to Sandy again. "Can you tell me how you would handle it?"

"You've got to try and give him a double message: that you love him, but that he's gone beyond the limits of what is acceptable. He is like a child now, and he is frightened of his own anger."

I walked towards the house. I was too scared to go inside. "Danny, I know you're struggling with something, but I just wanted to say ..."

"Fuck off!"

I knew now that I had to go to him. I had remembered what had worked before. I went into the house and walked into his room. He was now on a mattress on the floor. I flopped down beside him, as if chatting to a friend at the seaside. I put my hand on his shoulder. His words came like bullet: "Don't—touch—me!"

I picked up his teddy bear and hugged it and rocked backwards and forwards humming to myself, until I had lulled myself into a state of complete peacefulness. Because what I remembered was that if I was not afraid, his rage would stop. Sometimes.

His rage turned into a sort of howling and then into sobbing. I went on humming with the teddy bear. Finally he was quiet. I got up to go. "Would you like some tea?"

"Ja—I—would—like—some—tea."

I made him some and left him alone.

Half an hour later, Oliver and Danny met in the passage. They hugged each other. "I love you, Dad," said Danny. "I love you too my boy," said Oliver.

TO MAKE HIS LIFE WORK

On the Monday morning I stayed in bed. Danny was subdued. He brought me coffee and sat down for a chat.

"What would you like apart from getting your own band together?"

"A kitten and a 750cc motorbike. What would you like?"

"Breakfast in bed!"

"OK I'll bring you breakfast every day in bed. What would you like for breakfast?"

"Scrambled egg and toast and marmalade, and coffee."

So that's what he did for the rest of this year—and it made him feel good about himself. I was so genuinely pleased! I would wake him up at 8 am and bring him coffee. Even if I had woken up grumpy, I knew I had to go in bluffing that I was fine, and use a warm, cheerful voice. Then the rest of the day had a chance of working.

I found a kitten for him and he named it Dibbs. First thing after he got up in the morning was to feed Dibbs, clear the kitchen and bring me my breakfast.

My task now was to make his life work: within this place; within his mind. I could no longer rely on other people and other places.

Getting his driving licence was for him a worthwhile goal. But getting a learner's licence had become rather difficult. No more simple "yes/no; turn left/turn right;" answers. Instead the would-be learner-driver was faced with about 100 multiple-choice questions: four possibilities to each of 100 questions all in one session. I did not want him to feel the way he had in Hawaii when faced with their school-leaving exam: 100%

blank. I did not want him to feel as he had at Kahi Mohala when faced with an IQ test: anxious and fearful and tense.

I found a small shop in town which taught people how to do this test. Danny was happy to go. He was slowly taught the basics. Then the day came for his first trial test: he passed brilliantly and came home radiant. It might not be a B. Mus, but it was a start. He did a few more trial tests and then they sent him along the road to the official testing-place and he passed with 100%.

I arranged driving lessons for him. He loved these lessons. I feared he might be arrogant and sulky, since he had been driving for years, but instead he was happy and willing to learn. The teacher said: "I am teaching him not to have over-fast reactions. I've had a lot of these drop-out people, but he's by far the nicest."

After that last out-of-control episode until the end of the year, one of us was always in charge. Danny was reasonably willing now to try and be more adult, so we were working with a fairly reasonable person. We allowed him to carry on going to the Mean Machine, where he met friends and played pool, provided he only went for one hour and came straight home. There was no pot-smoking at this place—it had simply been where he met others who smoked.

We insisted on absolute accountability—little notes next to the telephone in the passage—about where he was going and when he would be back. One of us being in charge did not mean we could be there all the time. One night when I was staying over with my mother Oliver came back to find *"Gone to Mean Machine"*.

But no Danny was back after an hour. Oliver wasn't sure where it was so he went to bed. Later Danny wrote this message:

Dad—I lent Sandro my bike and didn't get it back again. I had trouble refusing, seeing as how he had to get home. Sorry. But please wake me tomorrow because I need to go and fetch it first thing.

Below this Oliver wrote:
If you want to suffer for your friends, the least we can do is to let you.

After that we said no more going to the Mean Machine on his motorbike. He could walk—it was only a ten-minute walk away.

There was a parents' evening at NA at the beginning of each month. Oliver and I once went together with Danny, then after that Oliver went with him on those open evenings and I stayed home.

With NA and our watchfulness established there was again a vacuum. What was he to do? He expressed an interest in karate. When he was seven he had been for a few months and achieved his junior Yellow Belt. We agreed to let him start again, but doubted his stickability.

The other thing at this time was that he was passionate about getting the big motorbike. In the end we put a programme together with the big bike as a reward if he stuck to the programme and didn't go near pot. He said, "So you mean if I do all those things—become reliable and healthy and so on—I will get the big bike by the end of the year?"

"Ja."

Lucy's diary: He has pushed two beds together and hung his skates on his board, and arranged his song-writings on a shelf—and he has incense and coloured lights. Now he is ready to start karate tomorrow. "Stan will help me," he says, with great conviction.

Stan Schmidt was both the owner of this dojo centre near us, and a South African karate champion. Danny assumed that since he remembered Stan so well from when he was seven, so would Stan remember him. He was disappointed when he didn't.

The second time he went to karate he did a double session by mistake—simply didn't realize that his session had ended—and came home very stiff.

I took him myself at this early stage, to be sure he got there. The times for his sessions were different on different days. I dropped him off and he came back by bus. He was still hopeless at remembering appointments. Later he went by himself, but with me prompting him about days and times. Only very much later could he do it all alone.

Danny did his 5th karate session and joined us downstairs for supper at a restaurant called Alan's Place. We were all mellow and he stayed with us. I got him to compare the pupils of his eyes with Oliver's. He was interested. His were big and he was sniffing.

I said, lightly, "So if you don't want us to know you've smoked, don't see Sandro, don't lock yourself in the garage, and don't sniff."

He said, ruefully, "Yes, I can see that."

For the first time since his breakdown he was able to go to Nicola's plays without talking loudly to himself all through the performance. He was very taken with her current play at the Market Theatre and went twice, seeing her afterwards.

After a few times at karate his usual problem came back—not feeling like going and letting himself off too easily. And about pot he was still saying to himself:

"If I have a little it won't matter."

"If I can get away with it ..."

"I need it ..."

"I deserve it ..."

"I can handle it ..."

So I made out a formal contract that he would get his big bike—a 750cc bike—after three months' regular karate, which meant at least four sessions a week, and after smoking no pot at all. We both signed this document.

I asked him, "Would you go to NA if we didn't say you had to?"

"Ja I think so—I would commit myself to once a fortnight."

"I wonder why you find it so difficult to give up pot completely."

"Yes, I wonder too."

"It seems like a rebellious thing rather than a craving—getting away with it behind our backs?"

"Yes, that's right. If I lived on my own ... not that I don't want to live at home ... but once I've come right ..."

"Do you think you can come right if you don't give up?"

"They go together."

The next day he worked all morning on a song.

"I feel so happy now. I feel so good."

"What's making you feel good?"

"My karate, my music. I finished my song this morning. It will make me famous."

"Don't you want to play it somewhere?"

"No. Only when I get my band."

Danny was starting to take an interest in South Africa and the world. One day in the car I asked him if he knew what a necklace was. "I don't understand the question. A necklace is an ornament that goes round your neck."

He had simply slept through the terrible times of the "necklacing"—when burning rubber tyres were thrown round the necks of supposed traitors.

"Am I defensive?" he asked one day.

"No—only when you are stoned."

"Well then I don't know what the hell I am doing."

Nicola visited. Danny played his new song to her. She was most impressed—felt he could do well on the Jo'burg entertainment scene. She also liked the way he looked. Alone with me in the car she said, talking of why she herself had given up pot:

"I felt I had a choice. Here was I with all these advantages of family etc. and who was I to throw them away? So I decided to be happy. The world is a dreadful place, so one just has to do the best one can, even if it's only for a short time."

Danny saw the big bike as something that would make it worthwhile for him to give up smoking dope.

"Yes it's for that—but also for keeping up your regular activities. I take it you mean that you aren't going to bring pot home, rather than that you won't smoke at all—even if someone offers it to you at a party."

"No—I mean that—that I won't smoke at all."

In a way he had given himself a new problem: disappointment with himself when he failed. One evening he missed his NA meeting. The next day he said, "Put it in the contract of the things I have to do."

I was going to stay with my mother to do some writing work. Oliver was free. He said he would take charge. "Oh God," he said. "I suppose there'll be all this trouble getting him up?"

"No actually—that's not a problem any more."

And there was no problem and Oliver was amazed—almost bemused. He had been going early to work so had not seen Danny making my breakfast and feeding the kitten.

I thought: And there is even a sign of breakthrough on the Mandela/Botha front.

A druggy girl phoned and said she had a "button". (a Mandrax pill). Danny told me about this and said he now had a key ring from NA which said: "JUST FOR ONE DAY", which he would look at if that happened again.

Although things were going so well he did still talk "garbage" at times. He would get carried away in a conversation and lapse into fluent-sounding sentences with real words, which meant nothing. But he didn't walk in an odd way any more, which meant that people didn't stare at him. He could pass for normal.

Lucy's diary: A real schizophrenic is cut off from "wanting", whereas Danny has passionate "wants".

Danny is not hostile to me any more except after pot—which he still has sometimes. As his behaviour improves and he gets more control over his life he is less bitter with himself.

Danny came to me and said, joyfully, "Dave and Chris from NA are going to be on Radio 5 on Thursday!"

"All the people who said it was tickets with you—I want to spit in their eyes!"

"Ja—I'll probably end up a better driver and a Black Belt (the final karate belt)."

In June he got his Yellow Belt—his first adult karate achievement. He said, "Me and another guy have to do 50 sessions instead of 35 for our Orange Belts. That's because I made a mistake. I had to counter-attack and my reactions went all wild."

WOW!! What a non-defensive admission.

On the night before the driving test he was a little mad—sitting at the kitchen table with an open pen-knife and laughing in a manic way. He had waited and waited for his friend Anthony to phone about a movie and he was also worried about the test the next day.

Early the next morning he left with Oliver for the test ground, and came back triumphantly at about 8.30. He had lost no points in the ground test, and lost only six on the open road. He was now a licensed driver.

He and I went to the Doll's House for lunch.

Danny: Check that Porsche!
Lucy: What would it cost?

311

Danny: About 60 grand.

Lucy: Would you like to drive one?

Danny: Yes, I really would!

Lucy: Well as long as that's not your only ambition.

Danny: I want to drive a Porsche and have my own pop band ... (softly) and have a girlfriend.

THE BIG BIKE

It was winter. The three months Danny had to do for the big bike were nearly over. He had done reasonably well. He had stuck to karate, which was the main thing we wanted him to do.

One day he came laughing out of karate: "I spoke to Stan. He said yes maybe he did remember me. And I'm doing so well. I'm so pleased with my karate."

His friend Mark came round when Danny was out.

Mark: I don't like his haircut.

Lucy: It'll grow.

Mark: Why did he do it?

Lucy: Karate-style.

Mark: You shouldn't give him a 750cc bike. It's a coffin on wheels.

Lucy: The guys at Honda have been giving him lessons. They say he's an excellent rider.

Mark: Believe me I've known guys ... It's the speed that gets to them.

Lucy: He's responsible about driving, and he's getting it for regular karate and quitting pot.

Mark: Danny just *has* to get stoned!

Lucy: He's changing.

Mark: A leopard never changes its spots, Lucy.

It was true that Danny had not entirely given up the dope. He had very few friends and those he had smoked dope. Anthony and Mark, his musician friends who tried to keep him away from pot (even though they both smoked themselves), were seldom available.

And the capacity for despair still lurked. The more his psychosis receded the more he was aware of having fallen way behind his sister and his American cousin, Cathy. She was the same age as he was. She had been accepted by the ten top American universities and had chosen Stanford.

Rage could still erupt. He would come back from an outing raging—and then explain to me the next day that he had been hurt, insulted and humiliated. Whether this was true or he had imagined it I didn't know.

But he was sticking to his programme—not only karate but also getting up in the morning and doing home chores and then going off in my car to do jobs for me and Oliver. He also painted a big yellow diamond on the bonnet of my car, very precisely. (I thought this was a good thief deterrent.)

"I got some white spray-paint as well to paint out that thing on the garage wall."

This was on an outside wall at the back and I had not noticed it. Now I saw it was a swastika, but Danny said that when he painted it on he had not known that.

He painted it out, then came to me and said, "You know Mom, the bike is a real incentive for me to give up smoking grass. I was looking for something which would make it worthwhile giving up."

The date of the bike approached. He had not gone the full three months without pot, but in the end we decided to ignore this. Everything else had gone well. He himself had found a second-hand bike which brought down the price considerably. A Kawasaki.

When the day came he and I drove to the Honda place and then I drove back behind him, watching him riding his Kawasaki big bike quietly and calmly back home, and he was controlled all day. At 3.30 pm he went off on his new bike to Anthony in Midrand for a rehearsal.

That night Oliver and I were chatting at supper. Oliver said, "I find it very disturbing that he is talking to himself all the time."

"Lately?"

"Yes—and he used to do it only when he was stoned."

(Oliver liked simple explanations. He had forgotten that Danny's talking-to-himself had started at Habilitat where there were no drugs.)

I explained to him my now clearly-formulated philosophy of not even *thinking* Danny mad, or an addict, or helpless, or hopeless etc.

Oliver went off to sleep. At 11 pm Danny was not home. I did not like to phone Anthony's parents at this time without a good reason. So I took a Normison sleeping pill and said cheerful sentences to myself and fell asleep about midnight. (The phone was next to my bed for emergencies.)

I woke at 6 am. Danny's room was empty. The bed was unslept-in. I imagined every horror. Then I went out to the garage for clues. There was Danny, sitting on the floor next to his new bike.

"Danny!" I exploded, "Haven't you been to sleep all night?"

"No. Me and Anthony rehearsed late late. And then I was just too fascinated by my bike. I couldn't leave it."

I thought: He is like a farmer sitting up all night with a horse.

Of course we were mad to give our somewhat whacky teenager a big bike. We did it because of our predicament. Looking back I am relieved that nothing that happened involved injury to other creatures or vehicles. For Danny the bike meant personal power. For us it was a holding device until he could develop himself further and not need that sort of power ever again.

Nicola now thought we were spoiling him, but it was more a matter of keeping him encouraged to go on trying. In St Paul's letter to the Colossians, there is an interesting verse (Ch 3, verse 21): Fathers, provoke not your children to anger, lest they be discouraged.

Here are three bike stories:

Danny was not supposed to go to the Mean Machine on his motorbike but he just couldn't resist showing off his new bike. On the fifth day after he got it he went to the Mean Machine at 1 pm and stayed till I fetched him at 6. At 4 he had phoned to say that someone was riding his bike and had not brought it back. He handled it all calmly. I praised him for this.

In fact many people had ridden his bike and it ended up at the Honda dealer where we had bought it. Danny knew these guys well from the free lessons they had given him. Three days later he drove me to Honda. Fred, Andre, Danny and I stood there looking at the red-and-black, panther-racehorse Kawasaki 750 motorbike. Damaged.

Fred said, "It's like your girlfriend. You wouldn't lend your girlfriend to anyone."

Andre said, "Do I wish I had one! You are so lucky. There are only a few in this country."

Fred said, "In a few years it will be a Collector's Piece."

The oily clutch rings were in a pile, one broken in several places. Fred explained that it was done by over-revving at the beginning of the ride: of all the rides. Fred asked, pointing to a mark on the seat, "What's this?" Danny answered, "Ja, I was wondering. But lots of people were riding it."

"If you borrow someone's girlfriend you don't look after her in the same way."

On the way home Danny said, "I felt so sad when I saw the broken pieces lying there. I'll never let anyone ride it again. I've learnt my lesson now.

Three days after he got his bike back came Lesson Number Two. I was phoned at 3 pm by Norwood police station. Danny had been charged with speeding: "119 km on Louis Botha Avenue". They said they would decide whether to keep him in for the week-end. Later they said I could pay the bail and fetch him. So I went there and paid R50 bail.

Danny said, "I'm very, very sorry, Ma. And you went to such trouble to get me the bike and everything. Well, it had to happen once. I didn't even realize I was going fast."

Always looking for the good, I said, "You have handled the situation well my love."

On the Monday I went with him to court. The magistrate didn't sneer. Danny said afterwards that he had been "neutral". He was fined R500. The magistrate said, "If you had been driving recklessly you would have gone to jail."

In our previous encounters with the police they had thought that Danny was disturbed. This time he came across as calm and sane. Oliver and I were immensely relieved by this.

The third incident was an accident. It was a week after the court case; mid-winter. Danny went for a happy, free bike ride, not going anywhere, just driving around joyfully. He went up to Glenhazel, a neighbouring suburb, and then was enticed by his exuberance onto a sandy road. He probably didn't slow down sufficiently for the different conditions: he skidded, lost his balance and he and the bike toppled over, the bike onto him.

He was badly grazed and cut and bruised and had pulled muscles, but didn't break anything. The doctor put on dressings and bandages and he went to bed. The next day he asked me to get him magazines—"Music, or cars … or girlie."

I was soon out of it. Oliver was having his school holiday and I went off to Cathedral Peak Hotel in the Drakensberg. I went for walks with the guests—up to the snow, and I wrote a story at the dressing-table in my room. I don't remember phoning home at all.

When I came back Danny was cheerfully on crutches. Anthony was having his university vac and was happy to chauffeur him around. Soon Danny was going on his crutches to the Mean Machine. Anthony would pick him up there, but didn't like going in. It was definitely not his scene. Oliver went in one evening to fetch Danny and said they were all sitting on the pool tables having a quiet chat! There was in fact a strong old black guy keeping an eye on things, and no alcohol was sold there. It was just the contacts he made there that were a problem. I picked up the phone in the other room one day and heard this conversation:

Girl (with "little girl" voice): Hey, Daniel?
Danny: Ja—Hi!
Girl: Will you come over?
Danny: Ja, OK, what's your name?
Girl: Karen.
Danny: OK, Karen, I'll be over.
Girl: I've got a button

I confronted him and he said he would have gone round but got out of the "white pipe" deal (pot plus Mandrax).

As long as Anthony was on holiday, Danny could go with him to his home at Midrand and they would play music. Anthony's mother, a speech therapist, said she noticed a difference every time Danny came. "And he's so gifted!"

Danny visited Nicky, who lived in Hillbrow with her boyfriend. She reported back to me on what Danny said:

Just when I think I'm independent then I think to myself: but I'm not as independent in my mind as Mommy.

I feel secure at home.

I used to feel scared all the time. That was because I was so heavily into the drug scene.

At Habilitat they seemed to put us all against each other. Griffin would come to me and say he had to teach me manners. People looked at you as if they cared nothing at all for you. You just had to think that they did really, and keep that idea in your head.

I can be more independent living at home.

I think about sleek cars and I'm in love with this girl on the cover of a magazine!

Danny was off karate for two months because of the bike accident. He had no more accidents.

Chapter Seventeen

BACK TO SCHOOL?

In this year of Danny being nineteen, 1986, life went on fairly well. When he had recovered from his motorbike injuries, he went to karate fairly regularly on his new big Kawasaki bike.

He made a demo tape with his Xmas band when they all had a few days free, and he felt strong and good about that. During the making of the tape he pushed himself in an intense and driven way. He had written most of the songs for this group. But Anthony was going to Israel for a year and the fourth member of the group, Jan K, got married! Danny went to his wedding rather unwillingly. Another wedding went better. It was of Nicola's friend Lesley.

Nicky told me afterwards, "Danny was unbelievable. He was so marvellous! My friends asked me who he was. He was witty. He talked appropriately. He didn't say *one weird thing* all afternoon."

During his bike injury, which had kept him away from karate, we bought a video player and I found him an afternoon art class. This was in a private house, with a large studio and serious art students. Danny brought home beautiful paintings.

He earned money by working for us and this he spent on renting videos. We felt he watched too many of them, but he said they kept him from pot. I praised him for winding back the videos and taking them back and so on. Any sign of initiative and responsibility I now noticed and praised.

One day he came back from art. I was making sandwiches in the kitchen and he was walking in and out with a cloth and a bowl. I asked him what he was up to.

"Cleaning the walls. The stuff I did when I was mad. Some of it is quite nice, but some of it is, you know, not so nice."

I visited Ria, his art teacher. She said, "He gets very involved. Sometimes frightened. But he is a kind and gentle person. He is religious."

"Well, not exactly. Perhaps spiritual?"

"Yes, that's it."

When he started karate again he got very stiff and often tried to get out of it. If he went and then was stiff, the next morning he tried to get out of getting up and making my breakfast. So I was still having to be his parent and to try to decide whether he should go or not, or get up or not. If I left it to him to decide he would take the easy way out.

When I first read about Grantley College, a remedial high school near us, I was enraged! Why had no one told me about it? All our helpers and advisers, and the schools which wouldn't accept him. They must surely have known; and I found out later that, yes, they had known, but just hadn't thought about it for Danny. "I thought it was for backward pupils," said a friend.

Now I thought: He could have gone there at 16; he could have gone there at 17. But to ask him to go there at 20 would be a bit much!

Nevertheless I went to see it. It was quiet and ordered. And possible. Mrs Simons, the sympathetic head, said, "We ask the more mature pupils whether they want us to treat them as adults."

I told Danny about it:

Danny: Oh no Ma that's not fair! You promised if I did art and karate ...
Lucy: Well not for *now*—for next year.
Danny: No. It would seem like a step backwards.
Lucy: It's a good course. You would learn from it.
Danny: No. I'm quite normal now. I can learn all the time.
Lucy: You have a lot of spare hours ...
Danny: I don't even think of them until you mention it.
Lucy: It would be good to be in a group.
Danny: I get that at karate.
Danny: Would you give me a Porsche?
Lucy: (not thinking!) Why not?
Danny: I'm not prepared to be dictated to ... except by you if you say I *have* to go back to school ... and then I think: What can I get out of it?"
Lucy: Well, that's honest anyway!
Danny: It might be quite nice.
Lucy: The physical science course is always very small.

Danny: Oh I'd love to do science again! And I do like being in a group
   at karate ... but I could do with more of that.
Danny: Do you like my hair? (which was dyed at the back).
Lucy: Well ... I liked the way you were looking before.
Danny: It helps me to differentiate myself.
Lucy: From others? Or yourself as you were?
Danny: From myself as I was.

He phoned his friends and went to karate. He came back rather
excited, saying he now likes the idea of school. "It's lekker. My friends
think it's a good idea. Anthony says why don't I go to the Arts School?"
(One of the schools which rejected him at 16 and did not mention
Grantley.)

"Well this school is helpful to people who have had any sort of
problem."

"So that will be best."

That evening he came in glowing. "I just went to the Means (where
his Standard 7 drop-out friends hung out). I told them I'm going back
to school—probably hey?"

"You really like the idea?"

"Ja."

"You'll have lots of new buddies."

"But that's good, hey?"

"Yes, yes."

"Ria says I must drive her round in my Porsche."

"Well I was being frivolous, my love."

"Oh."

A PORSCHE?!

One thing I was doing now was suddenly to do something kind which
he was not expecting. One morning, as no breakfast came to me in
bed—a luxury I was now very used to—I went in to him:

Lucy: It's 9 o'clock!
Danny: Oh please Ma—I'm so sore.

Lucy (very friendly): That makes no difference. It's my breakfast time—
and kitty's. (And he got up.)

Lucy: That's called "the overcoming of temptation".

Danny: (pleased)

Lucy: If you manage karate tonight I'll bring you breakfast in bed
tomorrow!

Danny (startled and joyful): You will?

Lucy: Yes.

Danny: I want to go skating but perhaps next week because I haven't
got any money.

Lucy (hugging him): Hey—aren't you good! No "Ah please Ma".

Danny (smiling): I'm good, hey?

We had decided to give him his own car—a second-hand one—for
going back to school. He was positive about everything—agreed to
have master-driving lessons in his new car and accepted that the car
probably wouldn't be a Porsche. He told me that he wanted to save his
work money to buy a radio for his new car. This was the first time he
had ever talked about saving money! Good forebrain stuff.

Lucy: I wouldn't give you a car for passing Standard 8—that puts a
wrong emphasis on the exams. You used to be carefree about exams.
That's the right attitude.

Danny: I had the wrong attitude to exams?

Lucy: No—the right attitude. You were very light-hearted about
them.

Danny: That's right! I managed exams easily.

After lunch Danny went to Oliver's studio to play the piano and I
to rest. Just before 2 o'clock, I heard loud angry explosive shouting in
his room. He refused to be comforted. He didn't want to go to art.

Lucy: Shall I make you some tea?

Danny: Ja, OK.

Lucy: Let's go shopping.

In the car I told him I thought he ought to be honest about whether he had smoked pot (very often a prelude to rage).

In a very subdued tone he said, "No I didn't." And I believed him.

"Well what do you think triggered the attack?" He didn't know.

We went to Sandton City and to the Waldorf for coffee. He seemed more relaxed. So I asked him in a very gentle, friendly way, "Do you have absolutely no idea what triggered off that attack?"

"Well you know Ma, I know it's not your fault and all that but I had set my heart on that Porsche."

"So you were terribly disappointed?"

"Yes I was."

"You've had so many disappointments. I suppose this one triggered off all the others."

"It just made everything right. I would have something to do from 8 to 1 and I would have style. It would make me feel right about myself. I wouldn't have asked for a Porsche if I wasn't going back to school."

"You can research it if you like. The family may just not be able to afford it."

He went shopping and I went to Exefit, where I was doing sessions of rowing, running and cycling. Then we met again at the Waldorf and had another excellent heart-to-heart.

"I will go to karate tonight. I could always stop if things really got bad."

"That's right. It's not the army."

"The trouble is that the Black Belts walk around seeing that you keep up."

"It's a difficult problem. You just somehow have to decide by yourself whether you can push yourself through a childish reluctance, or whether you really need to stop."

We were having tea and Black Forest cake.

"There's another problem with a Porsche and that's envy."

Danny grinned. He did not see it as a problem.

"I mean people can be quite nasty about it."

"Not my sort of friends."

"What would Nicola think?"

"Well yes, she would be envious."

"Would you think it fair—I mean she's *worked* for what she's got."

"But I deserve it after all I've been through."

After a silence Danny said, "*You* did it! *You* got me out of my psychosis."

As we walked away from the Waldorf Danny said warmly, "Thank you very much for the chat and everything."

Back home I talked to Oliver. He said, "If he got a Porsche it would be disastrous. It would be the motorbike all over again. And it wouldn't sustain him after the beginning."

"I don't know—he seems to need inspiration. The motorbike after all did get him going on regular karate."

"I don't know what to say. I just don't know what to say. Anyway you haven't got the money if you don't sell."

"It would be an investment in his education. And then when he is educated he won't value outward show as much as he does now."

The next day Danny went skating for the whole day. When he came back he said, "I skated all afternoon without my legs getting tired."

"Karate has made them strong!"

"That's right."

He rang up the Porsche place to find out the prices. They ranged from R25,000 to R300,000.

GRANTLEY COLLEGE?

There was a reliable Porsche dealer in Braamfontein. They felt they could find us a low-priced Porsche for him. It had to be red and look new—and the engine had to be reasonably reliable. It would take time for them to find—and it would take time for me to sell shares. In the meantime Danny would spend some time there and look around.

Danny: I can't wait for tomorrow! (to visit the Porsche place). I'm getting more and more enthusiastic about this plan all the time. To go back to learning and to do a standard I've never even done. And have a social life. (In his mind he had "done" Standard Nine at St. Martin's, and "Matric" at Habilitat. Now he would be going

into Standard 8—if they accepted him. He had only really passed
Standard 7 properly.)

Lucy: I wouldn't tell everyone that you are getting a Porsche for going
back to school.

Danny: No, I won't. I told my friends. At first they thought it wasn't
good because they wanted me for the band, but now they are
completely behind me.

Lucy: Plenty of time for bands.

Danny: I think so too.

In all this excitement—and our doubts—about the Porsche we
seem scarcely to have thought about the fact that Danny had not yet
been accepted for Grantley College. He had to spend two days there
attending school so that they could assess him, both for schoolwork
and for fitting in.

The night before school he was very nervous. "I didn't paint much
at Art. We just talked everything over."

At supper he said he felt sick and couldn't eat. He asked, slightly
aggressively, "Well, what will I be doing there?" I replied, "You are going
as a visitor."

Later in my room we chatted. I looked through a drawer of junk for
black laces. Found brown ones which he put in his black shoes. "I feel
like a veteran!" I told him about the ex-servicemen at 'Varsity.

"Will there be any other older people at Grantley?"

"I think so. Maybe not in your class. At Eden there definitely
are."

"I think this school will suit me very well. Eden is too big. But I
actually am a bit nervous."

After the first day he came home smiling. "It was amazing! I loved
it! No really Ma, I had such a good time. I've even got homework."

He wrote half an essay on "My Family"—half a page in the
afternoon. Then watched a video, then a short break on his bed, then
supper. Then he played the piano for a while. Then it was his turn for
a television programme.

Danny: It's all right if you watch telly now Dad, because I have to finish
my essay.

Lucy: You are being very conscientious!
Danny: Well I have to be to get into this school.

I heard him fussing around in the kitchen, playing with Dibbs the kitten. Eventually he went into his room for about an hour. Then I went in. He had just finished his essay.

The next day he came back radiant:

Danny: I really liked Geography. Perhaps I should do that?
Lucy: Well yes, especially as you are so keen on learning about the world.
Danny: All the subjects would teach me things. And I am quite able to do any of these subjects.
Danny: Mrs Simons is such a nice lady. We just talked and talked about all sorts of things. You know what? She has a daughter who is a mechanical engineer! In Art me and this other girl had to draw each other.

Days went past and I heard nothing from Grantley.

Nicky came to supper. Danny was at karate and NA. I confessed about the Porsche, first expressing all my trepidation to ward off the blows, but she struck nevertheless:

"It's the craziest idea I ever heard."

"Even if it gets him back to school?"

"What left is there to give him—a villa in France? He doesn't respect you. He just thinks: What can I get out of her next?"

But Oliver was very supportive of me, in spite of his own initial doubts:

Oliver: His motivation system is not normal. Before the bike idea he was doing nothing—nothing at all. I thought that idea was crazy—and some crazy things did happen—but basically I have to admit that it did change him.
Nicky: At least you could have given it in three years' time when he got Matric! What more can he live for?
Oliver: It doesn't work that way.

Lucy (to Nicky): I don't think you can understand the depth of his humiliation and despair. You and I have never really failed so we can't imagine what it would be like.

Oliver: It's the feeling of having altogether failed at everything.

Nicky: What he needs is someone who can stand up to him.

Oliver: It's only Lucy's persistence that has got him this far. I don't have the right temperament. I would have had to put him in an institution. His confidence is very fragile you know. A small thing can throw him off balance.

That afternoon Mrs Simons phoned. "I'm sorry," she began, and my centre plummeted. "I'm sorry to have taken such a long time to get back to you. The teachers all felt they could work with him. He was able to talk easily to the pupils. Some older ones are either braggarts or totally uncommunicative. Daniel is very welcome to come to Grantley College next year."

UPS AND DOWNS

Danny went with Oliver to look at Porsches. They didn't find an appropriate one and Danny was patient about waiting. But rages still came.

Danny: You said I could have it under my window.

Lucy: No, I didn't say that. It would be impractical.

Oliver: There must be something wrong with you if you think that. (Our driveway didn't go around the corner to this place under his window.)

He raged. I bathed. He kicked the bathroom door and his own door, and made many loud noises in his room. I went out. When I came back he was calm.

Lucy: I would never deliberately mislead you.

Danny: (silent)

Lucy: Something was not quite clear in the situation.

Danny (shouting): You just think I'm an asshole that I can't understand (bitterly) and you are my *mother*.

Lucy: No my love, I don't. Communication is not always perfect. I was saying something about the Porsche and in my mind it was sitting there waiting in the shop and in your mind it was sitting outside your window.

He calmed down and did a good kitchen clear-up.

"You'll have to stop giving me a bad time, or I'll fail my exams."

"OK, I really will, Ma."

This was September. I had Unisa English II exams in October and November. Three papers: Poetry, Plays and Novels. Sometimes I put quotes about male rage into my Danny Diary:

Ajax Telamon went mad and killed himself when Ulysses won the contest for the shield and armour of Achilles and was named the bravest of the Greeks.

(Anthony and Cleopatra): Anthony's rage has subsided into a deep melancholy in this scene. He expresses a profound sense of the illusory nature of all reality, even of his own identity.

Anthony's disappointment with himself becomes the principal cause of his subsequent defeat. He no longer has the will to fight with a winning vigour.

Finally a Porsche was available. Dennis (at the Porsche place) said, "It's one of the nicest I've ever worked with. Eddie knows its service history. It has had three owners, the last two elderly. The last owner was meticulous—only used it at weekends. He is selling it because he needs a large family car. It is red and looks perfect."

On October 16 he got his Porsche. I don't say anything else in the Danny Diary because I am busy swotting. Danny sold his Kawasaki motorbike, which of course was one of the conditions. He had advanced driving lessons in his Porsche, and spent a day at a skidpan place, learning to get out of a skid. He never had an accident in his Porsche—not so much as a scratch.

After this his life became rather dull. Anthony had now gone to Israel so there were no more band practices. Sandro from the Mean Machine had gone to jail—for dealing and possession. (We heard later that when he came out of jail he went straight.)

Danny smoked pot again. We had a meeting about it. All three of us very quiet. I stopped Oliver as soon as he talked too much.

Lucy: You did say you would give up pot altogether for the Porsche.
Danny: Now you are trying to make me guilty.
Lucy: Yes.

We talked about the great weight of misery which attacks him.
Oliver: Can't you tell us what makes you feel that way?
Danny: (silence)
Lucy: Do you know?
Danny: No. I'll just try harder to handle it. I'll just get in touch with my feelings. I'm feeling much better now.

On another day Danny talked to me about his rages: "It is an anger so strong it wipes out my character cells. I think I have an anger rate like Naomi Faz (woman next door) but I have learnt to control it. There was nothing I could turn to—I felt worse and worse. There is no block when I'm by myself. There just seemed to be no power that could help me. But now I will remember that last time I just sat there with my head in my hands and I didn't go wild and I got out of it. And I know I can come to you. In the past I did think there was a force in my mind—something like the Mafia."

"But it didn't really help you."

"Well—sometimes it seemed to."

"The only real power is in ourselves and each other."

"Yes, that's right …You know who helped me most with my rages?"

"Who?"

"Joaquin—when I first went to Habilitat. I was lucky to have him as my older brother. He persuaded me that I could be my individual self even at Habilitat."

"I think he gave you that winning combination of confrontation and absolute support."

From my Unisa notes I copied: "With awareness comes the possibility of asserting the will against the appetites."

Now was the time for peace and reassurance.

At supper:

Lucy: Well anyway Danny we are very very satisfied with how things are going.

Danny (softly): And will go on when I go to school, hey Dad?

Oliver: If you keep going on like this there won't be anything for us to do. You will do it all yourself.

Lucy: I only noticed yesterday how well you look after your records.

Danny: Ja well, I made a resolution.

He stayed home and in his room a lot of the time. He seemed almost afraid of going out. Perhaps because of the pot risk, or just because he was consolidating.

"I need security." He said. "The people in this town insult me."

Of Sandro he said: "I used to try to explain to Sandro about me—that pot makes me go mad, but he didn't seem to listen; his mind went off on all sorts of other things."

Peddie said, "I am bringing up Sammy very strictly. You were always too gentle with Daniel. You can't be blamed Ma, you tried everything."

Oliver was at last starting to moralize with Danny—giving him ideas of how to be: "Don't treat this as a major thing. It's only a small disappointment. Other people get over these things all the time. I will remind you next time."

Nicola and Danny were going up to Molozi:

Nicky: So what should I know? (Oliver and Danny came in)

Lucy: We can talk in front of him.

Oliver: Daniel knows—we've had good chats about it—that he can't behave badly and then say he is just sensitive.

Nicky: You see Danny, I haven't been here, and I don't know what the score is about pot—I mean I don't want to have to go behind your back ...

Danny (grinning): I'll bear that in mind!

Lucy: I don't like that.

Danny: It was a joke.

Lucy: Jokes about pot are not on.

Oliver: Danny—maybe we should be able to take jokes about pot but ...

Danny: Well, I apologize.

Nicola's report after Molozi: "He was fine. Completely stable. Didn't want to talk to me much. Very selfish. Never asked how *I* was. Slept 13 hours a night."

But when I was dizzy for a day, Danny took care of me—made meals, went twice to Norwood, made no complaints. In the evening I felt better and found him sitting in his Porsche:

"Thanks for all your help."

"It's a pleasure. If you're still sick tomorrow I can always do it again."

Jeff (the counsellor from Wits) nevertheless continued to think that Danny did have a biochemical disorder which accounted both for the over-reactions (lack of a barrier between mind and emotions) and for the withdrawal states and lethargy and lack of planning.

Jeff said, "At least we can say that he is a person who will have ups and downs."

GETTING IT RIGHT

After a gloomy period of staying in his room in the evenings and becoming almost agoraphobic—seeming to fear going out even with us or to Nicola—he met new and worse friends.

Danny: Derrick's brother has to prove with signatures that he has really got a job so that he can get his child back.

Danny: Derrick's brother's wife has been through such bad times—
heart operations, tubes in her chest. But she's like me—she never
loses her enthusiasm for life. I've taken her to town twice to this
restaurant where she works in the evenings.

Then there were another couple, Shane and Monique, who also
had a child who was in a foster home. Danny said, "Monique was in
a bad mood and she said she hadn't eaten for two days and I said I
understood. I invited her to our house for a meal but she said she was
embarrassed."

Danny: Shane and Monique spike you know.
Lucy: What's that mean?
Danny: They inject this chemical—not heroin, some other powder.
Shane wanted me to but I said NO!! He said he would give me one
for my birthday. I would turn them in for what they did to me. If
they lived next door I would ask you to turn them in, but I can't
be bothered.
Lucy: So you have to give up these friends, don't you.
Danny: I've given up so many friends.

He was silent and sad.
I told him about Prince Hal and Falstaff. He listened with interest.
It's not really a parallel because these friends are so new. He has no long
loyalty to them.

I was finished my exams by now, so could think of new ways to encourage
him. He had not read a book all year—had not been a regular reader
the whole of the five years since his breakdown. He looked at photo-
magazines and watched videos.
I went searching for easy books that would yet be interesting and I
found the Spirals. What a coup! They couldn't have been better. Good
young adult stories in short sentences. Scary, mysterious, funny. Danny
loved them. To get him going I said he now had to read a Spiral before
he watched a video. He was soon reading two or three at a time.
Nicola's old room was almost empty by this time. She really had
moved out. So I suggested that Danny have it. This spurred him to great
heights of clearing up his own things. He dumped all his own things

in Nicky's room and then started sorting them: to keep, to throw away, to give away.

And then: he threw away all this year's songs! "None of them are any good."

I think those songs were part of the hugely negative punk movement, where decadence was celebrated.

Oliver's pupils' exams were also over and Oliver was trying extremely hard never to be sarcastic and negative towards Danny. "I told him how impressed I was with the way he went to the porch to smoke without pleading to smoke inside. I said, 'The way you are going you are going to be a really useful member of society. A good guy.'"

Oliver and Danny bought a big new desk for his new room.

Danny: At my new desk I'll compose and arrange and draw and think all day. I'll be a philosopher.

Lucy's diary: His answer to the friend problem is to visit for very short times. Today he spent 20 minutes with Shane and Monique, then returned to work in his new room. I look in and see vast quantities of clothes everywhere and his huge box empty.

Danny: Right. I've done it. All these are for giving away (two-thirds). And all these are for washing.

Lucy's diary: The few remaining clothes are neatly folded in his cupboard. The new room looks magical. He could never make so many decisions before—he would have given up. If Danny can change, then who cannot?

It's 9.30 now and he is still at it—cleaning away at the mirror. A bit frenetic now. He has put some cushions and cuddly toys in the new room.

Danny: I don't want anything in my new room that I'm not using. This
    is my new image: clarity and simplicity—no muddle or mess.
Lucy: Sounds marvellous. You've ended up inspiring yourself.

We still had December and half of January to get through before school started. He had stopped karate and art "for the holidays". He had created his new room. He had read the 14 Spirals. What now?

And then I heard him on the phone: "I'm not like you 'Varsity guys who can do all these things. I have to fix myself up. I have to work things out. I could do keyboard in a recording-studio, but not on stage."

The next day Hedley, the band leader who had made this request to Danny, phoned me privately:

"Anthony said to take Danny, and I said I know he's good, but I don't think he can handle it. The last I heard him he used to play four bars OK and then go off on his own."

"Well he's much more together now."

"Would he listen to me, do you think?"

"He just might! I'll chat to him about it."

Hedley sighed. "Even when he was mad, the sensitive Daniel shone through."

I talked to Danny and he agreed to try playing keyboard for Hedley's band. So he was in a band not playing the guitar and not playing his own music. Everything went well, although sometimes Hedley had to be firm with him. This group were medical, dental and legal students. Not at all into the drug scene.

Danny said, "Tomorrow (Dingaan's Day or whatever it then was, now Day of Reconciliation) we are going to rehearse for ten hours. I'm really into that!"

Hedley phoned me one day and said: "I bawled him out for coming late. Then later I apologized, but he said: 'No you *must* shout at me—that's the only way I'll learn.'"

One of the band members, John, gave Danny his number. Danny phoned him up.

John: Come round. I'm just having a bath.
Danny: I'll just have some chow here.
John: No, wait—come here and I'll cook something for you.

I could hardly believe this. On Friday night he went to John who took him to dinner. Then John and the rest were going on for a late night. Danny felt this would be wrong because of playing on Saturday night, so he came home.

On Saturday Danny was nervous and excited. But then stayed calm listening to music in his new room. His American cousins were here (Neil who had smoked dope, and Cathy who was at Stanford) and they went to the concert. It was a big crowd and everything went very well.

Christmas Eve:

Danny: After rehearsal I'll just have Irish coffee with John. I really like John. I like Mark too.

Lucy: What about the girl? How does she fit in?

Danny: She's amazing! She has a very hard life, so she's just what we need.

Lucy: What do you mean?

Danny: She's like our Nicola—but she's had an even harder life. She lives on her own and has to earn her own living. I don't know why her family don't help her.

Lucy: So she's not spoilt—and she wouldn't mess around with drugs?

Danny: No. And she comes to rehearsals on time and she doesn't just want to do her own thing.

On Christmas Day my mother said, "Daniel sat here talking to me while he was waiting for Neil yesterday, and he behaved like a perfectly normal member of the family!"

Lucy's diary, New Year's Eve: The planet will disappear anyway, eventually—bombs or not, revolutions or not—but the boy in his new room is secure.

Chapter Eighteen

GRANTLEY COLLEGE
(AGED TWENTY, 1987)

Danny, aged 20, was going back to school. In his Porsche. Into Standard 8, where the average age was 15.

Advice to myself:
1. Continue being supportive. He is very inexperienced; needs a lot of encouragement.
2. Ignore bad behaviour. Walk away from tantrums.
3. Ask him first for solutions.
4. Encourage the slightest signs of initiative in solution-finding.
5. Use propaganda and foresight, not indignation.

At breakfast on the first day, Danny said, "I saw such an amazing movie last night. My favourite actor—he's won seven Black Belts. I had to keep saying and saying it until Dad agreed."

I said, "Can I give you a bit of motherly advice?"

"Ja."

"Be proud of being in Standard 8. If people are surprised, don't get defensive: that's what you are, and that's what is good.

"Yes, I will."

Off to school he went in his Porsche and home from school he came when school was over. "I must say it seems really nice. This Mr Jones—he's our class teacher, he's quite funny! But nice-funny—sort of buddy-talk. Very friendly.

But by the evening he was over-tired. He banged away in an uncontrolled way at his keyboard and broke it. Came and confessed after an hour or two.

"It's because I want to escalate. It's ridiculous. I must just learn not to do things when I'm tired. Otherwise I'll never get anywhere in life."

On the third day he was still thrilled, but very, very tired.

I gave him a hug. "I'm so very proud."

"And I haven't smoked dope either."

Oh dearie me, I thought to myself. Has he been offered dope at this school?

"Is it more like St Martin's or more like Damelin?"

"It's, it's—it's like a commune! Much more personal than both of them."

He has a new image of himself and he gives me quick looks to check whether I am disapproving or rejecting. He spends a lot of time keeping his room perfectly clean.

"I used to hate that brown carpet, but now I like it. It is so neat. I was noticing in my room last night how neatly it is fixed at the edges."

"Dad says your light was still on at 2 am."

"Well I like to lie there and look at my room."

A problem with Grantley was that there was no sport—except some occasional morning activity—and no after-school extra-murals. Danny was not going to karate—this one new activity was all he was prepared to do. But he had too much free time—and often didn't sleep well at night. And then the next day he would mutter and drift.

One non-problem was the Porsche. All my fears that he would be envied or scorned were unfounded. It was an uncomplicated symbol of who he was. A teacher said to me, smiling broadly, "Oh, he's the boy with the car."

We got back from a play one night at 11 pm and I found him still studying at his desk. He got angry when I suggested it was time to stop. (He had had a short sleep the night before.)

Walking into the kitchen after school the next day he said, "You know what! I got full marks for my Geography test. It was so easy, but that's because I learnt. I could do Zulu I at 'Varsity. I just say things over and over in my head and then I've got it."

He added, "I'm ahead in Art, so I have to draw myself from a mirror. It's very difficult."

It was Sunday at the end of his first week. Danny woke at lunchtime, finally recovered from all the sleeplessness.

At lunch he said, "It's a down-to-earth school. That's what I've decided. Tomorrow I play ping-pong."

"No religion?" I asked.

"None at all. You want to see all the work I've done!" (He showed me pages and pages of written work.)

I was impressed. "I can't understand how you've become such a worker."

"Well you see there's no way out of it."

I thought: It's the definiteness of the tasks.

Everything was going so well that we could hardly take it in. We were three new people.

First report, March 1987:
  English: The work he produces is of a very good standard.
  Afrikaans: Daniel is coping with the Afrikaans and works well.
  History: Daniel's test marks are disappointing.
  Geography: Daniel is doing well. He concentrates in class and is producing work of a satisfactory standard.
  Biology: He is attentive in class and has done well in tests so far.
  Art: Very creative—draws and paints extremely well.
  Head's observations: I am pleased with Daniel's progress so far—- both academically and socially. He is working well and has a good attitude towards his work and to school in general. We all wish him a successful year.

He got a certificate for coming second in his class.

It was five years since he had managed schoolwork.

RUSSELL and ANGELA

There were two Standard 8s at Grantley: one for people who had come unstuck in some way but who were expected to write Matric. Daniel was in this class. The other class was for people with real learning difficulties. Russell, aged 15, was in this other class.

Daniel and Russell became friendly. Russell lived very near us, so Danny was able to give him a lift home, and they visited each other.

Then Alfred our gardener told me that Russell smoked pot. He had seen him often doing this around our area. There was a house in our street where pot was grown in the garden and Russell went there to get it.

I was stunned—not for Danny, but for Russell. I felt there was no way I could keep this to myself, as was the fashion: the "don't interfere" fashion. Russell, who already had learning difficulties, was further damaging his brain by pot smoking.

I knew from my previous "telling" that it was wise to talk to the wife and mother during the day, rather than risk the father at night.

I phoned Russell's mother. She said, nervously, "But my children are not part of all that."

I told her everything I knew, and of the extent of pot-smoking among kids from good families. Pot crossed many boundaries.

Unlike the other mother I had told, who was desperate to keep the information from her husband, this mother immediately said, "I'll have to tell my husband."

Later in the day she phoned and asked if she and her husband could come round and see us that evening after supper. I agreed. When Oliver came home I told him. We were afraid that the father would not believe us and would be angry and feel insulted.

At 7.30 pm Oliver and I were reading the paper in the living room. Russell's mother and father walked through the front garden and we welcomed them in and offered them coffee. Russell's father was huge and broad—the biggest man I had ever seen at close quarters. He looked tough and aggressive.

Oliver said quickly, "I think I'll just go and make the coffee. My wife can fill you in with the details."

I smiled to myself. Then I explained why I thought Russell was smoking pot and the father asked some questions.

Then he said: "I am a miner. I've worked in the mines all my life. I have a simple solution which will confirm what you have told us—or not. When Russell wakes in the morning I will get a sample of his urine and take it to work. At work there is a large pot-analyser. All people coming to work at the mine have their urine tested when they first arrive. Then the ones who are tested positive for pot will still be employed by us—but never with machinery, and never in any position of responsibility." He paused, then added, "If Russell's tests positive then I will give him the hiding of his life. He will never touch it again."

I shrank at poor Russell's doom. But all this was done, Russell tested positive, never touched pot again, and eventually went to John Orr Technical School and did well there.

The fact that there was a pot test made me once again very aggravated, just as when I heard about Grantley. In the five years of Danny's breakdown, during which pot always made things worse, why had Sanca never mentioned this test? I now learnt that pot stayed for two weeks in the urine and was easy to test for. Danny in the first year of his breakdown had accepted our "Tough Love" conditions. This test could easily have been a part of them.

However, for the moment, Danny was enjoying school and not smoking pot.

One day Danny came to me and said, "I think I'm in love! But she lives in Bryanston and her parents are very strict."

Angela agreed to go out with Danny, but it had to be with parental consent.

"Angela felt a bit bad," said Danny, "a bit shy I think—about us having to phone her mother."

I did this, and it was arranged that Danny would fetch Angela and meet her parents and bring her back for lunch with us. Danny went in his black polished shoes and brought her here. He behaved with perfect manners and was protective towards Angela, who was pretty and shy.

The next time Oliver took them both to a movie. And then the third time they were allowed to go out alone. They went to *The Golden Child*.

The next day Danny told us, "Angela clung on to me she was so scared when the lizard came."

Then his day of triumph came when Angela came here and they listened to music together and she let him rest his head on her shoulder. She told him she loved him.

But she didn't want any more, and I don't think Danny did either at this stage. So the relationship went on in this innocent way.

POT, POOH-BAH, KARATE

The Easter holidays loomed as another great big blank. Hedley and the others, whom Daniel had played music with in December, were hard at work at university. His new friend Angela was away.

Danny came with me to visit Grandma, who had become an alcoholic in her old age and had to have her drinks controlled by us or by her domestic worker.

Danny: I feel so sorry for her.

Lucy: So you don't condemn her for her addiction? I suppose you understand that better.

Danny: Ja. I can understand withdrawal and craving. I go through two weeks of that and then I just get over-confident and start it up again. And then the rages come when I am coming down. But I will definitely go back to karate.

Lucy: Have you ever smoked pot after karate?

Danny: No! Not once. You get into something physical like that and you don't even feel like it.

Lucy: Now that you are fully sane I will consider you morally responsible if you throw our family into chaos again.

He looked a little startled—ashamed? caught out?—or perhaps just accepting the seriousness of it all.

But after two holiday weeks of doing absolutely nothing, pot must have seemed easier than starting karate again, so he bought a packet, which I found in the garage. He said, "I didn't know I was going to do it. I just felt depressed and did it."

We took control again and insisted on karate and on Sandy the therapist. I wrote a letter to Stan Schmitt the karate guru about Danny's breakdown and tiredness. Stan phoned me and was very encouraging. He said Danny could stop a session ten minutes early if he needed to. Danny was thrilled that Stan had phoned and started karate again the next day.

A few days later Oliver came back from work in a great state. The Arts School was doing the *Mikado*: everyone had been rushing around; a friend of mine (a teacher there) went to Chinatown for material.

Oliver was happy with his role as "the Mikado", which is a minor role which he had learnt easily in the first term. But now something had happened to Pooh Bah, the main character—a huge part. Oliver had been persuaded to take it on, but didn't know if he could manage to learn all the words.

Danny and I were talking about this and about Oliver's birthday the next day, for which Danny didn't have a present. The next day Oliver found this note on the table:

Dear Dad, you'll be happy to know,
that............
(and then on the other side):
I am offering to hear your part in the Mikado for as long as necessary....
HAPPY BIRTHDAY!!
from Danny.

And he did that, day after day, day after day, until Oliver knew it all; and the performances, later that term, were a great success.

So Danny went back to school the second term feeling relaxed and confident.

He left notes for Oliver asking him to help him with his Afrikaans homework, Oliver being the Afrikaans star in our household.

Danny wrote an Afrikaans essay on "What I Think of Adults."

"What did you say?" I asked him.

"I said I had a very strict upbringing when I was a child and then when I became an adolescent it was just the end of strict times and so they couldn't stop me. So I ended by saying I didn't think much of adults because they couldn't stop me becoming a drug addict."

"And are we forgiven now?"

"Yes. All is forgiven."

He took Angela for coffee after school in Yeoville. Her mother was shocked. "Such a sordid place!"

But Danny said in the car the next day, "Well one thing Ma, my relationship with Angela really is going well. I just can't believe how well it is going."

The Sandy sessions were a muddle. She would say, "That's what you *say*, but what do you really *think*?" I went with him once to see her. She said, "What do you think of your mom being here?"

"It's OK."

"But what do you really feel?"

Danny said on the way home that he didn't "really feel" anything in particular so didn't know how to answer her. He said that last time she had said, "That's not the real you speaking, Daniel," and it baffled him. Sandy had been wonderfully supportive and encouraging of his good self in the early days, but now she seemed to feel obligated to try and "break through" as her textbooks had told her to. So we stopped the sessions.

Stan—karate Stan—phoned Danny one day when he was out and I chatted to him about Sandy, and her wish to uncover Danny's "not OK" feelings.

"That's just pathetic," said Stan. "We want to build up his spirit— not break it down."

One day Danny felt too tired for karate. He said, "I'll go for the urine test if you let me off karate just for this time."

I had discovered that Sanca were now offering the dagga urine test themselves, but I also knew that at this moment Danny didn't need it.

He was nervous of going to a Grantley dance—said he'd pick up Angela afterwards. But in the end he was hungry and went to the dance to eat; and he danced with Angela and was happy.

"HIS HISTORY"

Danny was having difficulty with history, a subject which he had loved as a child, and in which he later got a distinction in Matric. But at this stage the language of history had passed him by. In his everyday talking I don't think he was now coming out with flows of meaningless abstractions—at any rate I don't mention them in the diary—but there was still a lot of junk in his brain competing with sense—and he still talked a lot to himself.

He was a lot more careful in speech now—and often silent in company. I think he knew when he was not following the conversation. Of a conversation I was having with his uncle he said afterwards, "It was interesting listening to how you and Alistair were talking. But your talk was on Level Three and mine is on Minus Six."

So his "disappointing result" in History was not because he wasn't trying but because the words didn't ring with real meaning. His solution was to stuff them in—learn them by heart—which got him through his next exam.

I still went to my writing classes with Lionel Abrahams on Monday nights. People new to the class were given two exercises: one was to describe peeling and eating an orange—but it had to be your own fingers and your own orange and your own taste buds—not some derived words. The other exercise was "Describe a room". Again it had to be what you actually saw, and not what you had read. I was not given these exercises, but I thought the "room" one would be quite interesting and one week when I didn't have a story in my head I decided to "describe a room".

And then I suddenly realized that I could describe two rooms—and then I would have a story after all: Danny's old room, and Danny's new room. I made it into a complete short story, but the parts I will quote here are what actually happened one afternoon. (Oliver was away.)

It is 3 o'clock on a freezing winter afternoon. This is the time that Danny and I study history together. I knock at his door. "Come in".

Danny-the-Good is sitting on his throne of cushions, with his orange karate belt looped like a halo over the cushion behind his head. Reading his history notes.

"I can manage this myself thanks all the same Ma."

"Good! Would you like some tea and toast?"

"Tea please. You know I don't eat toast in this room."

This is his new room. It shines pine-yellow with matching furniture. On the walls are pop-art pictures, clean and uncluttered. The one above his head has a huge red tomato with three drops of water on it, and seven white tomatoes on a cream-white quilt.

There is no heater in this room. A cord trailing over the floor would be inappropriate.

I wander into his old room with my notebook. Danny-the-Bad's room. The cupboard is pitted with a thousand holes. It was Danny's dart-board. The ceiling shows brown stains of long-ago spit. In the furthest corner a silver knife, bound with elastoplast, is stuck in the floor. I think of Danny in his pure new room, studying war and revolution.

On the window-sill of this old room is the pedal of a Kawasaki motorbike. I gave him that bike for attending karate consistently for three months. In another corner of the old room is a guitar, broken at the neck—the splintered wood spiking out of each part and strings flung out like crazy stamens. That was Danny in an explosive rage about his music and the frustration of not having his own band.

An hour has passed. Danny-the-Good still works in his cold room. I look in. He is saying history to himself. He is forcing it into his head in an ecstasy of concentration and he shouts:

"Don't disturb me!"

I put on a coat and gloves and wander round the garden. The cold wind numbs my brain. But I know that I have not yet finished with Danny's old room. I go back to it. I find a Christmas card: "To Tiger-Man Danny, the best, most wondrous, wacky, way-out, world-class brother, Merry Xmas!" That must have been the Christmas before the breakdown, when he was a precocious and over-confident fourteen. At the Battle of the Bands he was "Best Songwriter" and "Best Lead Guitarist". Swaying and singing, he'd point his guitar-neck now up to the ceiling, now down to the floor, while gum-chewing schoolgirls screamed for him.

I go outside again and look through his window. He is still saying history out aloud. I worry he is overdoing it, but I fear being shouted at again.

Two hours on I make coffee and take it to Danny's too-perfect room, where he is still at it. I take a hot-water-bottle to my bedroom and half doze. Danny's room is three shut doors away. I dream of beaches.

I awake to familiar strangled screams. I am angry: he must have got at pot again. These attacks come the day afterwards. I am upset: things seemed to be going so well. I am frightened: what will he do this time?

I go and sit on his floor. He pushes his flushed face at mine. For half an hour I'm in terror. I'm a bitch, a whore. Language is crude, violence is close, despair is total. I sit there quietly rocking with his teddybear.

He calms, and I go and sit in the kitchen. I look at the cold stew I had planned to heat for supper. I put it in the fridge and make boiled eggs and toast. Danny comes in.

He gives me a quick glance and an embarrassed smile:

"Sorry Ma."

"Perhaps you worked for too long."

"Ja, I think I did."

"Break it up into shorter periods next time."

"Ja, I will."

I wrote my story. It was published in the first *Frontline* magazine to go out with the *Sunday Star*. I got more feedback than ever before. There were many like Danny out there in this town.

But there was a downside to my success. A woman from the Schizophrenia Association pestered me to accept that Danny would never be independent and that we should join her association. I repeated every time she phoned that Danny had only residual symptoms and was not on any medication.

Eventually a man from the association phoned me and asked me to give a talk. It was a most depressing experience. I told Danny's story, and they asked questions. There were about 30 parents there. One after another they said that their child lived at home, was permanently medicated, was on a disability grant—and had no motivation.

CHOCOLATES AND MAURITIUS

Everything was going well. Sandy the therapist phoned me: "I would like to talk to you some time about how you get your good results."

I marvelled! I said to myself: All the time these analysts spend re-activating negative experiences is basically counter-productive. Danny has never come home from Sandy *glowing* like he did after the Biology test.

Other factors would be:

1. A strong holding structure—a programme, a syllabus, tasks to be done.
2. Success: karate, school, Angela.
3. My optimism and encouragement. Oliver's involvement.
4. Continuity. Us. This house. His music.

It was very cold. Danny gave R15 to Operation Snowball (blankets for the poor). He was not talking to himself and he was not withdrawing.

But the winter holiday was looming. He would again be doomed by nothingness and would smoke pot and be doomed yet more. Oliver would be on holiday too. He would be depressed and irritated by Danny.

I decided to send them both to Mauritius for two weeks. Oliver provided the income for our everyday lives, and I used my inheritance for these extras. Here alone at home it would be a holiday for me too.

I talked over Danny's pot lapses with him:

Danny: Pot is my security blanket.

Lucy: Well there's three weeks to go before Mauritius. I will give up chocolate if you give up pot for those three weeks.

Danny: I do know that it's not worth smoking pot because I have to work so hard afterwards to be normal. I can never relax. When I come down from a pipe I am aggressive and hostile—and then I just have to smoke again to feel better. (A pipe? Had he had dagga plus Mandrax at any time recently?)

Lucy: So what will you gain by not smoking?

Danny: Clear head, self-esteem, and I'll be able to relax properly.

A week later I was watching him eating chocolate. "Ooh—you don't know how deprived I feel."

"Oh Ma, here, have some. I'll let you off! After all you let me off so many times."

"No, no. I said I'd do it until Mauritius, and so I will. All I have to do is to give up a single pleasure at a single moment. What *you* have to do is to fill all the spaces that were taken up by pot philosophy and pot companionship."

Meanwhile he was overwhelmed by the thought of the mid-year exams. "I'm too stupid to know how to start."

I gave him some history pegs and now he was tackling it alone. I was able to discover him at it and be pleased.

But in a bad mood he said, "Why the hell should someone as special as me have to go to school day after day on icy cold mornings?"

However, he was delighted to find his name on the top of the Snowball donors in the Star.

Mauritius was fine. Oliver saw no sign of drugs anywhere. He said that he and Danny walked every evening and that they went to all the entertainments and that Danny played with the hotel band and had a long chat to an American model.

Oliver told me, "One morning he disappeared after breakfast. When he was not home by 5 pm I started to get worried. And then he walked into supper, exhausted but pleased with himself. I think he had been trying to walk round the island!"

"But there was one thing I hated," he added. "We had no conversations. He just didn't talk."

Oliver wasn't particularly good at initiating conversations (his family hadn't talked at meals) and Danny's mind was not yet re-stocked with "things to say".

LIPPING AND SMILING

Daniel passed his mid-year exams, including History, but I worried about how difficult it was for him and the way he had to cram without understanding. I took him to be tested at the Athol Desmond Remedial Centre. After the tests they said that Danny's overall ability to process words was good. "He has a high global verbal intellectual potential." However, Danny's "reading vocabulary" and "reading comprehension" were only at Standard Six level—that of the average 13-year-old. "He has deficits relating to clarity and definition of meaning. He needs to refine the precision with which he understands and uses words."

They said they could give him a special programme to help this, but Danny would have seen it as extra pressure, so I left it. He said to me, "I get scared that as soon as I manage a certain thing you will just ask me to do more. Then I will rebel again and smoke pot."

When he was relaxed with me Danny would make up a word or use abstract words with the wrong meanings. With other people he often stayed silent, being aware that he might make mistakes. Sometimes I thought he talked English like a foreigner—mostly correctly, but cautiously.

Danny went to see a dress rehearsal of *Othello* in which his sister Nicola played Desdemona:

Danny: She was very calabrific.

Lucy: What does that mean?

Danny: She gripped my attention all the time. It was quite eerie—you could think she was a real character of those times. Especially the scenes in bed.

Sometimes I could in the end make sense. His old friend Max came round and we talked in the kitchen. Later I said to Danny:

Lucy: I was interested in what Max said about belonging.

Danny: I would think it would be an attribute of level.

Lucy: What does that mean? Why did you say that?

Danny: I said it because it felt like what you were saying.

And later I realized that an "attribute of level" could mean that people on the same level tended to group together.

At school he found it easier to talk to the Standard 7s than to his own group.

"Angela saw me walking off and she was angry, but I was going to the Standard 7s because I feel comfortable with them."

Angela said to me when we were alone. "Our class doesn't like him. He does karate and sings between classes. They think he is quite mad."

But the teachers continued to appreciate him. They found him interesting and responsive. One day the Geography teacher said to me, "I saw him smiling, and I said, 'Come on Danny what's funny?'—and he suddenly went serious as if frightened and he said sorry. I could have bitten my tongue off."

The teachers knew his story and the kids did not.

He still talked aloud to himself when he was alone but usually controlled it in public. When not part of the conversation or when stressed he would now do what we called "lipping"—moving his lips silently.

Of his not talking Nicola said, "You mustn't try and make him like me and you and Dad. He's just not a talker."

But Terry, who was visiting, disagreed: "He was certainly a talker at Saheti!"

Danny decided not to go to camp with his class, saying, "I just want things to be smooth."

To myself I said: It doesn't seem to matter that he hasn't got a social life for the moment. His life has a pattern.

Danny was smiling and lipping one supper when Oliver was holding forth.

"Come on Danny!" I said. "Is Dad carrying on and on?"

"Ja ... something like that ... but I was listening."

One day Nicola visited when Danny was lipping. "Come on Danny," she said, "You can tell me what you are thinking."

Danny looked down, humiliated and ashamed. Caught out.

SCHOOLDAYS COLLAPSE

Everything continued well. Danny gave a dazzling display on the bass guitar to a small pupil of Oliver's. He did sometimes still say, "What am I doing at school when I should be working on my music?" but when he came home with good test marks he smiled with a "real-world" smile.

"I don't even *want* to be famous," he said. "I just want my own band."

Occasionally he thought of others. He got the video *Psycho III*.

"It's just what I wanted. Don't worry if I scream! I'm watching it early so that I won't disturb your sleep or anything."

Karate continued to go well.

To myself: Danny is practising karate in the garden. His speed! He looks very right doing it. Strong and controlled and swift. He says he will frame his next certificate.

"Twenty cigs is not bad, coming off zol and all," he said. "I want to cut them down myself. I don't want you to do it for me."

His relationship with Angela had cooled. She wanted to be "just friends". He raged at first, then said, "I don't want to worry about Angela because I want to concentrate on school and karate and self-improvement."

He told me a hair-raising story of how he assumed a car was going to turn left off the motorway.

Lucy (sweating, but "looking for the good"): Well, anyway, you gave
    me a very clear account of it.
Danny: That shows I'm not on drugs, hey.

In September he had "cycle tests"—just on the work that had been done that term. He was already dreading the final exams, which would examine the whole year's work.

And then quite suddenly there was a problem at our home which was not to do with Danny.

Lucy's diary: It's October now and something has happened to Oliver. He is very depressed, but can't give any explanation. He comes home white-faced and without expression.

There is total deadness between him and Danny. I make valiant efforts at supper, but they don't respond. Danny doesn't seem depressed—just doesn't know what to say. Easier to say nothing.

The karate belts went from white to yellow to orange to green. Danny had got his orange earlier this year and now got his green. "I can't believe how *smoothly* the grading went."

Before Oliver became depressed he and Danny had been having good history sessions. And Danny would say: "Me and Dad worked so hard at history today."

Danny now tried alone:

"Do you know what, Ma? I am beginning to be able to decipher a paragraph of history all by myself!"

He passed his cycle tests well. The teachers said he was fun to teach. But then the lead-up to the exams started and all was doom again. Danny no longer had written work to do and it fazed him just to have to swot. The task seemed too enormous.

We were only three weeks away from the end of the year.

Danny had a morning off to swot. Oliver was at home. They were doing history. I walked down the passage and heard a wrong situation going on. Oliver was back into his hostile, "You'd better learn this or else" tone. Perhaps his depression had knocked out all his new "encouragement" modes of being. What I was hearing now was his own youthful despair at himself, and his earlier despair at Danny. Whatever it was, it released absolute rebellion in Danny. He got up and walked out. That was it. No more school.

Danny did not go off the rails. He came back and talked to me about his plans for getting his own band together. The next morning he brought me scrambled eggs in bed and asked what he could do for me.

Lucy: I'm busy writing in the morning. You could help me by answering phones and doorbell.
Danny: Yes, certainly.
Lucy: I'd appreciate that.

That night:
Danny: I was thinking I might go jam on the roof tonight.
Lucy (laughing): OK.
Danny: It's such a hot night—and I haven't done it for a long time.

The next day Danny said:
Danny: Something good did actually happen in those last few weeks at Grantley.
Lucy: What?
Danny: I learnt how to talk to my own classmates—the Standard 8s.

The following August I asked Mrs Symons to write a report on Danny. Here it is.

This is to certify that Daniel attended the above-mentioned school from January, 1987 until late in the last term when he left of his own accord.

Daniel was placed in the Standard 8 class and followed this curriculum:

    English First Language
    Afrikaans Second Language
    History
    Geography
    Biology
    Art

He passed the first and second terms of 1987 but did not write the final Standard 8 examinations. Daniel's areas of potential were English and Art.

Daniel attended school fairly regularly and would have obtained a pass at the end of the year if he had written the examinations. His record marks were satisfactory.

It is the opinion of the school that Daniel is a talented student who has not yet reached his real potential.

J.M.Symons: Principal. Grantley Private School

Chapter Nineteen

DEPRESSED AT HOME
(AGED TWENTY-ONE, 1988)

I am surprised now that in the diary I say nothing regretful about Danny leaving school and not writing his exams. I think it was simply that he had moved on in his recovery, and this was what mattered most after six years. His current sanity was liberating to us. In my diary I wrote: "DANNY IS TALKING!!!"

This no longer meant that Danny was talking to himself. It meant that he had come out of his long silence.

Drummer Mark phoned up. I answered the phone: Mark said, incredulously, "He's starting to talk, hey? I suddenly realized. I know he wants to form his own band but I don't want to lose him for *my* band now that he's OK again."

Mark phoned Danny and asked him to breakfast:
Danny (very enthusiastic): I dig to!
Mark: So pull in like soon hey!

At supper:
Lucy: What are you going to call your band?
Danny: Gang-of-One.
Oliver: Doesn't that sound a bit as if only you count?
Danny: No. It's power to the individual. It means you can handle your life in an individual way.

Oliver had gone on anti-depressants towards the end of November and was now fine again, and delighted with Daniel.

But Danny's bad friends still lurked around.
Gary: Come over to that place and have a *skuif* (joint).
Daniel: No, I've got a rehearsal.

This was not quite "No, I don't smoke pot any more", but nevertheless impressed Oliver. "He is just amazing. He is behaving in a more adult way than anyone else. I'm lost in admiration for him."

Apart from Oliver and Danny being normal again we had a great project on the go, which kept us arguing and enjoying and having to work out how to live with chaos. Not the chaos of Danny's mind, but the chaos of the Good Building.

We had decided, some time in 1987, to stay in South Africa for the rest of our lives. There had always been some doubt about this. But South Africa was looking a lot more promising—people were not stopped from coming to town to look for work and there was a lot of work around when they came.

Nicola's work was totally involved with the evolving South African situation: she was either in local plays or writing her own cabarets. I too was writing within the South African context.

When we made the decision we did not think that Danny would ever be completely independent. So the plan was to break down the very old crumbling outbuildings and build a small two-storied place with a balcony for Danny, with two bedrooms so that friends and cousins could stay with him. Attached to the flat, where the old garage (Danny's den) was, would be a studio room which could be soundproofed for Danny and his band to rehearse. We didn't get planning permission for this pretty-looking two-storied place. Instead we built a tiny bachelor flat next to the new studio (which was approved as a "garage").

Oliver would have a workroom for woodwork and instrument-fixing. And we would have huge parking space for visitors and musicians and pupils. Up to now we had had only a single driveway and each one of us was constantly being blocked in by a pupil or by each other.

The work started in October 1987, and from the beginning Daniel and I were fascinated. Daniel's new speech was very concrete—he no longer attempted those convoluted intellectual sentences to try to keep up with the more educated. He watched everything that was being done, and often would come and fetch me to show me something.

We were lucky in getting an excellent building contractor, Louie, who handled the various people who came to work in a friendly, clear way. No white bossiness of blacks.

Danny and I had a big argument over whether we should get an electric gate. I had never lived with one and thought I would feel trapped when it didn't work.

Danny: I'm just not going to say any more about it. You and Dad just won't listen to me. Robert has electronic gates and they never gave any trouble.
Lucy: And their house burnt down.
Danny: Ma, what has that got to do with gates? Why don't you stick to the point?

The battle of the gate was won by Danny. It was put in later in 1988—and I've felt safe ever since. Another argument was with Oliver about parking.

"I'm telling you Dad," said Danny. "The *only* thing to do is to fill in the swimming-pool and have a round parking-place there."

That argument he lost. The swimming pool, which after all he used more than anyone else, was saved.

One day a huge vehicle with a crane drove down our muddy old driveway. It was to park there overnight. But after the driver left, it slowly toppled over onto our house. Our kitchen door and windows were blocked. This menacing thing, which looked as if it could push over our house, stayed that way all night. Danny got a bit hysterical about it.

We argued about what plants to cut down:
Lucy: But I love that bush.
Danny: You are just not thinking properly Ma. We are supposed to be doing things properly now.
Lucy: But my feelings!
Danny: What about my feelings? I loved that aloe. You had no right to make that decision on your own.
Lucy: The architect and builder were here and a decision had to be made, that's all.

I was keeping a special diary, "The Diary of the Good Building", which was going to include everything from the aloe to a political solution for South Africa. Peddie had chats about AIDS to the young

Zulu workers who were going home for Christmas. And then I wrote down what she and they had said.

Danny's cousin Hector was visiting from London. He stared at Danny with a silly grin on his face, not quite believing Danny's sanity. Then he came to me and said, "He's been talking about *my* life—that's so different!"

Danny turned 21 on January 24, 1988. We had a party for relations and our friends in the afternoon, and a party for his trustworthy friends in the evening.

And then most of the building was finished:

Lucy: This building that you've watched—you'll remember this as a joyful experience all your life.
Danny: Yes, I will.
Lucy: What are the sparks?
Danny: Welding. Mark says I'll know a lot about building. It's an advance on staying in bed, hey?

Oliver: That youngster is really pulling himself together! I told him so yesterday. I said: "Since your 21st birthday you've really been behaving like an adult."

DANNY'S DREAM

Danny's dream was never to be a star with someone else's band, playing someone else's music: it was simply to have his own band which played the music he himself composed.

A week after he left Grantley he was offered a job in a professional band. He turned it down. At that stage he didn't know just how difficult it would be for him to form a band that lasted, nor were we insisting on "going out and earning a living".

His band would earn—of that he was certain. "When the band is earning, then we would all be happy to pay you some rent."

His Porsche was costing us too much to repair, so he exchanged it for a workable Ford, and gave the balance to Peddie's son Sammy to go to a better school.

Danny's dream now had a real place where it could happen: his new studio. I had put down edge-to-edge carpeting so that it could double as a place where he could relax and entertain.

By February he "had a band". He had put adverts in newspapers and music shops and had finally selected people he felt he could work with. He and the singer, Sheri, were getting on very well, and went on dates together.

"How was last night?" I asked him.

And Danny, with a melty-wonderful grin, said, "Ag ... great!"

I thought: I have never seen anything as joyful as this boy when things are going well.

But in the end Sheri, who was a good singer, left to join a working band. And Dave left because he wanted a bigger share of the non-existent profits. And the other two were too unreliable to work with.

And so the day arrived when Danny once again had nothing to do.

EMPTINESS

By March Danny was disappointed and lonely. He didn't know how to start up again. He should have gone straight back to karate, but that was always difficult after a break. He was still talking clearly, and did not at first go back to drugs.

One day, a friend, Gary, phoned him. But Danny knew Gary was on drugs. Danny's own voice answering Gary got that whole drop-out failure tone.

The next day he said:

Danny: I don't think I could bring up children.

Lucy: In time you may be able to.

Danny: It's only now that I'm beginning to realize the damage I did to myself from drugs. It will take many years to be free of it.

Lucy: What made you change your attitude?

Danny: Things you said.

Danny: I've been sitting around all day with nothing to do so you should give me some money.

Lucy: Well Dad and I think you should earn it now.

Danny: But couldn't you just give me R5 for a cheap necklace or
    something.
Lucy: Danny, no! It's not my business any more to keep you happy.

He smoked a bit of dope. It did not make him mad again, but it
demotivated him even further. He was behaving reasonably well, but
just not effectively. If he now went back to regular karate he would have
to join an easier class until his stiffness wore off, and he didn't feel like
doing that.

Eventually, inevitably, he started linking up again with the Mean
Machine guys, who were fun and could take him out of himself.

It was the last week of March. I thought of Danny's craving for
a social life and the terrible isolation of the last years. At the Mean
Machine he found people he could relax and be himself with.

But things got swiftly out of control. He stayed out all night without
telling us. He came back another night without his car. And then he
stayed away without permission for three days and three nights.

Danny: I stayed with Byron and his mother. They live in style in a large
    double-storey. His mother goes out to work all day and we can just
    help ourselves to snacks any time we want to. Or watch videos or
    M-Net. It was a wonderful release. Byron has studied sociology at
    Wits and he's very interesting to talk to.
Lucy: But why didn't you tell us Danny?
Danny: Well ... Byron does pot and white pipes (Mandrax). I didn't
    think you would approve.

Chapter Twenty

TOUGH LOVE

THE BOOK

Of course Oliver and I had used a lot of "tough love" in the six years we had been trying to help Danny. We had been introduced to the concept by Jeff, our family therapist in the first year: consequences for bad behaviour; rewards for good behaviour.

But it had all been in the context of his psychotic breakdown. Now, since Danny was smoking pot and staying out at night without telling us, there were ordinary family rules to get established again. But there was also something more: we were no longer content for Danny to be completely dependent on us. We wanted him to start to be reliable and effective and to contribute both to the family and the world.

It was at this point that I found the actual book written by the founders of the Tough Love movement: *Toughlove* by Phyllis and David York, together with Ted Wachtel (1982 Doubleday).

I read this book with a feeling of astonishment—and warmth and gratitude. The parents, Phyllis and David York, were pretty much like us—kind and liberal and encouraging. They were in the caring professions themselves, and had started off believing all the theories: "analyse, sympathize, listen"—and had thought that any bad behaviour by children was the fault of the parents.

They went on sending their three problem daughters to therapy until the eldest was arrested for using a gun to hold up a drug dealer to get heroin for herself. When she phoned them from the jail they refused to bail her out—and from that moment the Tough Love movement began.

What the Yorks realized was that they were part of a wide cultural phenomenon. Children were cherished and loved; their needs were put before those of the parents: NOTHING WAS DEMANDED OF THEM.

Not all children in all families went wrong, but there were many who did. Their behaviour showed everything from nastiness and swearing at parents to actual criminal behaviour. Adult children in their twenties and thirties often lived at home and contributed little or nothing in the way of help or finance. And many took drugs and became even less able to control their impulses.

Children were disgusted with their parents; parents were anxious about their children: the atmosphere in the home was brittle and unharmonious.

Children spent years in one sort of talk therapy or another—and didn't change.

The action therapy of Tough Love produced change fairly soon. Not every sort of behaviour was tackled at once—but once one problem had been overcome the parents gained confidence and tackled another. Clear demands, clear consequences and the support of a community group were essential.

In the end Daniel changed so fundamentally that it's difficult to believe that Danny then and Danny now are the same person. At that point he was sane and cheerful when everything was going well, but had no coping strengths to overcome weaknesses and disappointments. And he had very little in the way of a value system.

With the help of the Tough Love book Oliver got over his liberal queasiness and I got over my extreme empathy.

But we didn't have the community support which the book says is so essential.

I found out that a Tough Love group had started in Norwood, near us. I immediately made an appointment to see Mary B, the therapist who ran the group. I told her Danny's story. She was shocked that I would even consider Tough Love. "He's a sick boy," she said. We should see him as fragile and likely to regress. Because of Danny's psychotic history she would not even consider putting me in touch with other parents in her group.

But I knew that Danny needed firm guidance *more* not *less* because of his psychotic breakdown. And we were not operating in a vacuum. We would be there with him, watching him.

None of our friends were willing to help. They simply didn't want to get involved. My sisters still lived overseas. In the end I found two people who were prepared to back us and to sign the contract: my uncle Jack, who lived on a farm, and Maureen, a pleasant Catholic woman who did errands for my mother. They would be told if Danny was not meeting our demands.

I typed out my Tough Love letters, and Oliver, having his Easter break, took Danny and the letters up to the Molozi farm, with some pages of the book which I had photocopied for Oliver to read.

Love was the other side of "tough love". But parents who had real solutions were more comfortable with themselves and likely to be more loving, not less. Everything you presented to the child was to be done firmly, but in a friendly calm tone.

LOVING PARENTS ARE ABLE TO SET BOUNDARIES AND STICK TO THEM.

FROM LUCY'S TOUGH LOVE LETTERS

Dear Danny,

From now on I don't want to be trapped into any situation which in the long run will make you weaker. So I'll write these letters stating our intentions clearly. I hope that clarity in us will give you the same feeling of security as do the new white walls! You may often feel uncomfortable, bored, a little anxious, tired—whatever. But the more of these small trials you have now the better you will cope in the future.

Love, Ma

Dear Danny,

I'm very sorry that "getting a band together" has not worked. But that's for the moment—it may be easier later. In the meantime we don't want to have a layabout for a son! You may think that because we are not giving you things any more we do not love you. This is absolutely not true.

About karate. In saying that your karate was a job, we did intend you to treat it as seriously as an adult would treat a real job in the world. You said, "You didn't really expect me to stop my socializing to go to karate, did you?" Indeed we did!

We expect you to go to karate 4 times a week, even if it's one of those boring days. Discuss your boredom with Stan, not with us.

It's impossible for us to tell whether you are "really tired". This problem was solved last year when we made the plan that you should go anyway, even if you only actually do karate for five minutes. Stan agreed to this plan last year, and he will again.

Because we value karate we will pay you R200 a month if you go 4 times a week. If you miss a session we will fine you R5. This is not a punishment but an incentive to make you consider how "really" stiff or tired you actually are.

You cannot live in this house and have our help in growing to maturity if you continue to smoke pot. I know you have intended to give it up, but this must now be definite. Once a week for the next 6 months you will have to have the urine-analysis test done at Sanca.

I am working out a job you can do for me and others in the mornings. You will be paid on Friday at lunchtime. I will lend you money for cigs and petrol in the first week, but after that you must handle your money on your own. Therefore:

i. You may not steal. This means not even one rand from Mom's bag.

ii. You may not sell any of your instruments or equipment in order to have money to live on.

iii. No borrowing from me or Dad or anyone else.

Maureen and Jack, who are your new instant fairy-godparents, say this is a very fair programme. They will give you every encouragement to stick with it. So you will be answerable to them as well as to us, and they will also give you support.

All the best,

Lots of love, Ma

THE PLAN BEGINS

Oliver and Daniel were still up at the farm. I was talking to Daniel in my head: "Tough Love is based on the idea that you are much more capable than you believe at present. In fact once *I* learn to say no to *myself, you* will be able to say no to *yourself.*"

Oliver on the phone from Molozi:

"This new regime will be difficult for him, but easy for us."

"Difficult for me though, because I have to crush natural sympathy."

"You can give him as much sympathy as you like as long as you don't give him *things*. And only money if he has earned it."

Lucy alone at home, suddenly bitter: Do you have any idea of how much I have given of myself to you without asking anything in return? Simply because of my own value system and my love of you.

On the whole though I thought that Tough Love would make us more able to be warm and friendly.

I visited my mother:

"What about Dr O (psychiatrist)? Shouldn't you check with him?"

I was shocked. "Pills? What for? How will that make him responsible?"

I thought: He has changed from mad to well but he has remained completely dependent.

From my mother I walked to my daughter. It was Good Friday. I had a hot cross bun and filter coffee and told her about the programme. She gave her support. (The support the Tough Love people were talking about was of the hands-on sort. We had plenty of well-wishers.)

Nicola said, "It will make him strong if he understands all that."

The next day Oliver phoned from the farm again.

"I had my first *real* conversation *ever* on Wednesday night with Danny. He read the letters in a flash. I said, 'Let's discuss it.' He said: 'It's quite clear.' Then he paraphrased the letters correctly."

Lucy's diary: I have sent in my work to the poetry competition. Now I will work with Danny for the next three months. He has to develop good work habits etc. Yes, but if we do "sink-or-swim" he will sink.

I care for Danny, but I also care for the good of the community, so my intelligence has to find a way to combine these two.

They came back in good spirits. Danny thought he still had money from the month before, when there was a different system.

Danny: Why didn't I have any money last month?
Lucy: You did, but you took us all out to supper with it.
Danny: Oh ja! I'd forgotten.

Lucy to herself: The idea of the job has really changed everything. Instead of Tough Love applied against him he sees the sense of working *for* me.

Danny: Dad said, "Buy your own batteries" and I just didn't know how I could.
Lucy: You were worried about earning *outside.*
Danny: Yes.
Lucy: That will happen very gradually. But I've already got some jobs for you to do for other people.

I thought: The most extraordinary thing is that he has completely accepted the urine test. I can't quite believe this yet.

I made a short simple commitment card for us both to sign:

1. **Urine test once-a-week for 6 months.**
2. **Job as personal assistant to mother for 3 months. (3 hours-a-day, 5-times-a-week)**
3. **Karate 4-times-a-week until Black Belt.**

NO BORROWING
NO DRUGGING

We both signed it.

Danny: Well I will try to picture this new way of being.
Lucy: Great living starts with a picture.

The next day I was in the passage talking to Peddie. Danny walked past in his swimming-costume:

Lucy: Isn't it so Danny—that if we are not lending you money Peddie mustn't either?

Danny (comfortably): Ja, that's so.

Lucy: So she's not going to be *unkind*. She's just going to stick to our conditions.

Lucy (to herself): He is saintly today.

Lucy: Thanks for the help, hey! You realize today isn't part of the job?

Danny: Ma! You know I would never take advantage of you in that way!

So all was going well. I don't think his bad friends realized he was back. They did not at first come around and he did not phone them.

THE URINE TESTS

The job started on April 11 and flew ahead. Everyone in my telephone book was helping me. Danny helped one grandmother write a letter and took the other (my mother) to visit her brother on the farm. (That was my uncle Jack who was now one of Danny's guardians.)

Grandma said afterwards, "He's an excellent driver—and so chatty!"

Maureen was Danny's other guardian and she did chores for Grandma—but these she would willingly give up, pretending to be ill, if Danny had nothing else to do.

Danny went to my disabled friend Lionel. He went nervously, but Lionel was funny as always and put him at his ease. He gave him the impossible task of finding a photograph he thought he'd lost for ever, but in the end Danny found it, and then he helped Lionel on with his jacket. This was in preparation for Danny holding Lionel appropriately when taking him to the dentist and the hospital on other days. Danny on that first day came back beaming:

"I'm so proud to have helped Lionel!"

Karate he had started the first weekend he was back. He went on Saturday and Sunday, partly I think to keep away from his dagga friends, since the scheme was only due to start on the Monday.

And now, on the first Wednesday, came the first dagga test. I wasn't sure whether he had really accepted it and taken it in.

"OK the job's finished. I just want to talk about tomorrow. You haven't said anything about the urine test."

He was silent, gave a slight, embarrassed smile.

"I know it's difficult—both giving up pot and the urine test. So I'll come with you and it can be an outing—we'll have some coffee and cake afterwards."

We parked and we were walking along the pavement. I didn't know which way to go but I thought he probably did, since he'd gone there to those NA sessions.

"OK," I said, "73 Loveday. You find it."

"But I don't know where from here ..."

I was tired of his helplessness so I sat down on the pavement, crossed my legs and arms and looked down.

"I suppose I could find it if I *had* to."

He went off and I went home. But once at Sanca he found that he just couldn't wee. I knew he hadn't done it on purpose so I just laughed. In a situation like that I often had the same problem. It was easily two weeks since the last pot and he was right at the beginning of his new self. So we had lunch at the Doll's House and talked amiably of other things.

The next weekend he again did karate on both Saturday and Sunday in addition to the weekday four. On Monday a special person came with Nicky to visit. This was Robert who loved both of them and often phoned Danny from Cape Town where he now lived. I say in my diary that Danny sat through a long evening with Nicky and Robert without talking to himself—so self-talk must still have been quite frequent. I heard him telling them about Habilitat: "I got so into cleaning the loos that I even did it at night."

The next day he said, "I hope my job is driving somewhere today. I love doing that!"

"Yes, it's taking Dad's clarinet—miles out."

"Good!"

"If you get lost it doesn't matter. I won't be cross. If you lose the clarinet however, well ..."

"You *will* be cross."

"Dad would be furious."

"Well I won't do that because I'm used to looking after my own instruments."

So off he went and it was bliss for me and bliss for Oliver (saved him a trip) and bliss for him too. He came back jubilant.

On the day before the next urine test Danny said: "I saw Byron yesterday and he said: 'Oh please won't you give me a lift to Orange Grove. I'll give you a button (Mandrax).' I just said no."

I decided to take his urine specimen in for him. I reminded him the night before, then in the morning I left a red jug on the toilet seat and a big notice on his bedroom floor. He put the red jug on my shelf and thereafter was not involved. We were going together to town. Nicky drove into the driveway while Danny and I were discussing expenses in the car.

"I like looking at you two," she said, "mother and son sitting there."

"We are doing expenses."

"God you are so organized and businesslike. I should do that."

Danny was very alive on the way to town.

"How many 5-star hotels do you think there are in Jo'burg?"

I thought two, he worked out five. We parted—he to a new address. "I'll ask when I get stuck."

I went to Sanca; he went to Oliver's accountant, Heather, with tax documents.

I sat in the Sanca waiting-room with my bag on my lap. The specimen bottle was secured next to *Bleak House*.

I saw the same woman who had counselled Daniel. Miss N. I explained about the wee. She explained why they couldn't test it. I patiently went over everything to do with it. Then I told her it would be almost impossible for Danny to "swop wee". His good friends would never do it—they knew about his breakdown and the importance of not touching drugs. His bad friends were addicts themselves. I told her how we lived and that Oliver and I were doing this together.

She refused to budge.

I said, bitterly, "Sanca has helped us not at all these last six terrible years. So many times Danny could have gone to Phoenix House, if only for a few weeks to give us a break."

"You are very angry."

"Yes I am."

To shift her mood I told her the Russell story (when the giant father came to see us). I laughed. Everyone else had laughed. Miss N stayed dead neutral.

She explained again, in great detail, why they couldn't do it. But I knew all that. I just wanted some flexibility. And some judgement of my credibility.

I walked my rage away and decided not to tell Danny. He was listening to music in the underground parking garage.

"That was great!" he said, enthusiastically. "We had such a nice chat. Heather said how nice it was that I was doing you this favour. I said: 'It's not a favour—it's my job!' Well anyway she said she thinks you need my help—since you are a writer and all."

On the drive home he said, "You know Ma, it's so *lekker* working for you! I used to get so aggressive and frustrated with nothing to do."

THE MAY CRIMINALS

I tried to find a place to take his wee: my doctor, the General Hospital, the mines even. Nothing.

On the first Friday when Danny got paid at lunchtime he bought me some chocolate but himself only fruit-juice. He said, "I have eaten only fruit and veg today. But I'm not going to use the rest of my money. I'm saving it for a BMW. I deserve a BMW for coming off drugs."

I thanked him for the chocolate and ignored his remark about the BMW.

The next week I sent him to Fordsburg—a busy Indian place, unfamiliar and far away. He was to go to *Frontline* magazine with a story of mine. He came back sulky and bad-tempered having not found it. "I got hopelessly lost—I don't even want to talk about it. It was overwhelming."

I ignored this.

Maureen, my mother's helper, came to visit me one afternoon. Oliver walked in.

Maureen said to him, "You should have seen Lucy in the passage—Daniel insulting her with his face right next to hers—and she just coolly walks away!"

"Well, I'm learning!"

Nicky came to supper:

Lucy (to Nicky): Do you think he's just weak?

Nicky: No—I don't think anybody's just weak, especially not Danny.

Lucy (to Danny): Do you think you are particularly strong-willed?

Danny: Yes, I am now. About dope. I've given it up for ever.

Oliver: It's easy to feel that now.

Danny: You should have seen me yesterday. I *took* them to score and I didn't score myself.

Lucy: Oh Danny! I don't think you should see those people. They are sad and sick people. For your second growing-up it is better to spend time with confident, happy, good people.

But these friends of his would not give up. They would chant his name loudly and heavily outside our house and kick on our new white wall.

On May 2 in the evening Danny came home wailing and with a bloodied face. I wiped the blood off and comforted him and tried to find out what had happened. Danny wept and was hysterical. I said he must calm down and talk quietly:

"But I was doing nothing *wrong*—I was just trying to be firm."

Whenever he tried to tell me the story he cried again, saying, "He's my buddy, he's my buddy, he's my buddy."

Then Oliver came in, took in the situation and was immediately strong and clear:

Oliver: We are going to report this to the police.

Danny: But Santino is coming to burn the house down if we go to the police.

Oliver: Let him!

At the Norwood Police station they reported the incident. Then they were sent to the hospital for a description of Danny's face: he was scratched and bruised but no bones had been broken and no teeth were missing. Oliver and Danny took the report back to the police station.

We never heard anything more about that case. We added "no druggy friends" to our list of demands. Danny recovered quickly and was back at karate a few days later.

What had happened was that Santino and Giovanni had phoned up Danny and asked him for a lift from town. Danny had fetched them. Then they asked to go to a place where there was Mandrax. Danny said no. They were at a robot. Danny was driving, Santino was sitting next to him. Santino suddenly turned and started bashing Danny in the face. Danny dropped them off and came home.

I had allowed the Mean Machine friends when I was afraid that Danny would go back into his head. But I was no longer afraid of that. He might not have a peer group, but he talked plenty to everyone else.

There was now a local informal anti-drug group near us—"The Drug Action Committee". Danny went to a meeting and was appointed Entertainments Manager. He got a sticker for his car and put it on his back bumper: "SAY NO TO DRUGS".

He went to see a movie about drugs: *Less than Zero*.

Danny: It was very heavy.
Lucy: Why?
Danny: He dies in the end. He owed all this money.
Lucy: If you had seen it when you were eleven would it have put you off drugs?
Danny: Definitely!
Lucy: The Drug Action ladies got it unbanned.
Danny: Ja I know—they told me.

At this stage we still had our old non-electronic gate which was easy to climb over. Giovanni came to the kitchen window. I was in the passage and heard their conversation:

Giovanni: So you want to pick me up later?
Danny: No I can't. I'm grounded.

Giovanni: Does your old lady know you smoked last night?

Danny: Ja—I had to tell her.

Giovanni: Why d'you have to tell her?

Danny: Because I'm having this test in two week's time. So I have to stay off.

We kept his car key now unless he was going to work or to this new group, Drug Action, or to karate. He brought it to us willingly, saying, "With money and a car and my tempting friends who knows what would happen late at night. But my intention is to keep off."

And then, on May 22 Danny confessed to me that Byron had been sleeping in his studio and smoking white pipes there. Byron and Giovanni had stolen R20,000 worth of jewellery and kruger-rands (gold coins) from Byron's mother.

I phoned Byron's mother and she fetched him. She had already told the police. I gave her the Tough Love number.

The next day Constable Goodman came to interview Daniel, who told him the truth. Later Danny said to me, "I'm fucking angry with myself for that. Because of what I said my buddy must go to jail for five years."

"Maybe it will save him—maybe he will be put on probation or something."

Nicky said Danny was still confused about drugs and theft. She told me that he said, as if it was quite OK: "Byron takes his mother's jewellery and sells it because he likes white pipes." And then in the next breath he says, "There's this nice lady Karen from the Drug Action Centre."

SECURE AT LAST

It was June. The new electronic gate was in. The pot tests had finally been arranged. We were secure at last.

My friendly doctor at Bagleyston clinic, Dr van N, just down the road, had found a method for me—and had no hang-ups about me bringing in the specimen. The Institute for Medical Research (SAIMR) delivered nitrous-oxide to the clinic on Tuesday mornings, and would pick up Daniel's sample—which I would deliver there on Mondays. So that's what happened—once a week or once a fortnight, from June to September, when the world ended.

I would get the results on Thursday or Friday. They were always the same:

Cannabis: negative

Nicola took him to a Japanese restaurant for supper. When he came back I heard shouting and was immediately in a panic. But he was being joyfully expressive because he had so enjoyed the Japanese meal with Nicky.

Nicky phoned me the next day and said, "He spent the whole evening trying to persuade me to tell my friends to come off dope."

Byron phoned. I knew from his voice that he was drugged. I decided to call Danny from his studio and listen in.

Byron: It was so cool seeing you yesterday. Can you come?
Danny: No.
Byron: What's going on with you? Are you grounded?
Danny: No. It's just that I have to have these tests.
Byron: Say you are visiting Andy—your karate mate.
Danny: Fuck, man, she knows all that stuff. Let's just leave it for a while. Once she starts to trust me again I'll be able to *jol* (go out for a jolly time).

Danny still got frustrated and resentful, and still got into rages, but he didn't threaten or kick or break things.

All the talk of doing his karate Blue Belt in May turned out to be nonsense, because he had lied to me about going in March and didn't have enough stamps. When I talked to him about this he looked down, red-faced. He had the beginnings of a conscience.

His self-control was improving. Sometimes he nipped off a rage as it started.

Oliver said to me, "I can see the beginnings of a yearning to be the sort of person he admires deep down. He will go inexorably towards becoming a real person. I had that feeling for the first time today."

And then Danny fell in love.

Lucy: How was karate?

Danny: There's this girl I like. She's in Brown Belt. Her name is Tasmin. She is so together—she's up there in another world.

His imagination soon turned this girl into the woman he would marry.

I told him about a now-clean couple in Cape Town who had a deformed child, which was thought to have happened because they had both been druggies.

"Don't worry about it Ma. I've taken care of that." (By stopping himself? Or by falling in love with a girl who had never done drugs at all?)

On a job which took him to Sandton City he came back later than expected. He explained. "I saw Tasmin in Sandton City with a guy. So I got in a panic. But then I went for a long drive—and I realized it must have been her brother."

I started gently to tell him that his view of it might not be real.

Danny: But I can't bear it. You are breaking my heart.

Lucy: I'm not saying she can't be your girlfriend. I'm saying she is not now your girlfriend.

Danny: But we have this understanding.

Lucy: Based on what evidence?

Danny: The way she looks at me.

Lucy: That's not evidence that she is your girlfriend.

Danny: I can't stand it. I was so popular with everyone—girls and boys.

Mark taught me how to talk to girls nicely, make them feel good.

Nicky came round:

Lucy (to Danny): Just say hullo to Tasmin.

Danny: But it will sound so silly!

Lucy: Try now!

Danny (defeated): Hullo Tasmin.

Lucy: Say it again in a relaxed way.

Danny (cheerfully): Hullo Tasmin!

Nicky: That's marvellous Danny—charming!

TWO GOOD MONTHS

June and July were two good months: the job went well, karate went well, the pot tests were negative.

Lucy: What did you learn from our trip together on Monday?
Danny: Not to assume things. Not to think I am always right. To sort
of ... check up.

Every week I gave him something a little more difficult to do, coaching him not to be fussed if he didn't achieve it. He could now get anywhere, always. I had bought a wall map which went with a spiral book map—of Greater Johannesburg. A winner: the page numbers of the book map were written on the wall map.

At the Doll's House I made certain that he knew north, south, east, west in the real space out there. (The Doll's House was a roadhouse which was especially good in these winter months, with the sun burning through the glass of the car windows; and the food was simple and inexpensive.)

The Danny who had liked things to be more complicated had returned:
Danny: Now let's do north-east and those.
Lucy: OK
Danny: Right—now on to north north east and that lot.
Lucy: No, no! I find those too complicated. And I've never needed them
in real life.

He went off to my mother's friend Hazel, who was disabled and whose sight was poor. She welcomed him, held on to him. He helped her make tea. She talked cars to him. He sat cross-legged on the floor, smiling at her. Then he went to the shops for her and put the milk in the fridge when he got back. All this she told me on the phone that night. She remembered saying:

Hazel: Why do they use legs so much in karate?
Danny: Well, legs can stretch further.
Hazel: I never thought of that! So you trip people up?
Danny: Yes, that's right.

Hazel: What I hate is wrestling.
Danny: Yes, I quite agree with you there.

It helped that it was winter. Not having friends and not going out at night were more bearable in these cold times. He sat on his bed cutting girlie photos out of magazines.
Danny: I'm finding better ways to live.
Lucy: But as soon as you have your car key you will find worse ways.
Danny: Well you must just keep on pressurizing me, that's all.

The boring part of karate when he had to do easy stuff to catch up was over. He was in the class that was preparing for Blue Belt.
Danny: I'm so enjoying my karate now—I really live for it.
Lucy: So the moral is: "Don't stop!"
Danny: Yes. I really appreciate you keeping me at it!
Lucy: Thanks.

Karen from Drug Action went to watch him at karate. "He looked so good doing his karate," she said. "And when he noticed me he said 'Hi' so naturally. I had this conversation with Linzi of Tough Love. She won't accept what you are doing. She says, 'But Daniel suffers from an *illness*'. But she's wrong. Danny is my favourite person. He's such a lovely guy."

Drug Action was run by older women who had themselves been drug addicts. They were getting more than 800 calls a day.

Danny drove miles out of town to meet Johanna who was to phone him once a week.
Danny: I must have driven about 100km to find that place!
Lucy: What was she like?
Danny: Such a lekker lady. She's also going to start a social club! Karen's going there this afternoon—but I would much rather be in Johanna's group. She's been 13 years on drugs, so she really can help me.

But I think this group didn't last. In the diary I don't mention it again.

Lucy: I just did a broadcast.

Danny: REALLY? What about? Your writing?
Lucy: No—you.
Danny: Me!
Lucy: Tough Love. Do you think you were too powerful?
Danny: Yes, definitely.

He could organize more and more of his life himself.
Danny: I still have to get another karate stamp—I was supposed to get it at the beginning of the year—but I just didn't read the rules properly.
Lucy: Well—you are taking on so much now. It's a lot to think about.
Danny: I'm just so glad that I can.
Lucy: That you can what?
Danny: Organize things myself.

Magic words.
Oliver told me, "I used to buy him hundreds of strings—I knew he *had* to have a working guitar because it was the one thing that kept him happy. He broke a string a day."
Now he came back triumphant with his Blue Belt certificate.

Danny: Look at my carpet: blue and brown.
Lucy: So?
Danny: Well! Blue Belt and Brown Belt together! (Him and his imaginary girlfriend.)

After Blue comes Purple—and then three Brown Belts, and then finally Black.
"It was *so easy*!! I really enjoyed doing it." He said. "I'm going to the advanced class now—to be with Tasmin. I'll risk it."
Lucy (to herself): Danny is the strangest of new-born creatures—he falls in love.
Danny's drummer friend, Mark, was working for his father's business now, but he still had a band, and he still loved it when Daniel agreed to play with him.
On one of these occasions Danny was in a particularly good mood. He came to me for a rub—which he had been doing without

embarrassment ever since Habilitat. I would rub his head and neck and upper back.

He was smiling to himself as I did so this time. Probably thinking of Tasmin.

Lucy: As long as you know it's a fantasy.
Danny: Oh I do, I do.
Lucy: And don't do it in public.
Danny: Sometimes it's so hard. And you know what Ma?
Lucy: What?
Danny: Sometimes I do think that you are mad!
Lucy: Why?
Danny: All these jobs you give me to do—like going far away and talking to your friends!
Lucy: Do you ever feel depressed doing these jobs?
Danny: No.
Lucy: Well then.
Danny: I could be reading.
Lucy: I think I do seem to be controlling you, but what I want you to do is to take over control yourself.
Danny: Become independent?
Lucy: Yes.
Danny: But I don't want to become independent.
Lucy: You just want me to stay your slave?
Danny: Ja. Why not? You are a queen mother goddess.
Lucy: What about when I am old and crippled?
Danny: Oh you will never be those things.

Off he went and got into his concert clothes. He came to say goodbye in his black jacket with silver zips and a pale baby-wool scarf around his neck.

The concert was a great success.

Chapter Twenty-One

GOING OUT TO WORK
AND OLIVER'S DEATH (1988)

I knew it was time for Daniel to go out to work. But where and at what? I phoned my active Christian friends: one did Meals-on-Wheels, another visited the elderly and a third ran an employment agency for black domestic workers. None of them could think of anything for Danny to do. But my fourth call was lucky: Eleanor Anderson said she had a friend, Denver Berry, who organized work for the blind in Soweto. Denver would certainly have ideas about where Danny could be placed.

Denver phoned me. He said he could do with extra help at the blind workshop south of Soweto, but that he couldn't pay much. He said it would be on a trial and error basis. If Danny fitted in and liked working there, then Denver would be glad to have the help.

I told Danny about it. He was curious and interested. We decided to go down there together and see the place and meet Denver. The drive there was interesting—through old mine territory and tired fields. Gummed wasteland. (What will be done with it? It could be so wisely designed for humans.) The workshop stood in the middle of nowhere. Danny was thrilled with this isolation. To work outside town and township appealed to him.

We each had a session with Denver. I can't remember what I told him about Danny's breakdown, but I probably told him that Danny had been working very well for us.

Going from our house at rush-hour would make the journey long and tiring, so it was agreed that Danny could leave home at 9 am and reach the workshop at 9.30. In the afternoon he could leave at 3.30.

Then Denver saw Danny alone and I looked around.

Then Denver called Marius, an Afrikaner who was in charge of the workshop. He had a nice smile.

"My Afrikaans isn't good," said Danny, "but I'm OK with simple Afrikaans."

"My English isn't good either!" said Marius.

Denver added, "The other person in the management is a black lady. We are non-racial."

On the way home Danny said, "I didn't realize it was for black people. I've always wanted to do something for black people—and if they are disabled, then that too I would like to help them with. I like working with people. Denver was very nice. He said I must come to him if I have any problems—not bottle things up."

"I didn't mention the dope."

"That's over anyway."

"I'll miss your help. People say you *can't* work for family—but you have done it so well, so generously."

In the lead-up to the job he went to visit Terry, his Saheti teacher, who was now assistant dean at the new mixed-race residence at Wits, Barnato Hall—situated where the old Show Grounds had been, where Danny as a child had had so much fun.

Terry was delighted and impressed with him. She said to me afterwards, "How many years since he last was able to have an effortless conversation? He is a sentient human being again. I remember that dinner we had at Baccarat when he was just talking to himself all the time. He was fascinated by the way the showground has changed. He talked about the 'aftermath' of the showground. I liked that! He uses words correctly now. We even talked about drugs."

The next day Danny said to me, "Terry was telling me how she hated it when John (ex-husband) and his friends all sat around stoned."

August came and off went Danny to work. No phone calls came for me so I began to feel it must be going OK.

Just after he came home that first day I saw him shouting into Oliver's workshop window. "So you *see*, Dad..." He came into the kitchen talking loudly to himself.

Lucy: Are you cross?

Danny: Not at all. It's great—it's really great. I'm just proud that I can do a day's real work.

Lucy: So you were saying, "So there!" to Dad?

Danny: Perhaps. But everything is so marvellous Ma. We had a great
   lunch—veal and salad. The people are GREAT.

All that first week he was somewhat out of control when he came
home. I think all his good focused self was going into the job. He soon
had a sore back from leaning over the work tables, but he refused to
take a day off.

The blind workers were putting plugs together. Danny had to see
that everyone was doing it properly, and to teach newcomers.

One day he was ready to go at 8. "But you'll hit rush-hour if you
go now!" I said.

"Ja, but you see I promised this new woman that I would be there
when she arrived. She's nervous and shy."

The next week, at supper, he said, "You know what! I'm a Quality
Control Manager."

"You did a lot of that when the builders were here!" I said.

"Ja," said Oliver. "You are a natural Quality Control Manager."

I thought the raging after work could have been pot related—I thought
he might have smoked some to calm down after the excitement of the
job. But the urine test showed him to be cannabis-negative. It turned
out that the stress came from *resisting* smoking pot—even though he
was somewhat overwhelmed by the job.

Danny shouted: "You see I had some zol here, but I didn't want to
smoke it, and last night I thought this has GOT to end and I chucked
that packet in the rubbish-bin. I was wrong—absolutely wrong—I
fucked my mind up. I didn't know what I was doing."

"People who can admit they are wrong are the tops," I said.

Danny was pleased, "You think that?"

"Ja, I do."

He knelt down—head on the ground like Pooh Bah:

"I swear to God I chucked it out."

"Since when did histrionics convince me?"

"Never."

So he put on washing-up gloves and turned the big black rubbish-
bin upside-down on the new paving and out came all the messy junk
and then right at the end out came the Nedbank cash packet with its
dope inside.

"So tomorrow you can come home sane instead of monsterish."

"Ja, OK. It's my mind working for my heart. You can write that down if you like."

SPRING: THE LAST MONTH

September was the second month of Daniel working for the blind: it was the last month of Oliver's life, but we didn't know that.

Some of the blind people spoke only Afrikaans, so Danny practised on us at supper.

Lucy: What's "suspicious"?

Danny: *Senuweeagtig.*

Oliver: *Agterdogtig.*

They shouted at each other. Then Danny looked it up.

Danny: You're right Dad. Why was I so sure I wonder?

Oliver: Well, everything you used to think of you then thought was true.

Danny: You just know EVERYTHING!

Lucy: Well Danny you know he's a bit of an expert in language. But not at everything!

Oliver: For instance I could never do what you do on the guitar: listen to something and then instantly reproduce it.

Marius phoned me from the workshop. "He sings to himself, but it's not a problem. He's performing very well at his work."

Danny: I had a long talk to Denver today. He said he is very proud of all that I have learnt.

Lucy: So you like work better than school?

Danny: No question. Sitting in those desks every day with the teacher glaring at you! This job has changed my life.

Danny went to a movie. I don't say in my diary what it was, but I have begun to use the word "moral".

Lucy: Was it a moral movie?

Danny: Oh yes, definitely—all goodies and baddies.

Lucy: Do you know why *Cry Freedom* was banned?

Danny: Just because it was such an old movie. They thought ...

Lucy: No, it's a new movie. They thought it might cause a riot. Nicky says ...

Danny: I can't think clearly right now.

Lucy: Well that's OK. Let's go for hot apple-pie and cold ice-cream at Grubs.

At Grubs:

Danny: So tell me now what Nicky thought. It's all right now.

Lucy: That anything goes—that nothing is really good or bad.

Danny: Oh. But I think they were right to ban the movie. Such heavy emotions.

Lucy: And you have the right to that opinion, though people may shout at you. It's not a fashionable opinion right now.

Danny: So maybe it's better not to say?

Lucy: Is that what you think?

Danny thinks, then says firmly: "No. I think I *should* say. After all what could they do to me? What? So I should just say and see what happens. But I *do* care about what the black people have suffered. After all I work for them. Denver says some of those blind people have to walk miles to the bus-stop, and it's cold. Marius always orders far too many plugs for our immediate needs. That's because once he ran out of plugs and the people who had struggled to come were depressed and restless."

And then a spring day came, and it was mild and the sky was clear. Danny went and lay on the roof and looked at the stars. When he came down again he said to us:

Danny: The thing about this universe is that you just can't conceive of it—and I like that in a universe.

OLIVER IN WONDERLAND

Oliver's last year of life was his best year ever. He was on a permanent high. I told people later that he died of "good stress". It worried me that he took on too much, but he did it because his depression had disappeared and he never wanted it to return. He no longer had migraines. His doctor said that he had slightly raised blood pressure, and Oliver himself knew that he should lose weight, but neither of these issues were considered critical. Oliver said he and Nicola would go to Weight Watchers "after Alice".

"Alice" was *Alice in Wonnerland*. A teacher at Die Kruin, the Afrikaans school for music, art and ballet, had translated *Alice in Wonderland* into Afrikaans—and then put it into verse. She gave it to Oliver on the first day of term in January and told him to write the music. Oliver had only ever composed pieces for pupils, but now he felt inspired and wrote all the music very quickly. The music teachers tried it out, and found that it was singable—and soon the whole school was caught up in it. They decided to put it on at the end of September.

Oliver was only supposed to train the singers and musicians, but got caught up in the production itself. The art department worked on surrealistic sets. The whole thing was coming together well ...

In addition to *Alice*, and all his usual teaching work, Oliver was also working every Thursday night at the Yard of Ale at the Market Theatre. This was a comfortably multi-racial restaurant with good simple food, where people ate before and after shows and met friends at any hour. Oliver's musician friend played an advanced keyboard which really did sound like an organ sometimes and a harpsichord at others. Oliver played his recorders or his flutes (ancient or modern)—whatever worked best.

Because life was so fulfilling, Oliver's negative side simply disappeared. People who met him for the first time this year thought he was the most delightful of humans.

Oliver had been pessimistic about South Africa and pessimistic about Daniel, but now he said, "We can always find a way."

Oliver was teaching white children at the English Arts School and white children at Die Kruin. At Die Kruin the staff had divided into two groups: *verkrampte* and *verlig*—the people who supported the government and the ones who wanted change. At break, Oliver sat with the *verlig* group who loved him and the way he would mock the government. They were devastated when he said he was leaving at the end of the year.

This was because he was finally going to fulfil his dream of teaching music to black children in Soweto. Mike Muller had started Pelmama, a black music school, and easily persuaded Oliver to join him. Oliver and I discussed it only very briefly. The school was in the heart of Soweto and therefore dangerous; the daily journey would be tiring; and it wasn't necessarily going to work out—which would leave Oliver without a job. But we were financially secure enough to risk it. We would find ways.

And Daniel was thriving. He loved the drive to work and back and he loved the job. And he had started karate again.

On Friday nights Oliver and I went out to dinner alone. We had been doing this for a few years by now. We never discussed Danny or South Africa at these meals. They were for our stability and sanity.

THE LAST DAY

Alice was performed on Wednesday 28 and Thursday 29 September. Nicola, Daniel and I went on the second night. Oliver was conducting his small group of musicians in the front of the stage on the right. I could see him—very tight and tense as if willing everyone to keep his somewhat difficult music together—which they did. Oliver had never done anything like this before.

The music and the production were strange and ethereal: it worked.

Afterwards we went home straight away and Oliver stayed to have a drink with everyone who had helped to put it together.

At home I left a note of praise for Oliver on the kitchen table and went to bed.

On the Friday morning Oliver went to Die Kruin to fetch his equipment. Then at home he loaded his car with things for the farm. Much to my relief he was going up to the pine farm for his week's holiday. He would have a good rest there. Philip, a young student who had helped with *Alice*, was going with him.

Oliver was packing the car.

Oliver: I don't want anyone opening that gate!

Lucy: When are you leaving?

Oliver: Tomorrow morning early—4 o'clock. Philip will sleep in the flat. (The new little outside flat attached to Daniel's new studio.)

That Friday—September 30—was the last day of my "Good Building" diary. I had written it every day for a year—from when the building had started—and now I was going to write a book based on it.

Peddie: Do you want the Sowetan?

Lucy: Yes, yes, let's see what everyone is saying. Buy the Citizen as well.

Danny returned from work. "I was helping this old lady to get the technique right. She didn't speak English or Afrikaans but I guided her fingers and she got it in the end."

He went out to his studio.

Oliver was walking down the passage and I met him coming the other way:

Oliver: Philip's taking me to the doctor—to get my blood pressure tested. He refuses to go to the back of beyond where they are no doctors.

Lucy: Why don't you just lie down for a while?

Oliver: I've been lying down for two hours—since lunchtime. It doesn't help. I've got chest pains and numb arms.

I gave him a hug and a kiss. "OK then—it's probably sensible."

I went to my bedroom. I suddenly felt panic. I knew those were the symptoms of a heart attack. I sat on my bed, bolt upright. The phone was next to my bed.

I wrote these final words in my "Good Building" diary: "Oliver with chest pains and numb arms taken to clinic by Philip. Me here frightened."

Half-an-hour after they went, our doctor phoned to say that Oliver had died. I screamed at him that it couldn't be true. I phoned Nicola and told her to go to the clinic. I fetched Danny from his studio and we went in silence to the clinic.

We stood in the doctor's room. Oliver was across the passage, lying on a clinic bed. We could see him there. We didn't know what to say or do. In the end I said to the children, "Give Dad a kiss and tell him you love him."

So we each in turn did that. Then we came home and sat in the kitchen. Oliver's sister joined us. Nicola said, "Dad would say it was a good way to go."

I lay shocked in bed. At some point Danny ran in—and I wrote down his words in the Danny diary: "I love you Ma and I always will and nothing will ever come between us again."

POSTSCRIPT

Nicky stayed with me for a while after Oliver's death. We ate nothing for four days. We met to weep; we met in the kitchen where we came to drink water; we answered the phone. We ignored Danny. He stayed outside in his flat.

After four days Nicky made supper for us. She invited a friend, and the four of us ate outside. She lit candles, which I said was foolish; but they stayed alight throughout the meal. We talked and felt a little bit normal again.

Nicky and I arranged the funeral, with a friend of hers working the sound system. Two of Oliver's most gifted pupils played flute and harpsichord. Nicky and I both spoke. I saw Danny sitting halfway back, slumped and ashen-faced. A lot of people came—our friends, who seemed almost as shocked as we were—and Oliver's pupils. I think the whole cast of "Alice" were there. Danny's boss, Denver Berry, came.

The following week Danny went back to work. Nicky and I were very envious. She was between jobs, and also between boyfriends. I couldn't write: I could scarcely read.

The next week Danny came to see me. He said, "I'm sorry I smoked dope—but I thought you would understand, since it really was a lapse. I really was stunned. The strong man in my life was gone—and you two women were too out of it to help me." He added, "By the way, Robbie phoned. He sends love."

Robbie wrote Danny a letter. It is both a message to Danny never to touch LSD, and an expression of his agony at Oliver being gone:

It was great on the phone the other night. You sounded so clear-headed. About 6 months ago I took some acid and went to the top of this very beautiful mountain and spent most of the trip up there. The trip was great but it took me about 3 months to become myself again. I felt as if my mind was sitting at a 45 degrees angle to my brain and things just weren't in sync, and it was a sad thing because in the last few years I had really become so together and had a solid heart and mind, and now all of a sudden it was a little flimsy. So now I have sworn that no matter how strong or how cool everything is I will never take that stuff again, and I urge you never to take that chance, please. Now I can't even have a beer because I can feel the ripples it creates in my psyche and you must understand what I mean by ripples because it is exactly that, the ripples that you create from throwing a cap of acid into your subconscious mind can last up to 18 years, according to some people, so fuck it, please just trust me blindly on this one ...

I now have a new understanding of the words to mourn someone's death. It is almost like saying goodbye to Nicola for the first time but without the self-pity that lovers experience. I can't say that in all my years I have felt this way. I have nearly cried a few times this week and I just don't feel like doing a fucking thing, as because God doesn't have a central embassy there is nowhere to take the protest that I feel, and so for the first time in my life I feel the silent shout of mourning in my chest. Now you can know how those Greek women feel, and they just let it out ... so it goes ...

Work at the Blind Institute went well. Denver would phone me from time to time to say how he was getting on. "His concentration has improved immeasurably—and there's no lack in brain-power."

One day I phoned Denver. Danny answered! "I help out with everything now."

So why, after Danny had spent a year working there, did Denver want to move him? "He needs new experiences," said Denver, who was also doing some other changes.

Danny was shocked. He said to me, "But that place has been my refuge all these months since Dad died. I know the place he wants to send me to—I've been there to deliver a message. It's a warehouse. I wouldn't be working with people. And these people love me Ma, and I love them too.'

But Denver was adamant, and in the end Danny left altogether.

His next job took him away from home and me for the first time since he had become sane. Robbie Robb's older half-brother, Larry Amos, needed a musician for his touring band. He didn't seem to know that Danny had been mad or difficult. He simply knew that Danny was a good musician. The band was called 'The Naughty Boys' and it went to Durban and the Drakensberg and all over the place. They played in hotels and got free rooms and free meals and Danny thoroughly enjoyed himself. He was not the star, but the music was near enough to his own music not to be too off-putting.

There was a write-up of this band in *Top 40* November 1989.

The Naughty Boys' sound is predominantly blues-orientated, as well as quite rock-orientated. Says Larry: "I've always played the blues, I can do it well. I only did one blues song in the early days, the rest is all original stuff. Blues is normally requested by the audience. I actually prefer to do rock and funk. From a live point of view, I wanna dance, move."

Daniel, the band's bassist is a regular virtuoso, being adept at drums, keyboards, guitar and bass! The guys spend a lot of time ragging each other, and word-play can get quite hilarious at times.

There was a picture of the four guys, and Danny looked like a professional musician. I was immensely proud of him.

Inspiration and Education

When the band job came to an end, Danny decided he was ready to put his own band together. They would play his own compositions. He didn't have many contacts in the music world, so he went back to his previously unsatisfactory strategy of advertising in music shop windows. Many phoned him up; many came for auditions, but those whom he thought OK musically and asked round to rehearsals proved to be inadequate in other ways. They came late, or didn't come at all. If there was a rehearsal they got frustrated easily and it would end in noisy argument and aggressive shouting. They are on dagga I thought. Dagga soothes while it is being smoked, and causes rages in the following days.

I told him to judge people on character as well as on musicality, and he agreed.

He went back to karate, and got his Blue Belt and then his Purple Belt, and the following year he got the first two of the three Brown Belts. After that would come Black Belt, but Danny did not quite have the stamina for high-level karate. He often got injuries and ached, so he felt that he had done enough.

Socially his life was difficult. He would visit cousins, or Nicola and her live-in lover and their friends, but he often just didn't understand what they were talking about. They had all been to university and he was aware enough to realize that he couldn't join in.

He did a typing course at a nearby secretarial school and became accurate and reasonably quick. I showed him the computer basics. He worked part time at an employment agency, putting the names of the job-seekers on computer.

Then he had some advanced driving lessons, and this time he got his Advanced Driving certificate, which he had not managed in his Porsche. He had all his certificates framed and he put them up around the living-room/studio in his garden flat.

And then came Francina—a warm joy to both of us for many years. One day when he went to Nicola's house and couldn't join in the conversation he went out into the back garden and there were six puppies. The gardener who lived at Nicky's house had found these puppies in a box at the Pick and Pay Hypermarket.

After that Danny often went to play with the puppies and found one whom he especially liked. He was allowed to keep this one, a girl puppy, and brought her home as soon as she was old enough. Apart from the bands he had tried to run, Danny had never had full responsibility for another creature. I stayed out of it—made no suggestions at all; and the puppy was loved and nurtured, and taken to the vet and for walks and to dog classes. All by Danny, who named her Francina. She grew into a lovely dog—very thin and very fast, like her owner—and with the same wild enthusiasms. She was light brown, but seemed to be some part greyhound. As a watchdog she was perfect: she would bark loudly at strangers, but never bit them.

A light golden cat jumped over our wall one day. I tried to find her owner but with no success. She became Danny's second pet. When Francina grew a little older she would lie on the warm paving in a semicircle, and Sylvie the cat would lie round next to her in the curve.

Meanwhile, in that year of 1990, I had awoken to a new world of fear and fright. I had had a lifetime of worry about South Africa, and six years of worry about my son, but now there was something even bigger to bomb and batter my soul: the planet. I had thought that environmentalists were taking care of environmental issues; they were, but only of a tiny part of the huge problem we were faced with.

I realized that behind all the other social and planetary problems was population growth. I found others, black and white, who thought the same way, and together we started an organization to look at population issues. We called it Sapler, which stood for "Splendidly Alive People within Limited Environmental Resources".

Danny was with me all the way. He didn't need to be persuaded—it made perfect sense to him. He decided to have a week's holiday all by himself at Molozi, the pine farm in the north, owned now by my sister and brother-in-law. He wanted to walk and think.

It was while driving home through the lowveld that he decided to become a vegetarian. This was both from a love of animals and from an understanding of how herds of cattle damaged the soil. I was happy with this decision. He had formulated something for himself that went beyond his family, and yet was not brain-damaging.

Sapler had formed a trust and gone public. We needed someone to do the outreach and the admin. In January 1992 Danny took on the job. He worked Monday to Friday, 9 to 5, answering the phone and sending out and receiving letters from all over South Africa and the world. He was very good. He never once asked for time off. He did the accounts well, and if there was something to finish after five then he stayed on until it was done.

He made friends with a man in Portland, Oregon who wanted the whole human race to die out. Les ran an organization called VHEMT, "Voluntary Human Exit Movement". People could join if they already had children, but after joining they made a commitment not to have any more. Danny and I discussed this endlessly over supper. Was he simply trying to win people's interest this way? Or did he really want a planet without people?

In the garden office which we had made from Oliver's short-lived work room, Danny phoned and was phoned. But he was allowed to read books on population and the environment when his other work was done. Very slowly, page by page, one page a day at first, he read—and we talked about what he had read at suppertime. The first three books he read were:

> *The Population Explosion* by Paul and Anne Ehrlich
> *Earth in the Balance* by Al Gore
> *The Third Revolution* by Paul Harrison

When he had finished these three books—the first serious non-fiction books he had ever read, he said to me one day, "I want to go to university."

He registered at Damelin for an adult Matric, with nightschool lectures. He had to do three subjects in one year and one subject the next year. He did Geography, English and Economics the first year. Geography and Economics went well with Sapler because his Economics teacher was not a businessman and had no vested interest in industrial development, so was quite happy to discuss planetary issues with Danny. His English teacher was Mr Riley, the dynamic teacher from Danny's fourteen-year-old time at Damelin. The next year Danny did History—and got a distinction. These subjects were all clearly taught. I don't remember Danny having any stress with them.

Nowadays I always enjoyed our supper conversations. If he got things wrong I could easily extend the conversation in ways which helped him to understand. I was his teacher/mother, not his many-degreed brother-in-law and colleagues, whom even Nicola had trouble with.

But there was a problem which even I had not been able to solve. This was word meanings. Even at 25, after several years of sanity, Danny still used some abstract words completely wrongly. He had his own idiosyncratic meanings lodged in his mind from his psychotic days. If I corrected him he hated it: he attacked me and defended his meanings.

What was to be done? If he was going to university he needed the real meanings. I put on my therapeutic hat and waited for a good opportunity. One evening he was in a particularly happy mood. I said, in a relaxed, warm way:

"That's not the dictionary definition of *orthodox*," (or *liberalism* or *motivation*).

"Oh," he said, in an equally friendly tone. "Isn't it?"

"Well, let's get a dictionary and have a look."

It was a breakthrough moment. He accepted the dictionary definition (or definitions) and he was hooked. I found him a dictionary to take out to his flat, and we had another one next to the table in the kitchen where we ate.

It was now 1995. For three years he had done the population job, and the last two years he had done Matric as well. He was now twenty-eight. He registered for a BA at Wits University. In his first year he did:

English I
Anthropology I
History I
Geography I

He was an extremely conscientious student, going to the library and reading all the suggested references. By the end of the year he was exhausted, and in a panic about the exams. I took him far out of town to an NLP therapist, who charmed him into a magic state, which he was able to take into the exam room. He passed everything. (Neuro-Linguistic Programming was based on changing negative brain patterns.)

But something else had happened towards the end of his first year. He had fallen in love with one of his English lecturers, and apparently she, who was the same age as he was, fell in love with him too. They talked and talked between the lectures, and Danny glowed at the supper table telling me about these chats.

But then she told him she was married, and she brought her six-year-old daughter to the last lecture of the year.

Danny was devastated. Tired out from all his studying and disappointed in this love relationship, he was very depressed at the beginning of the holidays.

My uncle had a job for him house-sitting. So he went to this very beautiful house in Sandton, with good art and two dogs and a swimming-pool, and came back refreshed.

Second-year University was his best year yet. He was much more relaxed about studying, and also managed for the first time in his adult life to put together a band which played his own music. It was now a three-piece band: drums, bass guitar and lead guitar. No keyboard or rhythm guitar or girl singer. He had found these two players for drums and bass guitar through music-playing friends, and they proved reliable. They rehearsed at our place twice a week throughout the year, and towards the end of the year they played in a Yeoville club.

Danny this year passed:
 English II
 Anthropology II
 History of Music I
 Comparative Literature I

And then his life changed.

Adventure

It was after his second year exams in 1996. Danny was 29. He had become kind and considerate and co-operative—a lovely person.

That winter he had taken blankets up to the people in Yeoville who slept on the pavements.

He visited both his grandmothers. Oliver's mother was now in the Jewish Old Age Home, frail and not making sense. But Danny said she recognized him and smiled. His other grandmother, my mother, was very impressed with him.

"He's become so articulate!" They did crosswords together.

Danny paid for First Year University himself, out of his savings. He enjoyed saving these days. My mother offered to pay for his second year.

And then she died. In her will all her six grandchildren got R100,000 each.

One evening after supper Danny came to visit me. He loved listening to my classical music CDs. We chose one. He turned upside-down on my relaxator chair and I listened in bed. The lights were off. At the end of the music we were silent, appreciating it. But on this particular occasion, Danny was probably thinking about what he was about to say.

"I've got something to tell you."

"Tell away."

"I'm going to live in Florida." I thought he meant Florida in Johannesburg—a far drive through heavy traffic. My insides collapsed, my outsides stayed put.

"It's because John is emigrating. His sister Lesley and her husband Steve live in Fort Lauderdale—Steve has a boat business and there is plenty of work on the boats for us. Martin is coming too, so the band can stay together." (John was his drum player.)

I felt immediately joyful. I didn't mind losing my good companion to a real adventure!

My friends were indignant. "You must be out of your mind! He'll never finish his degree now."

"It's really not my decision; he's an independent adult. And I think this is the only way he would leave the comfort of home. That's more important."

On Danny's 30th birthday we had a large supper party for the family, which included a new child, Nicola's son.

The next day at midnight he left on his complicated journey, which included a lovely day of sight-seeing in Amsterdam. John had gone ahead of him. Martin had backed out.

Danny left half his inheritance (R50,000) here at the very high interest rates we were having then. Eventually he bought a flat in Yeoville with this money plus some other savings. Outright. No mortgage. Danny never had debts.

John and Danny spent three weeks with John's sister. Then they found somewhere to stay and looked for work. Stephen had reluctantly told them that his partner was not prepared to employ illegals. They had no green cards. John had no spare money so he went after anything he could get—including playing the drums for established bands. Danny hired a rehearsal room and put adverts in a local band magazine.

Danny and John's flat was a tiny one in a single-storey, semi-prefab complex, surrounded by southern vegetation and nearby a big slow-flowing river. In the complex were elderly black people who couldn't stop their grandchildren playing and screaming into the night, so Danny made friends with the kids and established a time for the noise to stop.

Danny's life in Florida can be picked up from his letters home, so I'll leave the rest to him.

Later, he did finish his degree.

Daniel's letters from Florida
1997

I've no idea when I am going to finish or post this letter ... I've been dealing with a strange lifestyle in the course of:

    a. not having my own room

    b. constantly having people around

    c. having a multitude of things to do in the course of learning about American culture, immigrant culture

    d. trying to become more-or-less independent socially and financially.

Yes, we are on the verge of moving into our own flat! Complicated story, but we ended up with a one-year lease in John's name as he has a "full-time job" which is a bare-faced lie. Stephen can't let him work very much because they don't want to make out too many more "suspect" cheques. But we have this place—just wish I could have you and Silvie and Francina living up the road. Well, we can't have everything so we might as well just plod onward. Phambili! We've already got a sleeper-couch and a blow-up mattress which Steve and Lesley were cleaning out ... This he scored at a garage-sale for 5 dollars.

We are in a complex of which there are 3 in the area, just near a river—Rent? $104 a week

Otherwise, I have been watching horror movies on TV (horror-movie day, science-fiction week or something) and, wait for it, I eventually got an honest to god tattoo which I designed myself but which you'll have to wait to see—ha! (a mermaid).

So Buddhists only worshipped trees, huh? What about the Janists? They worship every little stalk and bug and movement.

Me and John seldom meet real Americans, mostly outsiders who think Americans are crazy.

Farewell from my strange world ...

Write lots!
Love,
Danny

How's life in the high-pressure zone?

About bicycles—I think it can't be that much worse than anywhere else—like Louis Botha with the taxis? It's just that everything here is so straight and so geared to easy motoring so people drive more—not to mention cars are cheaper and people have more money. About the only threat to motoring are cyclones and drinking. All avenues run north-south and all streets east-west—I think that's pretty clever.

So, America seems pretty hot on the environment; I'm keeping an eye out for specific examples. Everyone in this block has a blue plastic recycle bin for <u>everything</u> except metal. John tells me that the manatees (sea-cows) were brought from overseas to eat/clean up the excess of sea-weed in the rivers, but now their population is dwindling, I think due to death from motorboats.

My alternative radio station which constantly bombs its listeners with healthy, positive information, wait for it, <u>instead</u> of adverts, tells me this through an acted-out scenario of a manatee going whooahhhgg.

John isn't really doing roadwork anymore. Just today he started a private boat-sanding job in someone's back garden (a river). I might go and have a look with him sometime if I'm at a loss.

Population: I saw a TV thing called "Judge Judy" about a righteous but very human judge who argues her cases out with her clients—kitchen table manner! This time a man had for himself about 9 wives, about 4 of them under 20 years old. He argued that they were mistresses for which no marriage-licence was needed. They all had babies and most received state aid. Judy chucked him out—claimed he was irresponsible to place such a burden on the economy and on young girls—one to population!

John's moving back to his sister Lesley quite soon—he doesn't like close quarters with all black residents and lots of children—typical South African!

I wonder if they will have a World Population Day here. There are always "say no to early sex" messages floating around. There are refusal scenarios on my alternative radio station. Even on the commercial rock station a DJ discouraged an 18-year-old who hadn't finished school not to get married.

The weather here is just glorious, though pretty windy. It's like our weather with sun in the morning and cloudy later, but often as soon as mid-day. It's obviously good weather for animals, for this place is a zoo. Land animals include: squirrels, possums, racoons, lizards, snakes, alligators and a host of parrots, ranging from small, bottle-green wild ones to 3-foot macaws, which are usually pets. I even saw a monkey walking across a telephone line one day on a trip to a south beach.

I'm feeling a bit isolated so I'm going to pay the rent, shut myself in my bandroom for a few hours, then go out for a drink tonight—not that I'm feeling very rich, well, maybe just a walk to see what's going on locally— quite a lot I think because some big clubs have closed down, transferring many of the acts to my area. One block has six different clubs in it!

August

Well hi thar!—from the southern heatwave. It's been averaging 100 degrees in this area. The air-conditioner proved grossly expensive last month—it's an old-fashioned one, so I've been scared to touch it. But, either through die-hard concentration or genetic programming, I've managed to adapt and haven't really noticed, always having ice-water and fanning myself with music mags. I've just got back into my bandroom, for which I've purchased a small fan—so far so good.

The summer has delivered a macabre beauty to the mango tree in the form of 10cm+ spiders. They are very beautiful. A little boy told me these are babies! He says they are also poisonous. They do, though, seem pretty sedentary—two with webs like draped sheets with lots of flies. They have orange and black leg-segments. Me and a teenage female neighbour named Essence watched one, which was still slightly in its cocoon, drop a fly. She asked me for advice about what she should do when boys ask her to "go steady" after a brief conversation on first meeting. She didn't know at the time—just said "uhm". She also told me about her failure to be impressed by the "bad" (sinister) glare of a boy at school, as well as other gestures of male cock-headiness. They try to break her strength of principle by being dominating. Passion (my much younger friend) told me about times when she had been left at home alone the whole day.

I've just discovered there's a cactus growing out of my mango tree— wondrous.

Just now seem to have found sane people to play with. Feels like being an FBI agent—checking everyone out!

John's sister is going. Stephen has landed a top-paying job in Dubai (Asia somewhere). John will probably come and stay here again. He still hasn't found work, though guiltily looks every day. Stephen says the slump should be over by the time they leave. Who knows what will happen to us all. John and me will hopefully have our bands and each other—each to their own culture, which is what makes us unique, says Michelle Caruthers ("Why Humans Have Cultures").

John was a meat-eater and Danny a vegetarian. But in Florida he soon went back to eating fish, because it was cheap, delicious and not obviously bad for the environment. So John and Danny cooked separately. Danny used fish, dried beans, fresh cabbage and mangoes.

September

The weather is hot and rainy causing our toilets to break—something about the water-levels in the rivers rising too high. Someone threw shit-paper into my garden but it's okay—it'll contribute to compost when I plant things there.

John has moved out. This leaves me poor, but happy. I now have to try and move out the heavy carpets which Stephen bestowed upon us in all his gratuity and which are hot, causing sweat and dirt etc.

Oh yes, my beloved spiders have been brutally ridden by the annual hedge-trimming crew, all part of the management effort to please. I've still got my cat, squirrel, birds etc.

Otherwise, I've been generally practising a lot, haven't managed to read much, not that I haven't tried it, but the heat etc. Roll on winter! I do, though, want to go to this huge literature complex on Sunrise Boulevard to just look and maybe get some dictionaries—Spanish maybe?

Write lots!!
Love to everyone
Danny

In the second half of 1997, Nicola and her husband and two children (a boy and a girl) went to settle in Sydney, Australia. I visited them there. Danny wrote to all of us.

Hi, or should I say "G'dai"? Down under feels like a long way away from here, it's even further south than SA isn't it? Can't think what the weather is like there. Things are really cooling down here. The rain is good for my modest vegetable garden, in which are beans, swiss chard, tomatoes, lettuce and onions. The latter taste pretty funny around here—strong and soapy.

I hope your lives are all going well. Mine is once again an endless string of processes aimed vaguely at the music business. The band I had did not pull through, due to an inability to settle into a good compromise. We are still friends and could still jam if we don't find anyone else. I have though had a job offer from the guy John plays with—Chad—for a project churning out modern art works for luxury condos! Wow!

I went round to meet John's carpenter boss Mitch and his wife Amy on Halloween eve. They had a South African CD with Johnny Clegg on it. They are reasonably charismatic types, originally from New York, as are a lot around here.

Americans are generally nice people but it's often hard to get a word in edgeways. They are also pretty "close-culture". One probably just has to get to know people. It's not that there aren't the sort of universalities that you expect from a western country, it's that there are lot of non-universalities which, because Americans are so westernized, you are not ready for. There's a big article on drumming in south Florida which brings together many cultures—they reckon it's one of the greatest universals—it's definitely one of the simplest.

Two favours:

1.) What are Hannah's first words?

2.) What is the origin of Halloween—ja witch burning, but what country and why only a festival in the US? It's turned into a major holiday for adults as well as children—the flat was chaos with the kids playing my guitar.

December

I suppose you're getting back to normal after fire-wrought Sydney? I've had a "normal" response to my ad in the Rag mag—three drummers spread around a 40 mile radius, all interested, and one loskop bassplayer who goes to nightschool during the week and then disappears on weekends, his whereabouts and schedule oblivious to all known family—I think I might go back to the badge-sewing music enthusiast (Sal). I worked another day for John's band's boss. He was happy with what I did but it's John's job.

At the moment, John is re-attempting his idea of being "employed" by his band, the latter acting as an established company. A lot depends on

*whether he stays here or not. If not, I don't think I am going to come home
and then come back here again, but what I might do is stay here just sommer
illegally for a while. What I really need at the moment is to know where I
stand with my credit card. If you could find out for me simply:*

1.) *How much (in rands, if dollars are a hassle) I can draw each
month?*

2.) *How much I have left overall?*

*I would be extremely grateful for this info. At the moment it seems I'm just
blindly drawing money. John has had to borrow money from me because
his boss, who owes him over $700, has a "waiting period" with one of his
clients. I'll stop boring you now!*

*We are going to a real werklike "braai" held by this SA club. We don't
know anyone but it sounds like fun and a three hour drive; this happens
next Sunday. Xmas day looks pretty dead for us, but John has a gig on New
Year's Eve—his first paying gig! I'll go along.*

*The whole of Fort Lauderdale is elaborately decked out with lights. This
is done more by individuals in their gardens than the municipality. Trees
are covered—trunk, stems and all, sometimes twirly, sometimes flashing—
more than half the gardens have some creative, individualistic design. We
want to buy a cheap Polaroid disposable and capture some of this.*

Happy happy Xmas and love to everyone xxx
Danny

1998

April

*I'd been planning on a longer letter but I've ripped off my index fingernail
so…This is not so good, cause I've found someone to play with—but first,
more bad news—we got robbed! Very bad luck—through the front window
and money out of my room (less conspicuous to rummage in)—$140 rent
money and my deposit to the phone company. So even in Florida there is
desperation. It's good to suffer a bit—and it's only short term.*

*So eventually we all end up a little community of musicians. I've
even played keyboards for the old Creepy T's. Mark is pretty stable—does
computer research and we are hopefully playing with Dino—remember him*

from last year? The one who said I had gutzpah and gave me some clothes and a pair of headphones.

I miss our good talks like anything—though people here are pretty intelligent, if a little different.

I'm meeting lots of musicians and playing percussion for this 60's band with a guy and a girl. John calls it "surfer music", but I am inspired by the Latin-American feel in it. I figure this part of the world experienced some of the most dramatic "fusion" in music (blues, dance, marches).

I got my driver's licence last week. Your first DUI (drinking under influence) conviction results in a suspension of your licence for 180 to 360 days. My cop-buddy found that out the hard way. He's just been rejected insurance for the new sports car he bought, because of his DUI charge 40 years ago.

I spoke to an experienced drummer who has heard Robbie's band and has all his CDs.

Soon after this Danny put together a stable band, which lasted for a few months. The band was stable, but the bass player was not. He was an African American, Charlie, who had been in jail for five years for dealing heroin. In jail he had done all the electricity courses and was now a qualified electrician. Danny was helping him to settle in the outside world.

The third member of the band was a Brazilian, Luis. Luis had also been on drugs for a while, but was now completely rehabilitated and in fact ran a Narcotics Anonymous group. Danny went to this group for interest, but in fact he and John never did drugs. They knew they would be tolerated as illegal immigrants as long as they committed no other crimes.

John doesn't approve of the help I've given Charlie. You would, I'm sure be developing some health problems after hearing what I've been through but you remember the "Rolands" from other times. Charlie, like Roland, is charming, clever and loyal to serious music ambitions, plus all the problems of trying to survive—as was possibly Roland's case after having been cut off by his family. (I will leave you to devise your own plot, development and conclusion.)

Charlie couldn't settle to regular work and went back to jail, where Danny visited him.

Working on the Boats

Towards the end of the second year Danny was completely broke. He could come home on his open ticket, or he could draw money from the second half of his inheritance. But instead he went to a yacht fair and was taken on as a "yacht refinisher". His boss was another African American, and also named Charlie. But this Charlie was a man with a family and a business. The job was more than fulltime, because Charlie often had to finish boats at the weekends. And Danny worked right through the Christmas period.

Fort Lauderdale has concerts on a Monday night! In the aftermath of Halloween I suppose. (Will you look that up for me? My dictionary sucks on that.) Ja—me and John rode our bikes and saw the last number.

Hurricane Mitch has swung back east after its Nicaraguan devastation. Now only a storm, actually just rain. All that is threatened are the bits of teak on the boat I am working on. They are lying on top and could be swept away by the wind. I'm not riding up the river in the rain to save them, nor will my boss drive 15 miles from his motel. His cosy house in "Plantation"—a peaceful western suburb—was burnt down.

On my previous boat I met two South Africans. Both from Cape Town. Brian, who has heard Robbie, says, "I always like an optimist", about SA, when I told him about population and you.

I asked him for some of his bean recipes. He replied:

Lentils: Black beans and all lentils never need soaking, just cook on high exactly like rice. Same water, method etc.

Kidney beans and chick peas need an hour or two cooking or an overnight soak. Add chopped up veg—not too much. 1 cup max, and spices e.g. cloves, cinnamon sticks or curry spices providing variety. Add half tsp oil and salt, as in spaghetti. Mix till soft 'n juicy? Eat or offer to god of choice.

I'm glad you are happy I'm working. It's really tough, but weather has permitted the odd day off, due to Charlie's squeamish "warm-bloodedness".

He's a good guy and helps out quite a lot. He also runs me down quite a lot. I've helped him with some health problems (middle-age stress syndrome) beginning with digestion—brown bread and yoghurt (you brought me up good hey?). I have a large backlog of salary which will be paid when we finish the "big boat"—880 foot, high-quality aluminium (vis-à-vis fibreglass) yacht worth about 3 million. It belongs to a guy—someone Silverston who earns a million an hour. My bike got stolen so I have to walk. So one way and another my life's pretty full so I don't have much time to worry about band hassles. It either happens or it doesn't.

It's been a rough time for spare time not to mention spare money. But today my boss is giving me a lift and I'm sitting around waiting for him to come. I never know how long for—minutes or hours. If you ask me, he's an idiot with jobs. He can't concentrate on one job at a time and then, when under pressure from boat owners to finish on time, he hires extra help because it's too much. He has just lost more money because one of his crews broke some glass on the flying bridge. He doesn't know who. I wasn't even there on this big expensive one when it happened.

Most experienced boat workers are "hardened" to money issues and demand all their money every day or at least week. So, whether I stay with Charlie or not, that's what I'll do.

I've made a new veg garden, inspired by a new type of lettuce which is designed to fight Central Continental enemies: very bright hot sun and thin soil. The reason my last garden collapsed was because a branch of the mango tree was cut off, which, exposing the sun, frazzled the plants in 10 seconds flat. So when the mango tree got cut down for the new sewage system I got discouraged, but seeing later that the pithy plant-tree and vine-creepers had survived I was careful to let them grow to their full in order to use them for shade.

As for music, it's hard to care too much. I'm just happy to have my warehouse band room and my equipment. I'll advertise again some time in the Rag Mag, but even if I don't get a band there are many people I can phone to come and jam, and even possibly gig with.

My other short-term money goal is a new bike. It is essential to living here so I might have to draw some money for this, but it's a good "personal embetterment" cause.

I hope I have been sensitive and unboring in my assessments. I look forward to your book if you're still going to send it.

1999 Letters

Extremely sorry to hear of your trying holiday. Given it's tough having to go all that way just to put up with grumpy family et al. If we didn't have planes we wouldn't have to deal with having family in far-off places. Would they have crossed oceans on a raft?

We have entered the rainy season—two solid days of rain causing floods, but not loss of life. We can't work on the boats but Charlie has to pay my basic expenses anyway, so I'd rather not be working!!! Yesterday I collected 2 gallons of rainwater—for drinking in case they put a big dose of chlorine in the normal water.

One week later. No chlorine in the water but the mozies and fleas are out in full force. I've been working this week and I see a huge bank of clouds to the north. They look like a monument to the wrath of some sea-god.

I was just reading about someone saying that Florida, far from being a holiday place with trashy bars, is actually a natural haven with great historical interest. They see the modern buildings as enclaves in the jungle with the wildlife reclaiming developed land. This is true, except that thousands of people are moving here every day, and encroaching on the wildlife.

Well—Gore's serious about becoming president. He says he will keep the economy going while stepping up on environmental reforms, education and gun control. His opponent is anti-abortion and anti-gun control (Bush).

Back soon,
Love to all South Africans,
Danny

Danny came home at the end of 1999.

He remains stable, good-natured and thoughtful.

ACKNOWLEDGEMENTS

For help with Danny I would like to thank: Jeff Cumes, Sandy Gluckman, Joaquin of Habilitat, Stan Schmidt of the Karate Centre, Mrs Symons of Grantley College, Denver Berry, and my sisters.

I would also like to thank Mark and Anthony and Danny's other friends mentioned in the text. And Danny's cousin Hector.

I would especially like to thank the Yorkes who wrote the TOUGHLOVE book.

For their writings: Robbie and Danny and Nicola

For his observations: Grant

For the book: The first person to rejoice in this book was Christine Allen of New York. As I wrote the book I sent her the chapters. She is now sponsoring the book.

For copy-editing and proofing work and for computer help I would like to thank Mary Hazelton.

For the drawing of Danny on the cover: Greta Sadur.

For the final putting together of the book I would like to thank the people at Trafford Publishing.

As for TARA and SANCA, I would like to say that I have described only my experiences with particular people at particular times. I fully acknowledge that they have helped other people at other times.

Lightning Source UK Ltd.
Milton Keynes UK
05 July 2010
156562UK00009B/169/P